SELECTIVE
BRONCHIAL AND INTERCOSTAL
ARTERIOGRAPHY

SELECTIVE
BRONCHIAL AND INTERCOSTAL
ARTERIOGRAPHY

A. S. J. BOTENGA M.D.

H. E. STENFERT KROESE N.V. / LEIDEN 1970

Copyright 1970 by H. E. Stenfert Kroese N.V., Pieterskerkhof 38, P.O. Box 33, Leiden, The Netherlands

Published simultaneously

in the United States of America and Canada by The Williams and Wilkins Company,
428 E. Preston Street, Baltimore Md., U.S.A.

in Japan by Nankodo Company Limited, 42–6, Hongo 3 chome, Bunkyo, Tokyo.

Softcover reprint of the hardcover 1st edition 1970

Library of Congress Catalog Card Number 72–125543

ISBN-13: 978-90-207-0237-8   e-ISBN-13: 978-94-010-3156-1

DOI: 10.1007/978-94-010-3156-1

To my parents
To Lyberth

This study was performed in the Department of Radiology (Head: Prof. J. R. von Ronnen) of the Leiden University Hospital, The Netherlands.

Patients: Department of Lung Diseases (Head: Prof. J. Swierenga), Department of Cardiology (Head: Prof. H. A. Snellen), and Department of Thoracic and Cardiac Surgery (Head: Prof. A. G. Brom), Leiden University Hospital.

Histology: Department of Pathology (Heads: Prof. Th. G. van Rijssel; Prof. A. Schaberg), Leiden University Hospital.

Catheterizations performed with the aid of Miss J. C. Hensing and L. van den Boon, Department of Radiology, Leiden University Hospital.

Drawings prepared by J. Tinkelenberg and H. G. Wetselaar, Department of Anatomy, Leiden University Hospital.

Photographs by M. G. Popkes and C. Th. Ruygrok, Department of Radiology, Leiden University Hospital.

Translation by Mrs. I. Seeger, Leiden.

CONTENTS

I
INTRODUCTION

The lungs have two arterial systems, the pulmonary and the bronchial. The function of the pulmonary artery is the exchange of gases, the bronchial arteries have a nutritional function. The pulmonary artery has the low pressure of the pulmonary circulation, the bronchial arteries the higher pressure of the systemic circulation. The bronchial arteries, as the nutritional arteries of the lungs, are actively involved in all pathological processes, unlike the pulmonary artery, which undergoes only passive changes due to pressure or ingrowth.

After pulmonary arteriography became possible in 1931 (LOPO DE CARVALHO), its importance to cardiology was immediately evident and attempts were made to explore its applications for the diagnosis of pulmonary lesions. It was found that space-occupying lesions, *in casu* lung tumors, can lead to narrowing and displacement of branches of the pulmonary artery. These changes, however, were visible at such a late stage that the method offered no diagnostic advantages (STEINBERG AND FINBY 1959) and was discarded for the diagnosis of pulmonary lesions, although it is still applied to evaluate the operability of lung tumors.

Since it had long been known that bronchial arteries play an essential role in pulmonary pathology, it seemed important to find out whether a good picture of the bronchial vascularization of pulmonary lesions could be obtained and its diagnostic value determined. Some angiograms, which were originally made via the venous pathway, showed widening of the bronchial arteries. The first research concentrating on the bronchial arteries – done initially with aortography and later by selective arteriography – was performed in 1954 by NORDENSTRÖM (NORDENSTRÖM 1966b).

It need hardly be said that aortography is a simpler and less time-consuming procedure. With selective arteriography, however, there is a much better supply of contrast medium and much smaller vessels can be visualized. Furthermore, the superposition of intercostal arteries with their muscular branches and bronchial arteries, occurring on aortograms, makes evaluation difficult. We have therefore based our studies on selective catheterization, especially since we are of the opinion that only optimal visualization of these small arteries can provide a reliable basis for diagnostic conclusions.

Intercostal arteries are important because they may give rise to bronchial arteries and also because under pathological conditions intercostal blood can pass the pleura and thus reach the subpleural parts of the lung.

What is the present state of affairs with respect to the selective arteriography of bronchial arteries and intercostal arteries? Only a few medical centers apply selective bronchial and intercostal arteriography. Almost everywhere this method is still in the experimental phase, and it is certainly not applied routinely anywhere, in contrast to the selective arteriography of abdominal organs. There is still a high percentage of failures, and the method is considered to offer little or no diagnostic profit. As a consequence, in some centers the method has been discarded. Soundly based indications for its application have not been formulated.

The purpose of our research was to determine whether answers could be provided to the following questions.

1. Would a better understanding of the anatomy and improvement of the method make it possible to reduce the percentage of failures sufficiently to earn selective arteriography of bronchial and intercostal arteries a place among the accepted methods of selective arteriographic investigation?
2. Can indications for such selective arteriographical investigations be formulated?

The answers to these questions were considered to offer a basis for the evaluation of the clinical contribution to be expected of this method.

In designing this research project, we started by making a detailed study of the radiological and anatomical literature.

II
LITERATURE

II.1. PART I – RADIOLOGY

Wide bronchial arteries can be demonstrated by conventional radiological methods. CAMPBELL AND GARDNER (1950), CSÁKÁNY (1964) and KIEFFER ET AL. (1965) described characteristic pictures seen on normal X-ray's and RICHTER (1965) those seen on tomograms of the thorax. TAUSSIG (1947) and SEGERS AND BROMBART (1953) established typical impressions in the esophagus.

Some of these authors, including CAMPBELL AND GARDNER (1950) and GARUSI (1961), saw wide bronchial arteries on venous angiocardiograms, but direct study of the bronchial arteries can only be done by arteriography, which still has a rather brief history. Research has been done in dogs and in man; only the latter will be discussed.

NORDENSTRÖM was the first to make an arteriographic study of the bronchial arteries, for which he used thoracic aortography. As early as 1955 he used this method to visualize the human bronchial artery (NORDENSTRÖM 1960) but had to suspend his investigations because of the toxicity of the contrast medium.

Except for preliminary reports made by ALLEY ET AL. in 1958 and by PINET ET AL. in 1958 and 1959, the remaining publications date from the last eight years (GUNTHEROTH ET AL., 1962; VAILLAUD, 1962; WILLIAMS ET AL., 1962, 1963; MORAND ET AL., 1963; LEES AND DOTTER, 1965; MACK ET AL., 1965; MASSUMI ET AL., 1965a & b; PINET ET AL., 1965, 1966; DUSSAUT, 1966; FESANI ET AL., 1966; PADOVANI ET AL., 1966; VACCAREZZA ET AL., 1966; BENNET ET AL., 1966, 1967; GOFFRINI, 1967; HUTCHIN ET AL., 1967). GROEN ET AL., (1965, 1966) attempted to improve the picture by means of subtraction. All these investigations were based on the aortographical method.

Some investigators have attempted to retard the bloodflow by inducing hypotension, which leads to less dilution of the contrast medium and less stratification. As a result, more contrast medium can be introduced and the picture improves. The Swedish authors achieved this effect by increasing the intrabronchial pressure under general anaesthesia (NORDENSTRÖM, 1960) and the French, according to the reports of PINET ET AL. (1958, 1959) and MORAND ET AL. (1963), by the administration of the hypotensivum trimetaphane (ARFONAD). This gives a slightly better picture of the bronchial arteries, but there is only a limited gain with respect to the aortographical method without retardation of the bloodflow.

Better filling with contrast medium and finer detail were achieved by use of the balloon catheter (NEYAZAKI, 1962, 1964; NORDENSTRÖM, 1962, 1963, 1965, 1966b & c; CLIFFTON AND DHAN RAJ MAHAJAN, 1963; KOZUKA, 1964). By the use of one or two balloons, the aortic segment in which the bronchial arteries arise can be isolated. This method represents the closest approximation to selective arteriography. In one of his publications, however, NORDENSTRÖM (1965) says: 'The bronchial artery is better demonstrated during selective contrast injection than at occlusion aortography.' BLANK ET AL. (1966) came to the same conclusion on the basis of experimental results obtained in dogs.

VIAMONTE (1964) was the first to publish results of a selective investigation, which he performed in a series of 32 patients, and he is still the author with the widest experience (VIAMONTE, 1965a & b, 1967; VIAMONTE ET AL., 1965, 1966, 1967). Subsequently, a number of publications concerning small series appeared (SCHOBER, 1964, 1965; BOIJSEN AND ZSIGMOND, 1965; KAHN ET AL., 1965; NEWTON AND PREGER, 1965; NORDENSTRÖM, 1965, 1967; REUTER ET AL., 1965; DESILETS ET AL., 1966; E COSTA, 1966, 1967;

HALLER ET AL., 1966; BOREK ET AL., 1967; CHAVEZ, 1967; GERNEZ-RIEUX ET AL., 1967; OUTURQUIN, 1967; POLÁK ET AL., 1967; RÉMY ET AL., 1968; WIRTANEN AND ANSFIELD, 1968; DARKE AND LEWTAS, 1968; IKEDA ET AL., 1968; CICERO ET AL., 1968; NORTH ET AL., 1969). Although the high percentage of failures often led to disappointing results, it is evident from these publications that the method is feasible. As can be seen from the illustrations accompanying these papers, the detail obtainable with this technique far exceeds that provided by aortographic methods.

The development of the arteriographic investigation of the intercostal arteries has run parallel with the study of the bronchial arteries. A few publications have given special attention to the intercostal arteries (GUNTHEROTH ET AL., 1962; VAILLAUD, 1962; WILLIAMS ET AL., 1963; KIEFFER ET AL., 1965; VACCA-REZZA, 1966). With respect to the intercostal arteries too, selective arteriography deserves preference.

II.2. PART II – ANATOMY

II.2.1. Bronchial arteries

II.2.1.1. HISTORICAL REVIEW[1]

The first reference to the existence of bronchial arteries is made by GALEN in the second century A.D., although according to HALLER (1747) and PORTAL (1770) they had already been seen by ERISTRATUS in the third century B.C. and by the earliest Arabian physicians. The first known drawing of bronchial arteries is made by LEONARDO DA VINCI, but their existence is denied by COLUMBUS (1559) who writes: 'Ab aorta arteria ramus nullus, neque magnus, neque parvulus ad pulmones mittitur.' DE MARCHETTIS (1654) confirms their presence. The first detailed anatomical study was done by RUYSCH (1721)[2] who is unaware of the earlier investigations and thinks that he is the first to discover the bronchial arteries. RUYSCH denies the existence of bronchial veins. In 1743, FICKEL wrote a monograph on bronchial arteries and veins. HALLER, in his 'Icorum Anatomicarum' (1747) gives an accurate description of the origin and course of the bronchial arteries and is the first to discuss the anatomical variations, which he has observed in twenty-four autopsies. The discussions given by BOYER (1815) and BICHAT (1819) faithfully follow HALLER. In TIEDEMANN's 'Tabularum Arteriarum' (1822) bronchial arteries are portrayed as arising from the concavity of the aortic arch and from the proximal part of the descending aorta, and coursing anterior to the trachea to the corresponding surface of each primary bronchus. This highly unusual pattern is uncritically adopted in a succession of standard works on anatomy published between 1825 and 1942. A Russian monograph on the anatomy of the bronchial arteries and viens was published by SUSLOFF (1895).

II.2.1.2. ORIGIN OF THE BRONCHIAL ARTERIES

Because of the importance of certainty as to the origin of the bronchial arteries for the selective investigation, a detailed discussion of this subject is given here. This discussion is divided into two parts. The first part comprises a critical discussion of past research, and the second an anatomical classification based on the data yielded by this research, emphasis being placed on the practical use for selective arteriography.

CRITICAL DISCISSION OF THE DATA IN THE LITERATURE

Although almost all investigators of the bronchial circulation refer to the origin and course of the bronchial arteries, detailed descriptions are scarce. Systematic studies of the origin have been made by NAKAMURA (1924), CAULDWELL ET AL. (1948), SWIGART ET AL. (1950), LATARJET AND JUTTIN (1951),

---

[1] Based on historical data given by ZUCKERKANDL (1881, 1883), MILLER (1906, 1947), CAULDWELL ET AL. (1948), CUDKOWICZ (1953), FLORANGE (1960), CAMARRI and MARINI (1965).
[2] In the period between DE MARCHETTIS and RUYSCH, according to CAMARRI and MARINI, four authors refer to bronchial arteries: LANZONI (1688), SBARAGLI (1693), VERHEYEN (1693), and DIONIS (1696).

GIORDANI AND PINNA (1956), LAUWERIJNS (1962), and LIEBOW (1965). In the frequent references to these authors below, the year of publication will be omitted.

The work of CAULDWELL and (his) co-workers excels because of the superb analysis of the material, NAKAMURA's investigation is also well documented. LIEBOW's work was performed in great detail, but unfortunately the documentation leaves something to be desired. Despite some discrepancies between drawings and text, the investigation by GIORDANI AND PINNA is also fairly well documented. LAUWERIJNS gives only a limited analysis of his material. Rather poorly documented is the frequently quoted study by LATARJET AND JUTTIN. The investigation done by SWIGART ET AL. (of the same institution as CAULDWELL ET AL.) was primarily concerned with the vascularization of the esophagus. Although they indeed increased the material of CAULDWELL ET AL. to 300 cases, the bronchial arteries are, in our opinion, observed less exactly. This is evident from fact that as compared with the CAULDWELL study, the number of rare variants was hardly increased. For other reasons, too, as will be mentioned below, their data are not suitable for our purposes.

All these investigators divided their material into groups with a given number of left and right bronchial arteries. These classifications were based on the number of bronchial arteries counted on both sides at the level of the hili, and not on the number of sites of origin of the bronchial arteries. This latter point, however, is of special importance for selective arteriography, which is mainly concerned with the number of sites of origin and much less with how these arteries might possibly divide themselves during their further course. For this reason, the classifications found in the literature may be misleading or at least make the arteriographic investigation more difficult.

To illustrate this last point an example may be given of the way in which different anatomical situations are put in one and the same group in the literature.

1. One right and two left bronchial arteries with separate origins from the aorta.
2. One right and one left bronchial artery dividing immediately into two arteries: one for the left upper lobe and the other for the left lower lobe.
3. A common trunk for one right and one left bronchial artery and a separately arising left bronchial artery.
4. A common trunk for one right and two left bronchial arteries.

For the selective investigation this means that the investigator must find three arteries in the first situation, only one in the last, and two arteries in the remaining two situations, in order to obtain a complete bronchial arteriogram. We have therefore used the material of the macroscopical investigations to make a new classification based on the number of bronchial arteries counted at their point of origin. Consequently, some of the numbers given in the following discussion on the value of the earlier research do not occur in the original publications.

CAULDWELL ET AL. investigated 150 cases by means of dissection. By analysis and careful comparison of the data in their drawings, tables, and text we were able to find the answer to almost all of our questions. A minor shortcoming of their work is the fact that according to the diagram of the anatomical groups (Fig. 1 in the original publication) a right bronchial artery arose from an intercostal artery in 149 of the 150 cases, but in reality this occurred less frequently in their material (Table 2). In addition, according to this diagram only three common stems for left and right bronchial arteries were found, but in fact 44 stems were seen by the authors. This diagram is reproduced in the publications of SCHOBER (1964), BOIJSEN AND ZSIGMOND (1965), NEWTON AND PREGER (1965), GROEN ET AL. (1966) and NORDENSTRÖM (1967), and it serves as the basis for the anatomical considerations in the publications of almost all those who have performed selective studies. However, in this diagram the bronchial arteries were counted in the hilus and not near the ostium, and it does not appear from these publications that this is realized.

The desired information could also be obtained from the data of NAKAMURA, who also studied 150 cases by dissection. This author is the only one to provide complete documentation on the relationship between intercostal and bronchial arteries per case, but he did not consider the intercostal spaces traversed by the intercostal arteries giving rise to a bronchial artery and gave almost no attention to whether the bronchial arteries arose from the aorta ventrally or dorsally. The study of bronchial arteries with an aberrant origin is not possible with the technique he used. In 21 cases NAKAMURA saw a small branch arising in the aortic bulb (the part between the isthmus aortae and the origin of the intercostal arteries) and running to the carina and the tracheo-bronchial glands situated below it. He did not consider these to be bronchial arteries, although he could not exclude the possibility that small branches might go to the lungs. Since NAKAMURA found fewer bronchial arteries per individual than other authors, the chance seems to us to be great that these branches were indeed bronchial arteries. NAKAMURA excluded these cases from his material, which seems incorrect because this makes the rare forms relatively too numerous: these 21 cases all belong to the two largest groups of anatomical variants.

On the basis of NAKAMURA's data we have made two classifications (Tables 2, 3, 4, and 5: Nakamura A and B). In classification A these 21 small arterial branches are included but not in classification B. The method used to arrive at classification A was as follows.

Since it is not known whether the artery in question had sent branches to the right or left lung or both, we attempted to determine the chances of this according to NAKAMURA's data. In 13 of the 21 cases, besides the accessory branch one bronchial artery was present on the right (from an intercostal artery*) and one on left. If the branch in question is included, the following possibilities are to be considered.

a. One right bronchial artery from an intercostal artery* and one left and one right bronchial artery from the aorta (no cases in NAKAMURA's material).
b. One right bronchial artery from an intercostal artery* and two left bronchial arteries (35 cases in NAKAMURA's material).
c. One right bronchial artery from an intercostal artery*, one left bronchial artery, and one common trunk (5 cases in NAKAMURA's material).

By assigning the 13 cases proportionately to these groups we obtained: no cases in group a, 11 cases in group b, and 2 cases in group c.

In the remaining 8 cases, one right bronchial artery arising from an intercostal artery* and two left bronchial arteries were present. Inclusion of the artery now leads to the following possibilities.

d. One right bronchial artery from an intercostal artery* and two left and one right bronchial artery from the aorta (no cases in NAKAMURA's material).
e. One right bronchial artery from an intercostal artery* and three left bronchial arteries (4 cases in NAKAMURA's material).
f. One right bronchial artery from an intercostal artery*, two left bronchial arteries, and one common trunk (no cases in NAKAMURA's material).

Since the total of 8 is greater than the total number of cases in the groups d, e, and f, we assigned these cases, perhaps somewhat arbitrarily, as follows: 6 cases to group e and 1 case to each of the other two groups.

NAKAMURA found remarkably few common trunks in his material. We assume that his dissection was less subtle than that of CAULDWELL ET AL., so that smaller branches running to the contralateral side were missed. This assumption is supported by two other facts, i.e. that NAKAMURA found the fewest bronchial arteries per individual and saw no cases of bronchial arteries arising from the aortic arch.

* First right intercostal artery from the aorta.

LIEBOW studied 50 cases in casts in which the vessels were injected with coloured plastics, a technique by which very fine vessels can indeed be demonstrated. According to his calculations, which also were not based on the number of ostia, there were 3.68 bronchial arteries per individual. On this basis he stated that much finer vessels can be seen in his casts than could be discovered by dissection. Whether or not this is the case, it appeared from our analysis of LIEBOW's data that CAULDWELL ET AL. had found even more bronchial arteries (calculated from the ostia) per individual than LIEBOW, i.e. 2.77 per individual as against 2.64 per individual (Table 5). It is possible that finer lateral branches remained intact in the casts, but the extreme precision with which CAULDWELL ET AL. must have performed their dissections does not suggest that their investigation yielded less anatomical information. LIEBOW furthermore found a high percentage of common stems: almost 4 times more than CAULDWELL ET AL. and 9 times more than NAKAMURA (Table 3).

LIEBOW ascribes the 'virtual' difference between the number of bronchial arteries found by him and other authors to the fact that he found in his preparations a much larger number of small bronchial arteries arising high in the descending aorta or from the aortic arch. In his opinion, most of these small branches were missed at dissection. We are unable to agree with him, since he included in this group of bronchial arteries all the arteries arising from the aorta above the level of the intercostal arteries, whereas CAULDWELL ET AL. and NAKAMURA assigned to this group only arteries arising from the concave or convex parts of the aortic arch. The difference between the arterial counts does lie, however, in the greater number of common stems found by LIEBOW. How is this to be explained? As judged from the illustrations, LIEBOW assigned a bronchial artery to a common trunk if even one minimally small branch went to the other side, often only for the vascularization of the main bronchus. It remains possible that he saw these small branches more clearly in his casts. CAULDWELL ET AL. and NAKAMURA assigned bronchial arteries to common trunks only when they divided into at least one good-sized artery for the left as well as the right lung. By taking all these miniscule hilar branches into consideration, LIEBOW thought he had found more common stems for right and left bronchials (at the site of the pulmonary hili) than CAULDWELL ET AL. and NAKAMURA.

Because of LIEBOW's limited documentation it was more difficult to derive the number of bronchial arteries, counted from the ostia, from his data than from those of the other authors. We subtracted the number of common trunks from the total numbers of left and right bronchial arteries, and this made it possible to arrive at a reasonable approximation of the number of left and right bronchial arteries arising separately from the aorta, since according to the text, independent left and right arteries were counted from the ostia, i.e. only once. According to LIEBOW's table 1, the total number of left bronchial arteries amounted to 95 and the right to 89. After subtraction of the common trunks (totalling 52; LIEBOW's table 3) there remained 43 left and 37 right bronchial arteries (see our table 5). Presumably these values are still slightly too high, because according to LIEBOW's illustrations a few of the common stems were counted not as two but as three bronchial arteries (e.g., left superior, left inferior, and right inferior). Yet our further analysis of LIEBOW's data was based on the numbers of left and right bronchial arteries thus obtained and the results show reasonably good agreement with those of the other authors.

Although LIEBOW hardly mentions the site of origin of the bronchial arteries from the aorta, he made a thorough study of the course of right bronchial arteries with respect to the trachea.

LIEBOW furthermore found only once (2 per cent) the combination of a bronchial artery with an intercostal artery for two intercostal spaces. CAULDWELL ET AL. found this combination in almost 30 per cent of their cases, and in our material it was seen in more than 40 per cent. Since these arteries must certainly be visible in the casts, it must be assumed that in LIEBOW's material most of the intercostal arteries must have been torn off or ligated.

For his study of aberrant bronchial arteries, LIEBOW examined 100 additional casts.

The comparative analysis of these three most important investigations has shown that the differences between the results are much smaller than LIEBOW in particular had thought them to be. The remaining differences are, in our opinion, dependent – aside from the standard deviations arising from the analysis of series that must be considered rather small for the study of a type of artery with such a variable anatomy – on the following points, which also hold as a general tendency for the three best studies.

1. In LIEBOW's material slightly less so in that of CAULDWELL's, the finest structures were made visible.
2. Analysis of the material was done in the greatest detail by CAULDWELL ET AL. and in the least by LIEBOW.
3. The documentation of NAKAMURA's study is the most complete, that of CAULDWELL ET AL.'s almost equally so, but that of LIEBOW's leaves much to be desired.

The work of the other authors will be discussed more briefly. GIORDANI AND PINNA investigated 50 cases by dissection. They classified their material in several ways, e.g. according to the presence or absence of a common stem for left and right bronchial arteries. With respect to these common trunks they came to the remarkable conclusion that when this artery arises on the right side of the aorta the branch to the right lung is the most important, and if it arises on the left side the branch to the left lung. This opinion is based, however, on a small number of common trunks (eight, but with one exception). The documentation and analysis of their material is good, although less complete than those of CAULDWELL ET AL. and NAKAMURA. There is a disturbing discrepancy between the drawings and the text, especially with respect to the dorsal and ventral origin of the arteries. Almost nothing is said about the combination of intercostal and bronchial arteries.

LATARJET AND JUTTIN investigated 125 cases by dissection and injection with radiopaque material. Their analysis and documentation is so incomplete that many questions associated with our comparative study could not be answered. Here too, there are discrepancies between drawings and text, especially with respect to bronchial arteries arising from intercostal arteries. A detailed discussion is given of the course of the right bronchial artery in relation to the esophagus.

LAUWERIJNS investigated 48 cases by dissection and injection with plastic dyes. In spite of his classification (Table 2 of his thesis), we were unable to make a comparative study of his results because no mention is made of whether combined ostia for two or more arteries were present. Apart from CAULDWELL ET AL., only LAUWERIJNS discusses the intercostal spaces supplied by combined intercostal and bronchial arteries.

SWIGART ET AL. also do not report how the bronchial arteries were counted, which again made comparative study impossible.

ANATOMICAL CLASSIFICATION

The anatomy of the origin of the bronchial arteries is so variable that it is difficult to arrive at a classification that is both simple and logical. The literature contains incomplete classifications or fails to give a classification on the grounds that the origin does not follow any rule. CAMARRI AND MARINI do mention all the possibilities, but present so many groups that their classification leads to repetition and duplication, thus hampering a comprehensive view. We, at any rate, were unable to understand their classification. In addition, the nomenclature in the literature is confusing, the terms aberrant, accessory, abnormal, atypical, and heterotopic, for instance, being used alternatively for various types of artery. After ample consideration, we decided to present a new and simplified classification. This classification is based on the one hand on an evaluation of the material in the literature in the light of our own experience and is aimed, on the other hand, at usefulness for selective arteriography.

We distinguish in the first place two types of bronchial arteries, the *normal* and the *accessory*. Normal bronchial arteries are vessels with a relatively large caliber, supplying, in numbers varying from one to three per lung, important parts of the bronchial tree. Under accessory bronchial arteries is understood small arterial branches supplying structures in the vicinity of the hilus and playing an accessory role in the bronchial vascularization.

In the second place we distinguish a usual and an unusual origin, which we call the *normal* and the *abnormal* origin of bronchial arteries. The normal origin occurs from the descending aorta and a number of high right intercostal arteries. The abnormal origin comprises two forms, i.e. origin from the *aortic arch* and *aberrant* origin. Under aberrant origin is understood origins from all the arteries of the great circulation with the exception of the aorta and a few cranial right intercostal arteries.

Since for the discussion and analysis of the origin of the bronchial arteries the distinction between normal and accessory bronchial arteries cannot always be made, these two types will first be treated together and then a separate discussion will be given of the accessory bronchial arteries and their highly variable origin.

a. Normal origin

In this section we shall discuss not only the two normal modes of origin but also the anatomical formations resulting from them and the numbers of 'normal' sites of origin. The occurrence of common trunks for left and right bronchial arteries will also be dealt with here, since this concept is indispensible for a clear presentation of the macroscopic anatomy and would otherwise be taken up too late in the discussion.

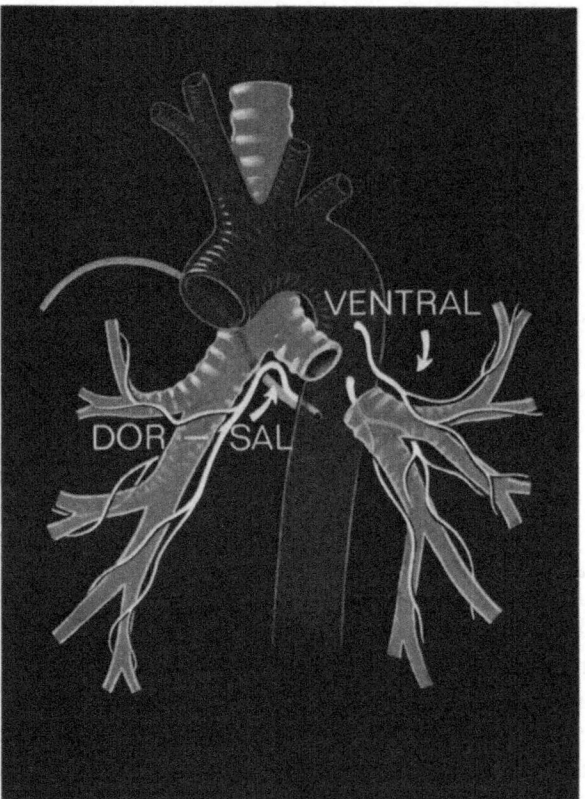

Fig. 1. This anatomical situation occurs most frequently: 1 right and 2 left bronchial arteries. The right bronchial artery usually arises from the first right aortic intercostal. Fig. 14 shows this situation *in vivo*.

The 'normal' anatomical situation

There is considerable justice to the claim that the highly irregular structure of the bronchial arteries makes it impossible to speak of a normal anatomical situation, but a certain regularity can nevertheless be distinguished within the variations. Right bronchial arteries usually arise jointly with right inter-costal arteries, and as a rule left bronchial arteries arise directly from the aorta. As for the combination of a right bronchial artery with a right intercostal artery, most authors speak of a truncus intercosto-bronchialis or intercosto-bronchial trunk. Although this term is not entirely accurate – in view of the question: parent stem and derivative – it is convenient and its application in the literature is consistent.

The most frequently observed situation is that in which one intercosto-bronchial trunk and two left bronchial arteries, arising directly and ventrally from the aorta, are present (Fig. 1). This formation is found in more than one-third of the cases, and the percentages[1] do not differ greatly (CAULDWELL ET AL.: 38.7 per cent; NAKAMURA (A): 34.7 per cent, and (B): 30.7 per cent; GIORDANI AND PINNA: 40 per cent; LATARJET AND JUTTIN: 40.8 per cent; LAUWERIJNS: 37.5 per cent (see table 4: 'NORMAL ANATOMY' I). This is the largest group in all the material except that of NAKAMURA, who saw the situation with one right bronchial artery (truncus intercosto-bronchialis) and one left bronchial artery arising from the aorta more often (A: 33.3 per cent, and B: 41.3 per cent, table 4).

a.1. *Origin from the descending aorta*

It is important to know whether the bronchial arteries arise anteriorly or posteriorly from the aorta, and the level at which the origin is situated must also be determined. These data are shown in table 1.

Dorsal – ventral

The following rule of thumb serves here. All the bronchial arteries arising directly from the aorta have a ventral origin. The literature contains only one mention of a single bronchial artery arising directly from the dorso-lateral aspect of the aorta (CAULDWELL ET AL.). GIORDANI AND PINNA do state that 24 per cent* of their left bronchial arteries arose dorsally from the aorta, but since these authors did not consider the relationship between bronchial and intercostal arteries these must in our opinion be arteries in association with intercostal arteries, since the combination of left bronchial arteries with right intercostal arteries also occurs. Nevertheless, this percentage is remarkably high and must in our opinion be explained as due to the frequent counting of branches to the left lung (arising from a single bronchial artery) as separate bronchial arteries.

According to CAULDWELL ET AL., left bronchial arteries arise on the ventral or right ventro-lateral side of the aorta and seldom on the left ventro-lateral side. According to GIORDANI AND PINNA, 70 per cent* of the left bronchial arteries arise on the ventral or left ventro-lateral surface of the aorta and 6 per cent* right ventro-laterally.

Right bronchial arteries arise right ventro-laterally according to CAULDWELL ET AL. and according to GIORDANI AND PINNA in 12 per cent* ventrally and in 8 per cent* right ventro-laterally (the re-maining arteries arising from intercostals).

Cranial – caudal

CAULDWELL ET AL. give a detailed discussion of the level of origin of the bronchial arteries (their tables IV A and IV B). As reference point they took the thoracic vertebrae. For purpose of orientation, they refer to the corresponding levels in MORRIS's anatomical atlas:

---

[1] These percentages derive from our comparative analysis. In the groups of CAULDWELL ET AL. and GIORDANI AND PINNA, it is possible that not all the right bronchial arteries arise from intercostal arteries. The two percentages given for NAKAMURA belong to the division into A and B made in this author's material as described above (page 11). The percentage given for LAUWERIJNS is taken directly from his data and possible does not depend on a classification according to the site of origin.

* Percentage taken from author's classification, not based on the ostia.

Th 3: highest point of the aortic arch

Th 4: bifurcation of the trachea; second part of the aortic arch; beginning of the thoracic aorta

Th 5: most cranial portion of the heart

Th 6: commencement of the aorta and pulmonary artery; end of the superior caval vein

Since the bronchial arteries shown in table IV B of CAULDWELL ET AL. were not counted on the basis of the origin, an exact calculation based on the ostia could not be performed, but an acceptable approximation could be reached.[1]

Data on the level of origin are also to be found in GIORDANI AND PINNA and in the radiological literature in VIAMONTE ET AL. (1965).

Of the data tabulated in table 1 some points will now be brought forward. In 95 per cent of the cases the segment of the aorta from which the bronchial arteries arise is limited by the cranial and caudal margins of two adjacent vertebrae and in 38 per cent by one vertebral level (CAULDWELL ET AL.).[2]

In 70.7 per cent (CAULDWELL ET AL.) to 78 per cent (GIORDANI AND PINNA) of the cases all the left bronchial arteries, including common trunks, arise opposite the combined levels T5 and T6 and for the right bronchial arteries these values are 84.2 per cent and 90 per cent,[3] respectively.

Of the total number of isolated left bronchial arteries, 76.5 per cent (VIAMONTE ET AL.) and 85.4 per cent (CAULDWELL ET AL.), and of the total number of isolated right bronchial arteries 93.9 per cent[3] (VIAMONTE ET AL.) to 95.1 per cent (CAULDWELL ET AL.) arise opposite the extremes of T5 and T6. Therefore, the left bronchial arteries seem to be less constant than the right with respect to origin, which is indeed expressed in the wider range of their points of origin (Table 1 II). Of all the bronchial arteries taken together, 86.3 per cent (CAULDWELL ET AL.) to 90.5 per cent[3] (VIAMONTE ET AL.) arise opposite T5 and T6.

Consequently, the greatest number of bronchial arteries is to be found in the segment of the aorta facing T5 and T6.

a.2. *Origin from intercostal arteries* [4]

The majority of the right bronchial arteries do not arise directly from the aorta but from an intercostal artery, usually the first right intercostal, which takes its origin from the aorta. This artery supplies, according to CAULDWELL ET AL., the first (but very rarely), second, third, or fourth intercostal space, most frequently the third (43.6 per cent). As a rule, the artery in the first and often also that in the second intercostal space arise from the innominate or the subclavian arteries. The right bronchial artery seldom arises from the second intercostal artery, which arises from the aorta (7.3 per cent in the material of CAULDWELL ET AL.) and very seldom from the third aortic intercostal artery. The last possibility was seen only once by CAULDWELL ET AL.

According to NAKAMURA, an intercosto-bronchial trunk sometimes bifurcates immediately into a bronchial and an intercostal artery, but more usually 6 to 10 cm beyond its origin.

In contradiction with the opinion of VIAMONTE ET AL. (1965), NORDENSTRÖM (1966), E COSTA (1967), and MILNE (1967) a bronchial artery is never given off by a left intercostal artery; the examples in their publications concern muscular branches of intercostal arteries. If these authors had made lateral exposures, they would have seen that these branches supply the muscles of the back running outside the thorax. O'RAHILLY ET AL. (1950) give the only description of a case in which an artery was followed to the left hilus after being derived from a second left intercostal artery arising on the left cranial surface of the aortic arch. Since this artery could not be followed further than the left hilus, it does not

---

1 The number of left and right bronchial arteries in their Table IV B was reduced by subtraction of the number of common trunks and the number of arteries arising from the aortic arch.

2 With the exception of the arteries arising from the aortic arch.

3 This percentage also includes intercosto-bronchial trunks. Separate calculation was not possible.

4 For data, see table 2.

provide conclusive evidence of the existence of such an artery. In cases of *situs inversus viscerum*, however, an intercosto-bronchial trunk with a left intercostal artery may occur (CAULDWELL ET AL.).

Right intercostal arteries in association with left bronchial arteries or common trunks are rare but have been described in both the anatomical (CAULDWELL ET AL.; NAKAMURA; LIEBOW) and radiological literature (VIAMONTE ET AL. 1965; KAHN ET AL. 1965; BOIJSEN AND ZSIGMOND 1965). Unless explicitly stated otherwise, the term intercosto-bronchial trunk or truncus intercosto-bronchialis will henceforth be reserved for a right bronchial artery from a right intercostal artery.

Two intercosto-bronchial trunks also occur (CAULDWELL ET AL.: 3.3 per cent; NAKAMURA: 5.3 per cent; LIEBOW: 12 per cent). The lower intercostal artery often provides a left bronchial artery.

One or more intercosto-bronchial trunks were present in 92.7 per cent (CAULDWELL ET AL.), 84.7 per cent (NAKAMURA), 77.6 per cent (LATARJET AND JUTTIN), and 74 per cent (LIEBOW) of the cases. These percentages vary rather widely. Only NAKAMURA's could be calculated directly and is therefore the most reliable. The proportion of intercosto-bronchial trunks among the total number of bronchial arteries shows more agreement (CAULDWELL ET AL.: 34.4 per cent; NAKAMURA A: 35.2 per cent, B: 37.2 per cent; LIEBOW: 32.6 per cent).

Of the total number of right bronchial arteries, 86.7 per cent (CAULDWELL ET AL.) to 89.6 per cent (NAKAMURA A) arise from intercostal arteries.

The occurrence of trunci communes[1]

Common stems for left and right bronchial arteries were found in many of the cases, LIEBOW: 84 per cent, CAULDWELL ET AL.: 27.3 per cent, GIORDANI AND PINNA: 18 per cent, and NAKAMURA: 10.7 per cent.

The reason for the wide variation in the percentages of common trunks found in the various studies has already been discussed. In our opinion, it has no anatomical basis and must be ascribed entirely to differences in interpretation and methods. LIEBOW, for instance, used the term common trunk for a bronchial artery providing a minimally small branch running to the other side for supply of the main bronchus. If, however, it is demanded for a common trunk that at least one macroscopically visible branch must be traceable in the opposite lung, the percentage given by CAULDWELL ET AL. may be considered representative. This definition is also appropriate for the selective investigation; the artery will be called a *truncus communis*.

Generally, a truncus communis is incomplete, which means that still other bronchial arteries are also present. In a small percentage of the cases (CAULDWELL ET AL.: 3.3; NAKAMURA: 6; GIORDANI AND PINNA: 6) a truncus communis is complete. These are at the same time the cases with only one bronchial artery (Table 5). For the selective study, it is unfortunate that this situation is so seldom seen. LIEBOW, curiously enough, found a complete truncus communis much more often, i.e. in 22 per cent of the cases. We are unable to offer an explanation of this difference.

Cases with two trunci communes were not found in the materials examined by NAKAMURA and by GIORDANI AND PINNA, but CAULDWELL ET AL. saw three (2 per cent) and LIEBOW ten (20 per cent). This again is a question of definition.

The occurrence of a truncus communis as an intercosto-bronchial trunk has already been mentioned. On this point the data of CAULDWELL ET AL. are divergent. In their table IVB, which includes all bronchial arteries arising directly from the aorta, 21 trunci communes are listed. According to their table III, which includes all the trunci communes, there were 39 in all. From this it might be concluded that 18 trunci communes arose from intercostal arteries, but is is explicitly stated in the text that there were 3 of these. Since the latter figure is much more probable, we used it for our comparative study.

---

[1] For data, see table 3.

Only in rare cases does a complete truncus communis arise from an intercostal artery, but LIEBOW saw this situation, again unexplicably, rather often, i.e. four times (8 per cent).

Other anatomical situations[1]

Somewhat less frequently than the situation described above as normal anatomical situation, one bronchial artery is seen on the right (intercosto-bronchial trunk) and one on the left arising ventrally from the aorta. Other arrangements are seen much less frequently.

In the material of the macro-anatomical studies, our analysis (based on the site of origin of the bronchial arteries) showed the occurrence of eight different groups of left and right bronchial arteries and eleven combinations of trunci communes with left and right bronchial arteries i.e. a total of nineteen anatomical variants. Even then the presence of an intercosto-bronchial trunk is not yet taken into consideration; when this is done, it can be calculated from NAKAMURA's data that this number of groups of anatomical variants still almost doubles (classification 'NAKAMURA II').

The number of cases per group could only be calculated from the documentation of CAULDWELL ET AL., NAKAMURA, and GIORDANI AND PINNA.

From the point of view of selective arteriography, it is important to estimate how many cases can be expected with one intercosto-bronchial trunk and one to two arteries arising from the ventral aspect of the aorta. These latter arteries are usually left bronchial arteries but can also be trunci communes or right bronchial arteries. The high percentages in which this situation was encountered show good agreement, CAULDWELL ET AL.: 80.7, GIORDANI AND PINNA: 80, and NAKAMURA A: 70.7 and B: 76. So this combined anatomical situation proves to occur in almost eight out of ten cases. In connection with the percentages of CAULDWELL ET AL. and GIORDANI AND PINNA it should be remarked that it is not certain for these cases that all the right bronchial arteries arose from intercostal arteries.

Numbers of bronchial arteries[2]

All the authors consistently found more left than right bronchial arteries. In LIEBOW's material the differences between the two were small.

The numbers of right bronchial arteries correspond strikingly well in the different investigations, CAULDWELL ET AL.: 38.0 per cent, NAKAMURA A: 37.5 per cent, B: 39.1 per cent, GIORDANI AND PINNA: 39.6 per cent, and LATARJET AND JUTTIN 39.1 per cent.

Some discrepancy was found only for the numbers of left bronchial arteries and trunci communes, possibly because some authors included left bronchial arteries with a small branch to the right among the trunci communes and others put them among the left bronchial arteries. It is also possible that these small branches were missed in some of the investigations.

The number of right bronchial arteries arising directly from the aorta is very much smaller than that found for the left bronchial arteries.

The highest number of bronchial arteries found per individual is five. Our search of the literature yielded five cases with five bronchial arteries.

With the exception of NAKAMURA, the authors found 3 bronchial arteries in half or more than half of their cases. Two bronchial arteries were found in at least 25 per cent (by NAKAMURA, however, in more than 40 per cent).

The average number of bronchial arteries per individual varies in the different investigations from

---

[1] For data, see table 4.
[2] For data, see table 5.

2.42 to 2.89. Calculated for the combined material of all the authors (525 autopsies), this value is 2.70 bronchial arteries per case.

To answer the question of how many left and right bronchial arteries are possessed by the average person, we formed two groups, one omitting cases with trunci communes. In the other these cases were included and counted as one left and one right bronchial artery. Only the second group, therefore, comprised all the cases.

The material of CAULDWELL ET AL. proved to have about twice as many cases with two left bronchial arteries as with one left bronchial artery and about twice to five times (Group II) as many cases with one right bronchial artery as with two right bronchial arteries. NAKAMURA found slightly more cases with one than with two left bronchial arteries, but between 14 and 26 (Group AII) to 43 (Group BII) times more cases with one than with two right bronchial arteries. GIORDANI AND PINNA found slightly more cases with two left bronchial arteries and five to seven (Group II) times as many cases with one right bronchial artery. LATARJET AND JUTTIN found more than three times as many cases with two left bronchial arteries and more than four times as many cases with one right bronchial artery.

In total, three cases with four bronchial arteries on one side are known: two with four independent arteries and one with three right bronchial arteries and one truncus communis.

b. Abnormal origin

b.1. *Origin from the aortic arch*

Bronchial arteries arising from the aortic arch are rather rare. The published percentages vary between 0 and 16 (Table 6), but they are not comparable because the investigators did not clearly define the borderline between the descending aorta and the aortic arch.[1]

The exact determination of this borderline is of importance for the selective investigation, however, because the arteries arising above the horizontal tangent plane of the concave part of the aortic arch cannot be catheterized.

The demonstration of these often small bronchial arteries is dependent on the technique employed.[2] In his material NAKAMURA, for instance, found no bronchial arteries originating from the aortic arch.

This artery is seldom an important component of the bronchial vascularization of the lung. Only CAULDWELL ET AL. saw in one case a complete truncus communis and in two cases a bronchial artery, supplying the entire left lung, taking origin from the lower aspect of the aortic arch.

According to the literature, the arteries, where mentioned, arise from the ventral part of the aortic arch, with the exception of one case described by O'RAHILLY ET AL. (1950) in which a truncus communis arose from the dorsal side of the right portion of the aortic arch.

b.2. *Aberrant origin*

The normal bronchial arteries do not always arise from the aorta or intercostal arteries. In very rare cases they take their origin from other arteries of the great circulation: the subclavian, internal mammary, innominate, superior intercostal, inferior thyroid, and in one reported case, from the vertebral artery. In the literature, which has been reviewed by HOVELACQUE ET AL. (1936), CAULDWELL ET AL. (1948), and CAMARRI AND MARINI (1965), these aberrant origins are usually mentioned in case reports.

Anatomical studies concentrated on aberrant origins have been performed by CAULDWELL ET AL. (1948), O'RAHILLY ET AL. (1950), EL ASSAL (1956), and LIEBOW (1965). For this study LIEBOW increased his material from 50 to 150 cases. The most frequently seen aberrant origin was that from the subclavian artery (the literature on which up to 1962 has been exhaustively reviewed by CAMARRI AND

---

[1] See also the general discussion of LIEBOW's study (page 12).
[2] See also the general discussion of NAKAMURA's study (page 11).

MARINI). In fact this was the only form of aberrant origin seen by CAULDWELL ET AL. and LIEBOW (although the latter does not explicitly say so), who observed this form in 2 per cent and 2.7 per cent of their cases, respectively.

Accessory bronchial arteries and anastomoses

Under accessory bronchial arteries is understood small arterial branches playing a supplementary role in the bronchial vascularization. They supply structures in the region of the hilus and parts of the pleura, seldom penetrating the lung tissue. They often anastomose with the large bronchial arteries. Some of these small branches occur in normal circumstances, others probably only under pathological conditions; these two forms will be discussed separately. The classification used here is based on topographic and functional factors, and cannot be applied too rigidly because so little is known about most of the vessels in this category. The literature offers very little guidance on this point due to the lack of uniformity in the use of terms and concepts and because no comparative study of the occurrence of these arteries under normal and pathological circumstances has been performed.

Normal accessory bronchial arteries and anastomoses

Although these small arteries have been described by many authors, we found a special investigation of their origin reported only by CAULDWELL ET AL. Accessory bronchial arteries were found to arise from all the arteries of the great circulation passing along or in the vicinity of lung tissue. In the region of the hilus they almost always send small anastomosing rami to the branches of the large bronchial arteries.

Some authors have described anastomoses between other arteries of the systemic circulation and bronchial arteries. Although there is of course an anatomical difference between these anastomoses and anastomosing accessory arteries, this difference has no importance for the present study. Furthermore, it is often difficult to determine whether the artery in question is an branch of a large bronchial artery anastomosing with another artery of the great circulation or an anastomosing accessory bronchial artery. Therefore, these two forms will be discussed together.

Like the normal bronchial arteries, the accessory bronchial arteries can arise from the

1. descending aorta (e.g. MARCHAND ET AL., 1950)
2. aortic arch (e.g. NAKAMURA and LIEBOW)
3. internal mammary artery (CAULDWELL ET AL. consistently saw shunts between the right superior bronchial and right mammary arteries)
4. subclavian artery (CAULDWELL ET AL. describe two types of shunt: one directly between the right superior bronchial artery and the subclavian or superior intercostal artery, and the other occurring indirectly via collaterals, between the intercostal artery of an intercosto-bronchial trunk and a superior intercostal artery)
5. inferior thyroid artery (LUSCHKA, 1863),

but they have also been described with an origin from the

6. inferior thoracic and abdominal aorta (e.g. BENNET ET AL., 1966)
7. esophageal artery (CAULDWELL ET AL.; SWIGART ET AL.; SWEET, 1950 – according to CAULDWELL ET AL. present in all individuals)
8. pericardiacophrenic artery (e.g. CHRISTELLER, 1916; VON HAYEK, 1952; LAUWERIJNS)
9. phrenic artery (e.g. LATERJET AND JUTTIN; HOVELACQUE ET AL., 1936; PAUL AND KAHN, 1967); these accessory arteries running through the pulmonary ligament
10. coronary artery (e.g. HUDSON ET AL., 1932; SCHOENMACKERS, 1958); recently reattracting interest

due to the detailed anatomical studies of PETELENZ (1965), ARVIDSSON AND MOBERG (1966), and MOBERG (1967) as well as the angiographic investigation by BJÖRK (1966)

11. vasa pulmonalis (PARK AND MICHELS, 1965)
12. thymic artery (BOIJSEN AND REUTER, 1966).

Thus, most of the accessory bronchial arteries (the ones indicated under points 3–12) have an aberrant origin.

Abnormal accessory bronchial arteries and anastomoses

Under pathological circumstances the normal accessory bronchial arteries can become wider. In addition, the anastomoses may become so wide that the normal bronchial arteries seem to be supplied via them. It then becomes difficult or impossible to distinguish between an accessory and a normal bronchial artery with an aberrant origin.

Some accessory bronchial arteries and anastomoses are probably relics of a phase in the embryonic development (TOBIN, 1952), persisting because of a need for a much greater bronchial blood supply than is normally required, for instance in congenital cardiac defects with pulmonary stenosis or atresia (DANKMEIJER, 1964, SNELLEN ET AL., 1962), but they are also found in cases of congenital bronchiectasis and infected bronchogenic cysts (LATARJET, 1958). They arise mainly from the low-thoracic and high-abdominal aorta, phrenic artery, and pericardiaco-phrenic artery. CAMARRI AND MARINI called them heterotopic bronchial arteries with an abnormal distribution in the lung. They distinguish six groups and give a very detailed review of the literature largely comprising case reports. This classification on the basis of the data in the literature is, however, very complicated and lacks clarity. Analysis would be facilitated by considering these arteries as a single group, but this involves the risk of oversimplification.

Separate mention must be made of the abnormal accessory bronchial arteries in sequestration. These arteries arise from the descending aorta just above or below the diaphragm or from the phrenic artery (PRYCE, 1946; VALLE AND WHITE, 1947; SANTY ET AL., 1952; SWIERENGA, 1952; LATARJET, 1954; AINSWORTH, 1958; GERARD AND LYONS, 1958; DELARUE ET AL., 1959; GEBAUER AND MASON, 1959; KAFKA AND BECO, 1960; TALALAK, 1960; KILMAN ET AL., 1965; RIBAUDO ET AL., 1966; RUBIN ET AL., 1966). Their presence is probably dependent on a disturbance of embryonic development (e.g. PRYCE, 1946).

In cases of sequestration or lung cyst the use of the term accessory is questionable, because in these anomalies the supplying bronchial artery is an essential and not an accessory artery. We have included them here, however, because normal bronchial arteries are found in the normal parts of the lung.

c. Conclusions of the data in the literature on the origin

A study of the literature on the origin of the bronchial arteries yields conflicting results. Critical analysis shows that most of these differences are not real, and that the remaining few are a result of differences in the technique applied.

In a new, simplified classification, two types of bronchial arteries are distinguished (*normal* and *accessory*) and two modes of origin (*normal* and *abnormal*). The normal origin is from the descending aorta and high right intercostal arteries. The abnormal origin occurs rarely, and comprises the origin from the aortic arch and the aberrant origin. Under aberrant origin is understood origins from all arteries of the great circulation with the exception of the aorta and a few cranial right intercostal arteries. The most important conclusions are:

– Most of the bronchial arteries arise from the descending aorta, always from the ventral surface.
– Despite the wide range between the extreme points of possible origin, more than 80 per cent of the bronchial arteries arise opposite the fifth and sixth thoracic vertebral levels.
– More than 85 per cent of the right bronchial arteries arise from the cranial right aortic intercostal

arteries. This combination is defined as intercosto-bronchial trunk. Normally, no bronchial arteries arise from left intercostal arteries.

– Common stems for right and left bronchial arteries occur frequently, but a complete truncus communis, i.e. only one bronchial artery, is seldom present.

– Although the possible anatomical variations are legion, in more than 75 per cent of the cases there is an intercosto-bronchial trunk with one to two bronchial arteries arising from the ventral aspect of the aorta. This represents a major simplification of the complex anatomy.

– The average number of bronchial arteries per individual is 2.7, and there are more left than right bronchial arteries. The highest number observed in one subject is five.

– A large number of accessory bronchial arteries are known, all of them making an insignificant contribution to the bronchial vascularization and usually supplying only structures in the hilar region. In pathological conditions these arteries may become dilated.

II. 2. 1. 3. CENTRAL COURSE OF THE BRONCHIAL ARTERIES

The most extensive investigation in this field is again that of CAULDWELL ET AL. In the following, where no source is given, the data are taken from their results.

Because of the left-sided position of the descending aorta with respect to the trachea, the left bronchial arteries reach the corresponding main bronchus over a shorter distance than do the right bronchial arteries.

Left bronchial arteries almost always run to the left of the esophagus. Only in a small number of cases (2.7 per cent) is the esophagus passed on the right side. In such cases the artery too passes along the right side of the trachea.

Right bronchial arteries arising from intercostal arteries run anteriorly to insinuate themselves between the vena azygos and the vertebral bodies and pass the esophagus on the right, whereas the right bronchial arteries coming independently from the aorta may pass the esophagus on either the right or left side (but usually the former is the case). A truncus communis usually runs to the left of the esophagus, the right branch running anterior to the esophagus or the trachea to the right main bronchus.

According to LIEBOW as well as LATARJET AND JUTTIN, right bronchial arteries course to the left of the main bronchus and then anterior to the trachea much more often than was found by CAULDWELL and his co-workers, but they included in their counts the right bronchial arteries from common trunks, which LIEBOW in particular found in large numbers of the cases (Table 3). A separate count can only be made for LIEBOW's data: the number of isolated right bronchial arteries on the left side of the esophagus is then much lower and the percentage barely differs from the numbers reported by CAULDWELL ET AL. (12 per cent of LIEBOW's material and 8.7 per cent of CAULDWELL ET AL.'s).

As a rule, the bronchial arteries reach the main bronchus on the postero-superior margin at the site of the attachment of the dorsal membrane and send out small branches to the anterior aspect of the bronchus (e.g. HOVELACQUE, 1936; LATARJET AND JUTTIN). In the loose network of the peribronchial connective tissue the motility is so great that the changes in the shape and location of the bronchial tree during respiration can be easily followed (FLORANGE, 1960).

Right and left bronchial arteries are connected by fine mediastinal anastomoses. When more than one bronchial artery is present on one side, shunts are also found between them in the hilar region.

AMEUILLE AND LEMOINE (1935) saw cases in which a bronchial artery traversed a hilar gland. In lymph-node pathology such an artery may show secondary changes.

II.2.1.4. INTRAPULMONARY COURSE OF THE BRONCHIAL ARTERIES

The comprehensive studies devoted to this subject chiefly concern the microscopic anatomy (e.g. MILLER, 1906). Because, in connection with the limited possibilities for visualization we are only interested in the macroscopic anatomy, the discussion of the intrapulmonary course will be brief.

The bronchial arterial branches run along the bronchi peripherally, at least two branches per bronchus, and provide for their blood supply as far as the bronchiolus respiratorius. The alveolar region is supplied by the pulmonary artery. The capillary networks of these two systems are connected.

II.2.1.5. FUNCTION OF THE BRONCHIAL ARTERIES

The structures supplied by the bronchial arteries will be briefly discussed in succession.

1. Bronchi: The supply reaches as far as the bronchiolus respiratorius (MILLER, 1906).
2. Loose peribronchial and perivascular connective tissue.
3. Trachea: In the recent literature MARK ET AL. (1965) describe an abscess in the trachea and RHEIN-LANDER ET AL. (1966) necrosis of the trachea after experimental selective perfusion with cytostatics in the bronchial arteries of dogs.
4. Esophagus: The blood supply of the middle third of the esophagus is provided by the bronchial arteries either directly or via anastomoses (CAULDWELL ET AL.; SWIGART ET AL.; TOBIN, 1952). This should be kept in mind when the evaluation of selective perfusion of lung tumors with cystostatics is undertaken, since HOCKMAN AND MARK (1964) and MARK ET AL. (1965) found esophagitis with ulceration of the mucous membranes after experimentation in dogs and RHEINLANDER ET AL. (1966) even saw perforation of the esophagus.
5. Visceral pleura: The supply of the visceral pleura has been studied by many investigators, including ZUCKERKANDL (1883), MILLER (1906), HOVELACQUE ET AL. (1936), VERLOOP (1948), MARCHAND ET AL. (1950), CUDKOWICZ AND ARMSTRONG (1951), VON HAYEK (1953a), LAUWERIJNS, and FEDEROVA (1965). It appears that the mediastinal and diaphragmatic visceral pleura are supplied by superficially running twigs of the bronchial arteries, the other parts of the visceral pleura being supplied by pulmonary arteries. Deep branches of the bronchial arteries supply the interlobar pleura almost as far as the the costal pleura; according to MARCHAND ET AL., these derive from the vasa vasorum of the pulmonary arteries.
6. Vasa vasorum: The blood supply of the aortic arch (HOVELACQUE ET AL., 1936), the pulmonary arteries (e.g. CUDKOWICZ AND ARMSTRONG, 1951, and MILNE, 1967) and pulmonary veins (e.g. VER-LOOP, 1948) is provided by branches of the bronchial arteries. CLARKE (1965) demonstrated that only the pulmonary trunk is supplied by another source, i.e. by branches of the coronary arteries.
7. Lymph glands: Paratracheal, carinal, and hilar lymph glands (CUDKOWICZ AND ARMSTRONG, 1951; TOBIN, 1952) as well as the intrapulmonary lymph nodes and lymphoid tissue (LAUWERIJNS) are supplied with blood by the bronchial arteries.
8. Nerves: The vagus and broncho-pulmonary nerves are accompanied and supplied by fine rami of the bronchial artery (e.g. CUDKOWICZ AND ARMSTRONG, 1951; VON HAYEK, 1953a).
9. Parietal leaf of the pericardium: CAULDWELL ET AL. saw large branches of the bronchial artery running to the pericardium in 10 per cent of the cases. According to HOVELACQUE ET AL. (1936) only the dorsal and part of the lateral side of the percardium are supplied by this artery.
10. Prevertebral muscles: HOVELACQUE ET AL. (1936) consistently saw one or more large branches being sent to the prevertebral muscles.
11. Thymus: LATARJET (1954) saw a small twig disappearing into the thymus in some cases.

II.2.2. Bronchial veins

The bronchial veins were discovered by the Leiden anatomist JACOBUS RAU (1658–1719). The most fundamental anatomical study is still the work published by ZUCKERKANDL in 1881.

The drainage of the blood carried by the bronchial arteries is a complex anatomical situation shown, with some schematization, in fig. 2.

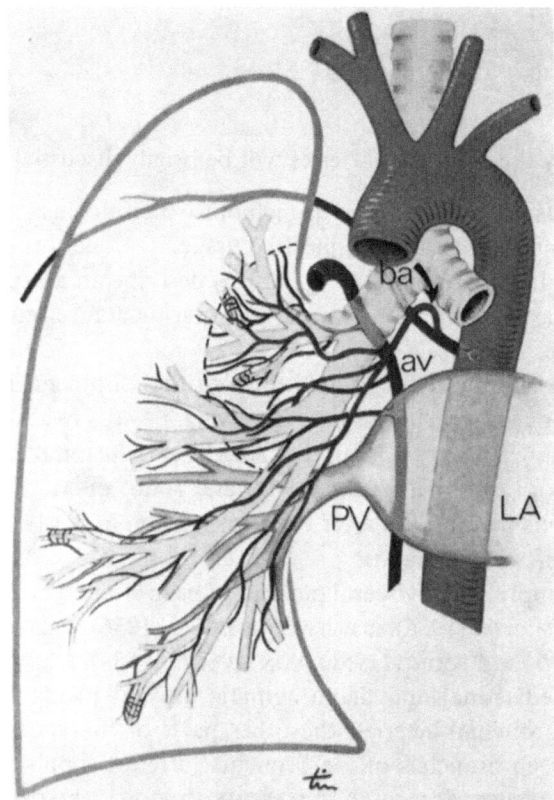

Fig. 2. Diagram of the bronchial venous system. In the hilar region (inside the dotted line) bronchial veins drain a small part of the bronchial blood into the azygos (av) or hemiazygos veins. In the lung, however, the greater part of the blood supplied by the bronchial artery (ba) is drained by the pulmonary veins (PV). LA: left atrium.

A distinction must be made between a central and a peripheral system of bronchial veins, which will be discussed separately.

In the periphery the venous drainage occurs via a venous plexus in the bronchial wall, situated on either side of the tunica muscularis (MILLER, 1906), the two being connected by anastomoses (CAMARRI AND MARINI, 1960). From the bronchiolus respiratorius as far as the segmental bronchi the blood is drained into pulmonary veins and by veins called by some, following LE FORT (1859), broncho-pulmonary veins and by others, following MARCHAND ET AL. (1950), true or deep bronchial veins. According to ZUCKERKANDL (1881) the drainage into the pulmonary veins occurs continuously via multiple small connecting veins. According to MARCHAND ET AL. (1950), each lung has one large collective vein emptying into a large pulmonary vein just before the latter enters the left auricle or emptying directly into the left auricle. This true or deep bronchial vein has numerous anastomoses with pulmonary veins.

The drainage of the central bronchi (bronchi of the 1st, 2nd, and sometimes of the 3rd order), of the other structures of the central supply region of the bronchial artery[1], and of the mediastinal and interlobar visceral pleura (SCHOENMACKERS, 1960; FEDOROVA, 1965) occurs in a different way, as follows:

a. Via the venae bronchiales anteriores and posteriores of ZUCKERKANDL also called the pleuro-hilar veins of MARCHAND ET AL., the blood is drained into veins of the great circulation.

On the right side these veins generally drain into the upper part of the azygos vein (according to MARCHAND ET AL. usually just before the latter's entrance into the vena cava superior) or directly into the vena cava superior. According to SCHOENMACKERS (1960) they sometimes empty into the vena cava inferior.

On the left side the venae bronchiales anteriores empty into the venae bronchiales posteriores, which in turn generally drain into the superior hemiazygos vein, the inferior hemiazygos vein, or the superior intercostal vein.

These bronchial veins have seldom been reported to drain into the innominate vein (MARCHAND ET AL.), the subclavian and other brachiocephalic veins, the intercostal and internal mammary veins.

ZUCKERKANDL and other authors have reported finding multiple anastomoses between the venae bronchiales anteriores and posteriores and the large pulmonary veins. The largest of these connecting veins empty into the central pulmonary veins or directly into the left auricle.

b. Via the venae recurrentes of ZUCKERKANDL or the T-shaped veins of LIEBOW (1953), another portion of the blood is drained as it were backwards into the intrapulmonary portion of the pulmonary veins.

Between the central and the peripheral systems of bronchial veins there are intercommunications first described by LE FORT (1859). According to MARCHAND ET AL., these two venous systems are connected by a few small anastomoses; according to ZUCKERKANDL, they are connected almost continously by numerous anastomoses.

Anastomoses

In addition to the communications with the pulmonary veins, still other anastomoses of the bronchial veins have been described, i.e. with the esophageal veins and via them with the portal vein system (CALABRESI AND ABELMANN, 1957), with the pericardial and tracheal veins (e.g. LIEBOW, 1953), and further with the coronary veins, the venous plexus around the aorta, and the prevertebral veins (SCHOENMACKERS, 1960), all of which drain into the azygos-hemiazygos system. According to the latter author, small veins from the diaphragm, esophagus, pericardium, and parietal pleura, besides direct drainage into the azygos vein, also empty into the venous plexus around the aorta.

Discussion

Thus, part of the blood in the bronchial arteries reaches the left atrium via the larger peripheral venous system; the rest arrives, via the smaller central system, at the right atrium. Experiments in dogs, in which the anatomical relationships are roughly the same as in man, have shown that the part received by the left auricle represent about two-thirds of the total flow (BRUNER AND SCHMIDT, 1947; AVIADO ET AL., 1961; MARTINEZ ET AL., 1961). According to the results of a lung-perfusion study done by AVIADO ET AL., this quantity was 62 per cent and according to experiments with heart-lung preparations performed by MARTINEZ ET AL. 68 per cent. About one-third, therefore, enters the right atrium. In some diseases there is an extracardial exchange of blood between the atria (FERGUSON ET AL., 1944; HURWITZ ET AL., 1954; SCHOENMACKERS, 1963; VIAMONTE, 1967b).

[1] See under Function of the Bronchial Arteries (page 23).

II.2.3. Intercostal arteries[1]

The upper one or two intercostal arteries arise from the superior intercostal artery. The others arise in pairs dorsally from the descending aorta. According to ENNABLI (1966), left cranial intercostal arteries arise a few millimeters higher and closer to the median line than the corresponding right intercostal arteries. In the caudal direction the sites of origin become more symmetrical and the vertical distance between them amounts to 6–8 mm. Some intercostal arteries provide for the supply of several adjacent intercostal spaces.

The higher intercostal arteries arise from the aorta, the more cranially they are directed. This observation has contributed to the technique used for catheterization.

From their origin the intercostal arteries run over the prevertebral muscles to the costal groove. After remaining for a short distance in this groove, they enter the intercostal space and divide after a few centimeters to form two branches. The upper branch is highly developed and runs along the upper side of the corresponding rib. The thin lower branch runs on the upper side of the next rib. Both branches have communications with the rami intercostales of the interal mammary artery.

Intercostal arteries send branches to the spinal cord and prevertebral muscles, dorsal back muscles (rami dorsales), intercostal muscles, and the parietal pleura.

The superior intercostal artery arises separately or together with the deep cervical artery (truncus costocervicalis) from the subclavian artery.

II.2.4. Intercostal veins

The intercostal veins run on the upper side of the intercostal arteries and empty into the azygos-hemiazygos system and in rare cases into the left innominate vein. Ventrally, the intercostal veins have anastomoses with the internal mammary veins.

---

[1] Where no reference is given, the anatomical data derive from the anatomy textbooks by SPALTEHOLZ, RAUBER KOPSCH, and CORNING.

III
TECHNIQUE

III.1. METHODS APPLIED FOR THE ARTERIOGRAPHY

THE CATHETERIZATION

Refinement of the methods used for selective radiological investigation of blood vessels is required for the catheterization of the smaller arteries such as the bronchial and intercostal arteries. These narrow vessels are occluded by the usual catheters, so that new types had to be formed.

Catheterization was performed after percutaneous puncture of the femoral artery, under local anaesthesia, according to a modification of the SELDINGER method (VAN VOORTHUISEN, 1967). We used the red KIFA catheter, made of radiopaque polythene (ÖDMAN, 1959), initially with the shape applied by VIAMONTE (1964). A slight caudal curve presses the point lightly against the wall of the aorta. Cranially (toward the tip of the catheter) comes a more acute curve of about 110°. We draw the point out longer than is usually done, resulting in a smaller inner diameter (0.5 to 0.7 mm). Fig. 3 shows one of these catheters and, for purposes of comparison, a catheter used for selective arteriography of the kidney. For the introduction of our catheter, we were unable to use a flexible guide wire of normal caliber, and those of the smallest caliber, such as are used for catheterization of children, proved to be insufficiently rigid. We therefore use a solid stainless steel guide wire 1.5 m long (Fig. 3, inset 1), which is introduced into a wide catheter later replaced by a thin bronchial catheter, the guide wire being held in place – stretched and without movement – during the exchange, to prevent injury to the vessel.

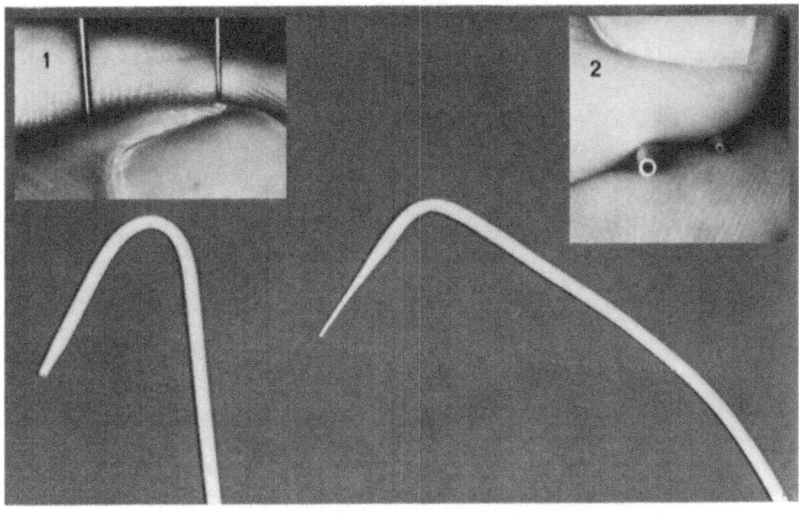

renal catheter   bronchial catheter

Fig. 3. Catheter adapted for bronchial arteriography compared with the catheter used for selective renal arteriography.
Inset 1: Thin solid guide wire used for the introduction of our catheter compared with a flexible guide wire of normal caliber.

The catheters for the investigation of the right and left bronchial arteries – actually intercosto-bronchial trunks and the other normally arising bronchial arteries – must be given different shapes.

Fig. 4*a* shows the anatomical situation on the right side. Since the right bronchial arteries usually arise (see page 16) from the upper right intercostal arteries and these high intercostal arteries run in the cranial direction, the cranial curve in the catheter must be 135°. The tip is slightly curved upwards. The length of the straight part to the tip must be chosen in proportion to the caliber of the aorta, so that the point is not going to float freely in the lumen of the aorta. The slight caudal curve must hold the point in the proper position in the vessel.

For the left bronchial arteries (and the others with a normal origin) catheters must be shaped differently, as shown in the lateral projection in fig. 4*b*. These bronchial arteries arise ventrally and perpendicularly from the aorta. The tip of the above-described catheter could still reach the vessel in the descending part of the thoracic aorta, but in the aortic arch the point would slide along the ostium. To permit catheterization, therefore, both the cranial and the caudal curves of the catheter must be more acute. Unless the shape of the catheter is adapted to the above-described anatomical conditions, the results of arteriography of left bronchial arteries will be poor (Fig. 13).

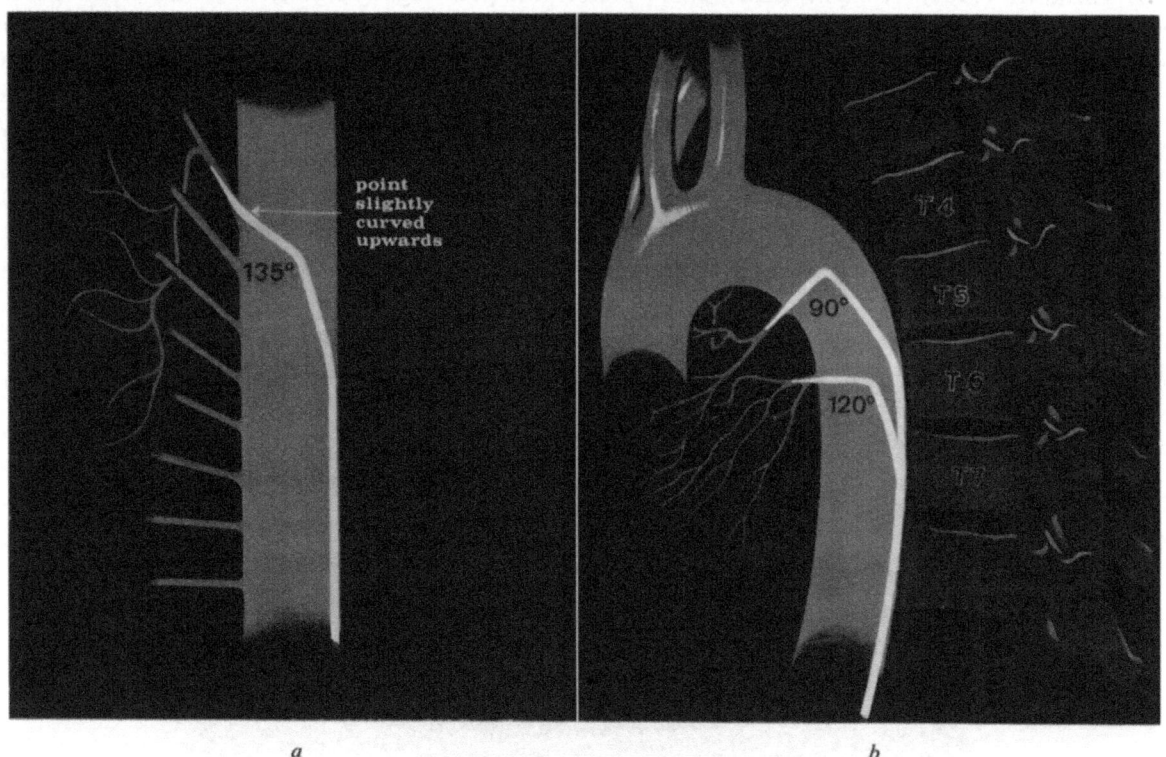

a   *b*

Fig. 4. Diagram illustrating the anatomical basis taken for our technique applied for the catheterization of bronchial arteries.
a: Catheterization of right bronchial arteries (actually high right intercostal arteries).
b: Catheter for left bronchial arteries (actually all bronchial arteries directly arising from the aorta).

The catheter is introduced high into the thoracic aorta. The upper border of the 5th and the lower border of the 6th thoracic vertebrae are marked by lead pellets previously applied to the patient's back. The wall of the aortic segment between these markers is systematically searched, since most of the bronchial arteries arise in this segment. This search is done under fluoroscopic control – image amplifier – television circuit. If a complete bronchial arteriogram is to be made, a catheter with an inner diameter at the point of 0.7 mm and curved for use in right bronchial arteries is introduced. The uppermost right intercostal arteries are sought. After this search, in which an intercosto-bronchial trunk is usually found, the ventral wall of the aorta is probed by moving the point of the catheter up and down with a zigzag movement between T5 and T6. It is not necessary to turn the patient during this procedure, because the entrance of the catheter point into at branch of the aorta gives a distinct optical effect. This effect is even more distinct when use is made of the electronically enlarged picture. If no bronchial artery has been found after two minutes at the most, the catheter is exchanged for a pre-formed catheter for the investigation of left bronchial arteries, which has a smaller inner diameter near the point (0.5 to 0.6 mm). The systematic search of the ventral aortic wall between T5 and T6 is then repeated with greater precision.

If the mobility of the catheter is not impeded, the point can usually be seen entering an artery within a few seconds. When the catheter is less maneuverable – due to marked tortuousity of the pelvic arteries and aorta or spasm in the femoral and external iliac arteries – the catheterization may require much more time. Each time an artery has been found, 0.1 to 0.5 ml of contrast medium is injected into it.

Intercostal arteries and large bronchial arteries are easily recognized on the monitor of the image amplifier. The patient experiences a burning sensation in the back after the injection of contrast medium into an intercostal artery and an urge to cough[1] or a burning sensation in the throat after injection of a bronchial artery. An injection of contrast medium into small bronchial arteries often cannot be seen on the monitor but is always following by a fit of coughing. When a small bronchial artery arises from an intercostal artery, the burning sensation in the back often masks the cough stimulus, but the patient usually still notices the burning sensation in the throat.

THE SERIAL ARTERIOGRAPHY

Depending on the caliber of the catheterized arteries, 3 to 12 ml of contrast medium was injected. To prevent the catheter from jumping back out of the vessel the injection was done under low pressure (1.3 to 1.7 atm.; GIDLUND injection apparatus), the lowest pressure of course being used for the narrowest vessels. The average injection time was 3 seconds. Exposures were made for 6 to 12 seconds, starting at the beginning of the injection. In the arterial phase the exposure frequency was 2 per second and in the venous phase 1 per second. For radiography a film changer was used (ELEMA-SCHÖNANDER, film size 35 × 35 cm).

Series exposures were usually made in the antero-posterior and lateral directions.

RADIOGRAPHY

For the exposures a roentgen tube with a rapidly rotating anode and foci of 0.6 mm^2 (AP) and 1.2 mm^2 (L) was used. The focus-film distance was chosen at 100 cm. A grid with 24 lines per cm, ratio 10, was applied.

It took a considerable amount of time to find the optimal tube tension. If the kilovoltage is too high, the contrast differences are too small to visualize the small vessels, and if it is too low the differences between the lung fields and the mediastinum are disturbing. We finally chose 75 kV as the most satisfactory. Since the contrast difference between the mediastinum and lung field increases after inspiration and decreases after expiration (Fig. 5), it is preferable from a technical point of view to make the exposures during expiration.

---

[1] The cough is not pathognomonic of bronchial arteriography. According to BELL ET AL. (1959), it also occurs after wedge arteriography of small branches of the pulmonary artery.

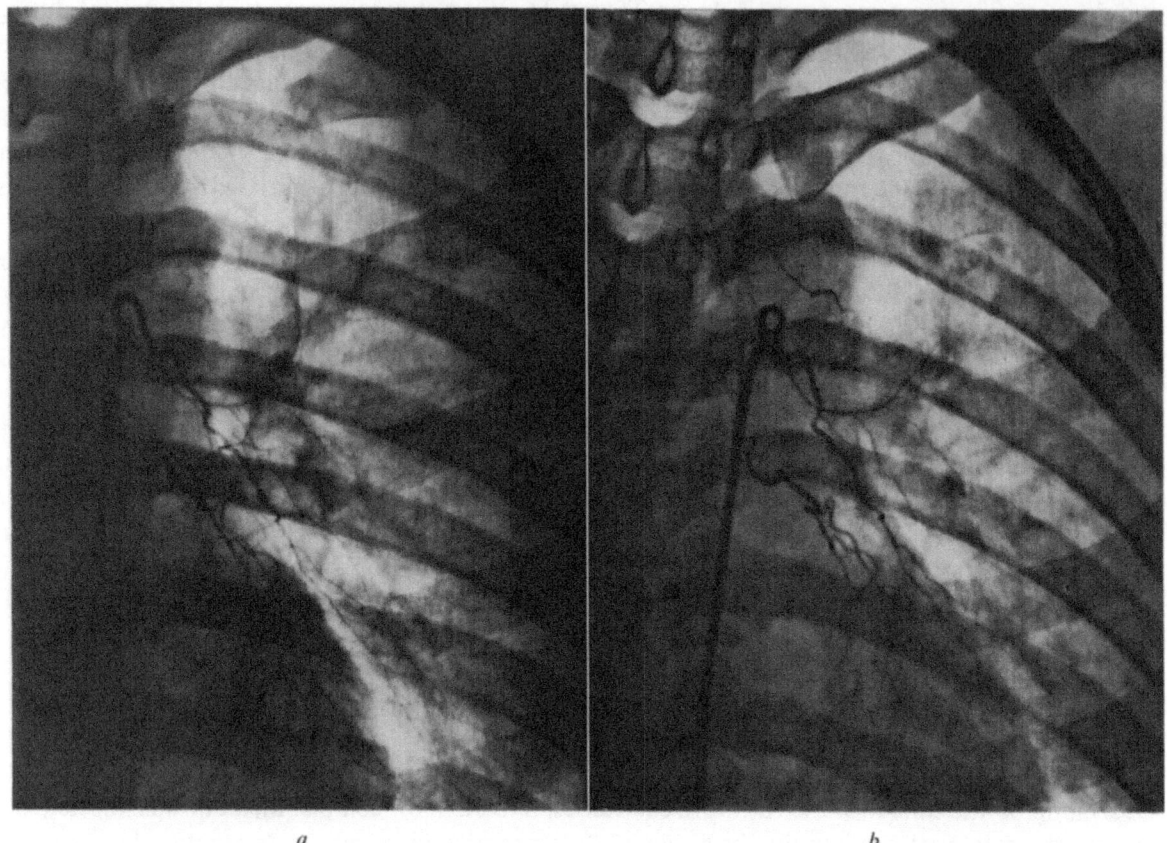

a   *b*

Fig. 5. The contrast difference between the mediastinum and the lung-field increases after inspiration (*a*) and decreases after expiration (*b*).

THE CONTRAST MEDIUM

As contrast medium Isopaque 60 per cent was used because its low viscosity facilitates injection into small vessels.

III.2. COMPARISON OF AORTOGRAPHIC AND
SELECTIVE ARTERIOGRAPHIC RESULTS

In 40 per cent of the patients in our series, aortograms were also made. Most of these aortograms were made during VALSALVA's maneuvre, because the investigations of NORDENSTRÖM (1960, 1966e), LUDIN (1963), and FOX ET AL. (1966) have shown that this leads to an appreciable retardation of the bloodflow, thus enhancing the supply of contrast medium.

Under a pressure of 7 atm., 50 ml Isopaque 60 per cent was injected through a catheter with a large number of holes, the tip lying at the level of the origin of the left subclavian artery. The injection time was 0.5 to 1 second, and series exposures were made for 6 seconds at a frequency of at most 2 per second. The patient was in the supine or prone position or on his side.

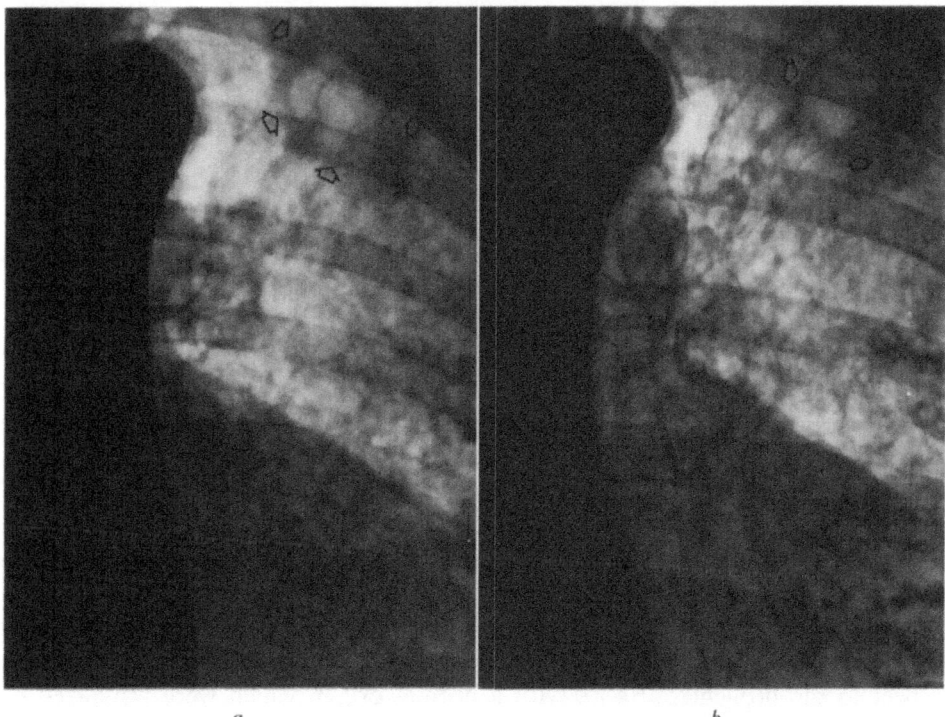

a   *b*

Fig. 6. Comparison of aortograms made in the supine position (*a*) and in the prone position after 10 seconds of straining (*b*).
a: In the supine position the best picture made during the arterial phase shows only two vaguely visible branches of the bronchial arteries in the region of the left hilus.
b: The X-ray in the prone position shows three distinct bronchial branches in the central region, as well as vaguely fine twigs which can be followed into the area of the lesion (arrows), located cranially in the axillary field.

The aortograms made in the prone position after 10 seconds of straining gave the most information and the 'normal' aortograms made in the supine position the least (Fig. 6). Aortography done with the patient in the lateral position – either with or without straining – also gave very little information.

3

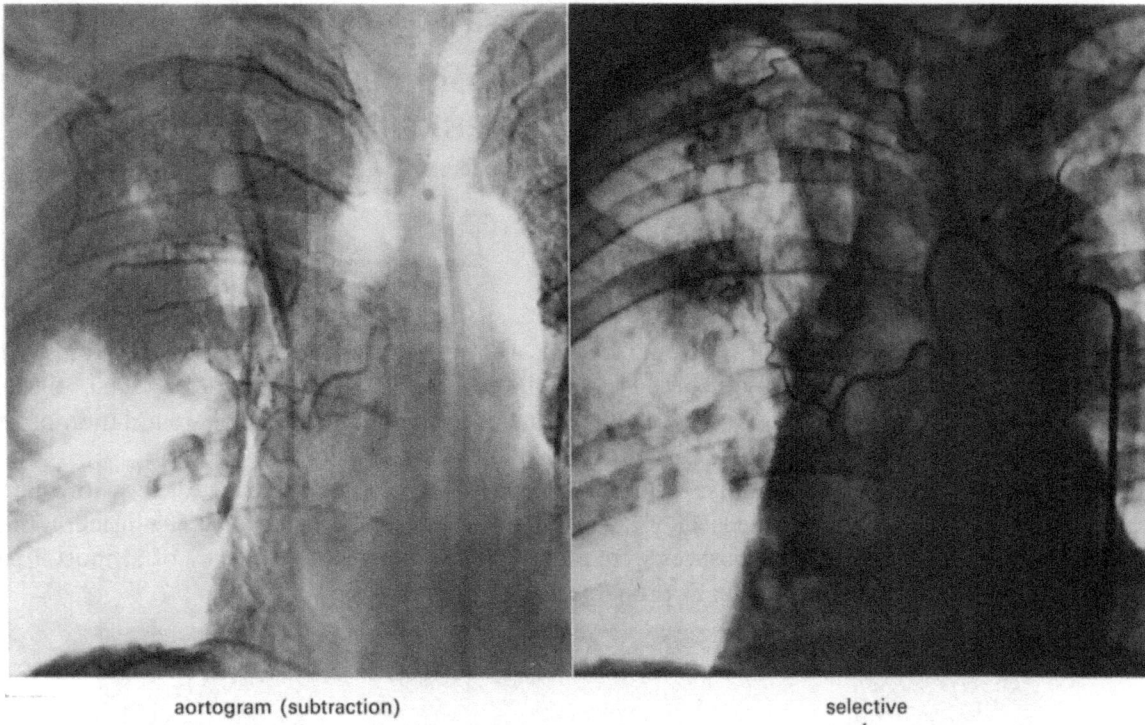

aortogram (subtraction)   selective
a   *b*

Fig. 7. Comparison of aortography (*a*) and selective catheterization (*b*). Patient with recurrent tumor in the right upper lobe. Only the selective picture shows vessels in the region of the tumor. Subtraction was applied for the aortogram.

Bronchial arteries of normal caliber were seldom visible outside the parahilar region. Dilated bronchial arteries could indeed be observed on the aortogram, but these vessels can always be found by selective arteriography. Comparison showed that with selective arteriography arteries with a caliber two to four times smaller can be visualized than with aortography (Fig. 7). More than 15 per cent of the already selectively catheterized bronchial arteries could not be observed again on the aortograms of the same patient. There were, however, a number of bronchial arteries that could only be demonstrated aortographically, i.e. all those with an aberrant origin and 9 per cent of the bronchial arteries with a normal origin.

In some anomalies, i.e. congenital heart and lung diseases with an increased bronchial circulation, the number of bronchial arteries with an aberrant origin is very high. In these cases an aortogram provides important additional information. For other reasons too, as will be discussed in the relevant sections, it is advisable to perform a supplementary aortography in patients showing congenital heart disease with increased bronchial circulation.

With respect to the bronchial arteries with a normal origin, which were visualized only on the aortograms, it may be remarked that the picture was too poor to yield diagnostic information. For acquired pulmonary diseases we therefore consider that there is no indication for supplementary aortographic investigation.

III.3. APPLICATIONS OF SUBTRACTION

GROEN ET AL. (1965, 1966) obtained good results by applying subtraction to the aortographic method. It therefore seemed useful to us to explore the applications of subtraction to selective arteriography.

In a number of cooperative, well-immobilized patients, in whom the position of the ribs and diaphragm indicated that respiration had not occurred during the serial exposures, subtractions were made.

a. We first investigated the extent to which the smaller arterial branches in the region of the pulmonary lesion could be visualized more distinctly. In spite of all the precautions taken, these small vessels were found to shift slightly, which made it impossible to obtain a satisfactory subtraction (Fig. 8). It need hardly be said that for very small vessels only the smallest amount of displacement is sufficient to make subtraction impossible. For the peripheral regions of the lungs, therefore, subtraction has no applications.

b. In the hilar and mediastinal region, however, use of subtraction gave considerable improvement in the results. We use the method mainly for the visualization of bronchial veins. Fig. 9 shows an example of a subtraction as well as the original picture, in which the vein is very difficult to distinguish.

c. Subtraction is also useful for the demonstration of a small quantity of contrast medium in large vessels, such as pulmonaries (Fig. 10).

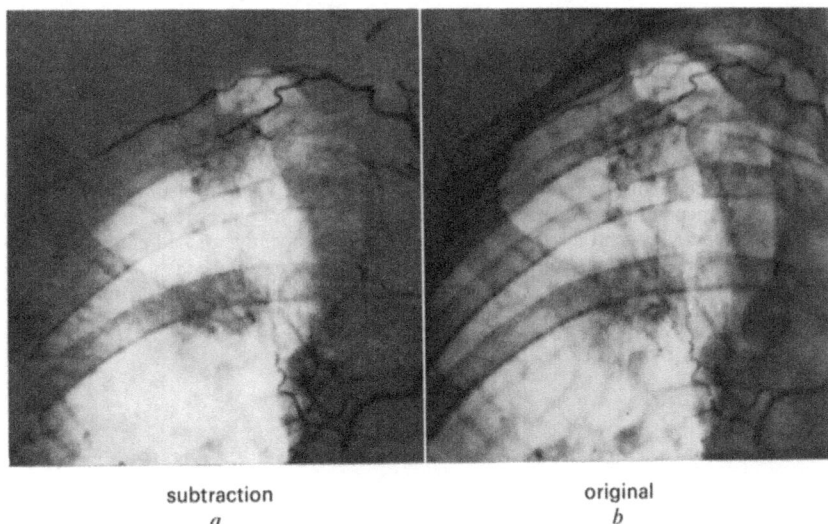

subtraction   original
a   b

Fig. 8. Comparison of a subtraction (*a*) and the original X-ray (*b*). The tiny vessels in and around the area of the tumor are less clearly visible on the subtraction. Same patient as in Fig. 7.

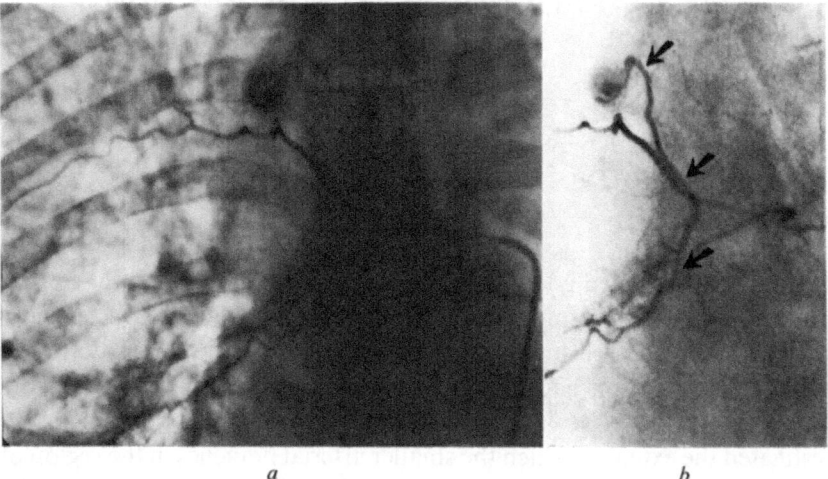

Fig. 9. The subtraction (*b*) shows a bronchial vein (arrows) hardly discernable on the original X-ray (*a*).

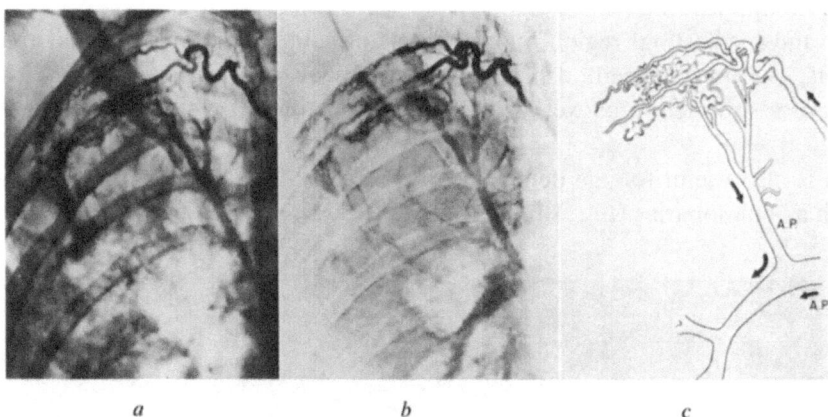

Fig. 10. Intercostal arteriogram in a case of histiocytosis X. Via transpleural anastomoses, the contrast medium has reached the pulmonary artery of the upper lobe (*a*). Retrograde – from peripheral to central – the hilus is reached; subsequently, a small amount of contrast medium has flowed into the pulmonary branch of the lower lobe (arrows in schematic representation *c*). This last observation could only be made in the subtraction (*b*). AP: arteria pulmonalis.

III.4. CONCLUSIONS

1. By using differently shaped catheters for the investigation of right and left bronchial arteries, the chance of a successful and complete selective arteriographic investigation is appreciably increased.
2. There is no indication for supplementary aortography during investigation of the bronchial vascularization of *acquired* pulmonary diseases, but for *congenital* heart and lung diseases accompanied by increased bronchial circulation aortography provides valuable supplementary information. Aortograms made in the prone position after 10 seconds of straining give the most information.
3. Subtraction is useful for the visualization of bronchial veins and for the demonstration of small amounts of contrast medium in wide vessels (e.g. pulmonary vessels), but has no value in the peripheral regions of the lungs.

IV
RESULTS OF THE PRESENT STUDY

Introduction

The discussion of the literature has made it evident that the anatomy of the origin of bronchial arteries is extremely complex. Although it is possible to state general rules [1], the anatomical data offer little encouragement for the undertaking of an arteriographic investigation of the bronchial arteries; the chance of obtaining a complete selective bronchial arteriogram indeed seems small. Furthermore, the bronchial arteries with an abnormal origin cannot be reached selectively via the groin. There are, however, a few favorable circumstances:

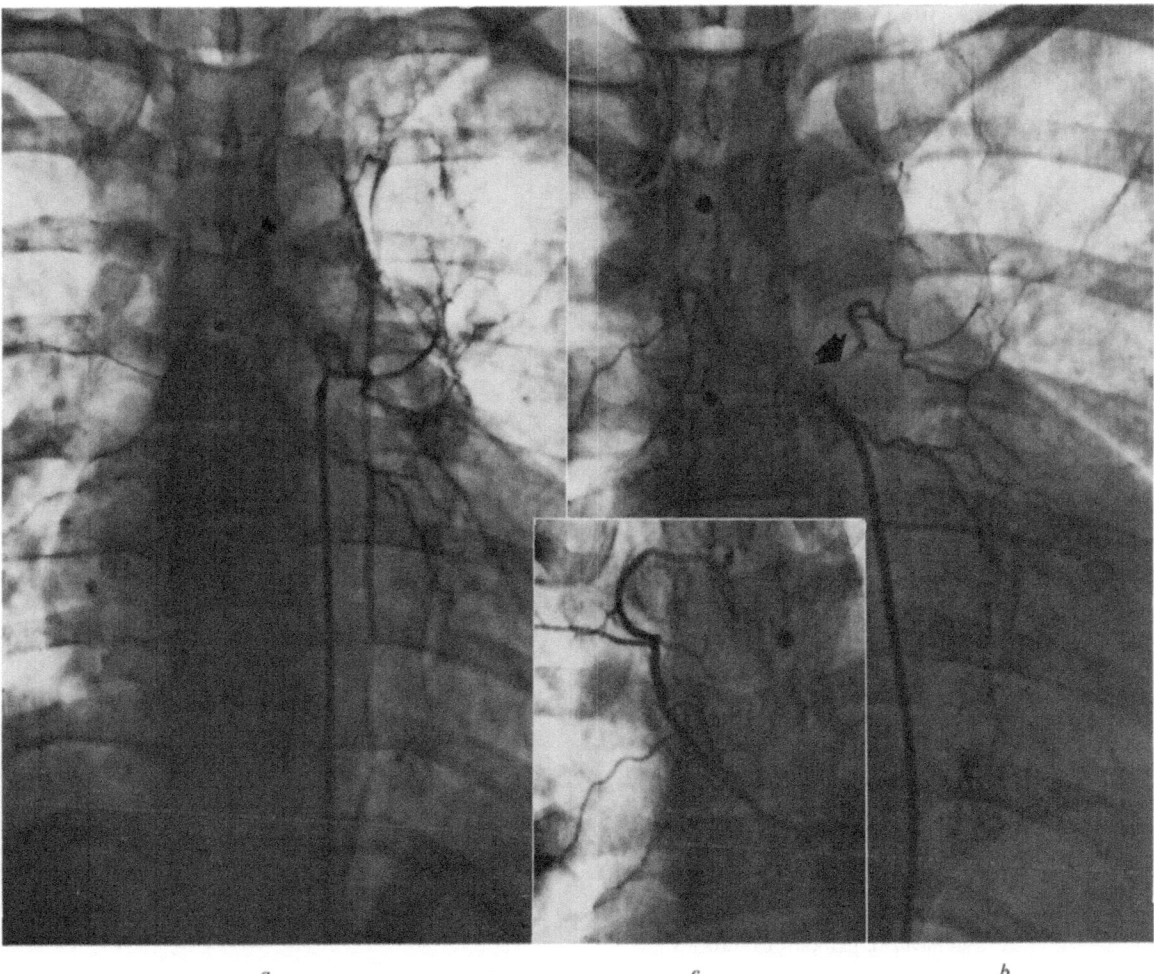

a   c   b

Fig. 11. The bronchial arteries are connected by fine anastomoses.

a: Injection of contrast medium into the left superior bronchial artery. Via collateral vessels, scarcely or not visible on the X-ray, the left inferior bronchial artery is filled as well as an accessory bronchial artery on the right side, arising from the aortic arch (arrow). The left internal mammary artery also shows collateral filling.

b: Arteriogram of the left inferior bronchial artery. Collateral filling of the left superior bronchial artery. As a result of the injection pressure, the latter vessel is visualized up to its aortic origin and there is even a retrograde flow of contrast medium into the aorta (arrow). On the right side occurs filling of a fourth bronchial artery, again via invisible anastomoses.

c: Arteriogram of the fourth artery, which after selective catheterization proved to derive from an intercosto-bronchial trunk.

[1] See under Literature, Origin Bronchial Arteries, Conclusion (page 21,22).

a. Fine anastomoses between bronchial arteries are known[1], and via these anastomoses, which are often almost or completely invisible on the arteriogram, bronchial arteries other than the catheterized one can be filled collaterally (Fig. 11). This made it possible in a few patients to obtain a picture of the vascularization of a pathological process even though the supplying bronchial artery had not been found. It is remarkable that there is no reference in the literature to this fortunate aspect of collateral filling.

b. The artery supplying a pathological structure with blood is usually easier to catheterize than the other bronchial arteries, because as a rule such a structure requires more blood than the same volume of normal lung tissue and therefore the vessel has a wider caliber making it easier to find (Fig. 12). BOIJSEN AND ZSIGMOND (1965) have also pointed this out. Even more important, in our opinion, is that the flow in the vessel is also increased, as a result of which the tip of the catheter is so to speak sucked in and thus tends to remain in place.

c. Bronchial arteries arising from the aortic arch and from other arteries of the systemic circulation are almost always accessory bronchial arteries, thus playing an accessory role in the bronchial vascularization.

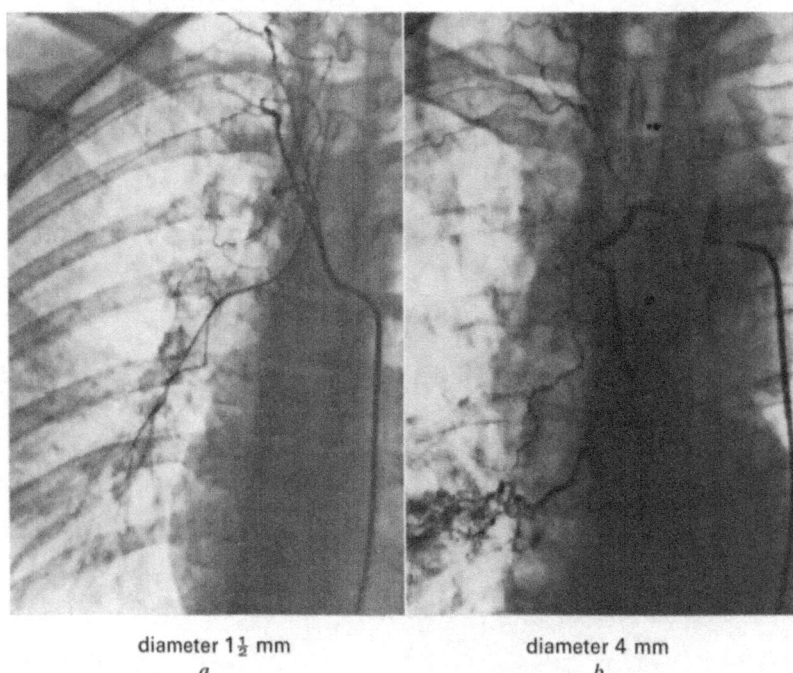

diameter 1½ mm   diameter 4 mm
        a   *b*

Fig. 12. Bronchial artery of normal caliber compared with a dilated bronchial artery supplying a pathological process.
a: The normal caliber (1.5 mm on the original film).
b: Strongly dilated artery in a richly vascularized pulmonary tumor (4 mm on the original film).

_____

[1] See under Literature, Central Course Bronchial Arteries (page 22).

a

truncus intercosto-bronchialis 59 (49)

b

arteria bronchialis sinistra 51 (17)

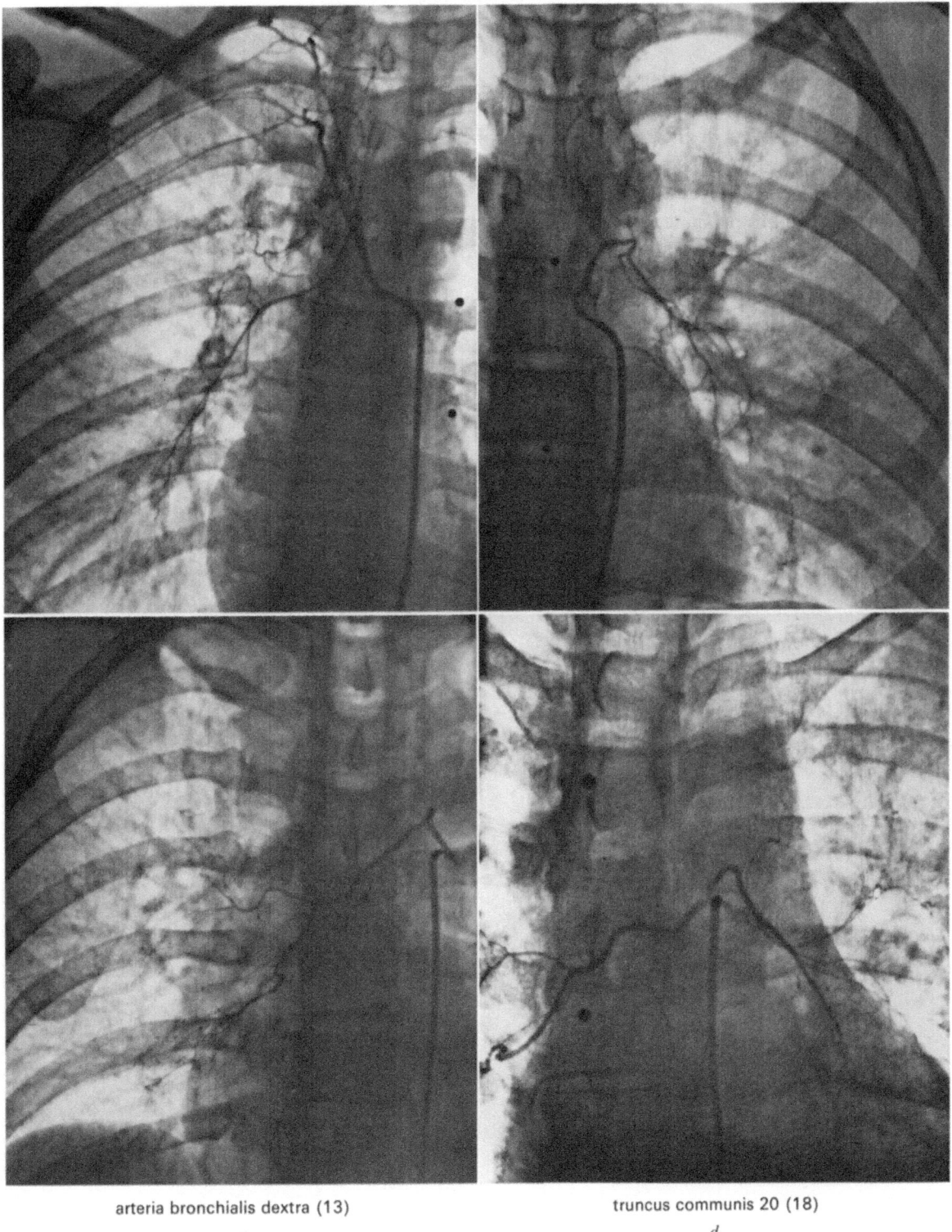

arteria bronchialis dextra (13)

c

truncus communis 20 (18)

d

Fig. 13. Anatomical classification of 143 selective bronchial arteriograms. The values between brackets refer to data of VIAMONTE ET AL. (1965) (see also Fig. 28). The values pertaining to the left bronchial arteries show a striking discrepancy.

Material

In eighty-four patients an attempt was made to obtain a complete arteriogram of the bronchial arteries. This resulted in 143 selective bronchial arteriograms (Fig. 13) and 120 selective intercostal arteriograms. In seven of these patients no bronchial arteries could be catheterized. In the other seventy-seven, 216 bronchial arteries were visualized, 73 of which – 216 minus 143 – had therefore been filled collaterally or during aortography.

The discussion on this material will be divided into two parts: Anatomy and Pathology. The seven cases in which the investigation failed will be discussed separately (page 163).

IV.1. PART I – ANATOMY

In this chapter an anatomical classification based on the present patient material is given. This may be useful for other investigators, since the classification is based on data obtained by catheterization *in vivo*. Supplementary information can also be given on some points. The present findings are compared with the anatomical data in the literature, which are based on autopsy material.

IV.1.1. Bronchial arteries

In this section our material will be treated in the same sequence as applied in the anatomical section of the review of the literature (page 13–23), and the same nomenclature will be used.

IV.1.1.1. ORIGIN OF THE BRONCHIAL ARTERIES

For the study of the origin of the bronchial arteries, we first determined the number of patients for whom a complete bronchial arteriogram had been obtained. We included not only the selectively catheterized bronchial arteries but also all those aortographically and collaterally filled arteries whose origin could be demonstrated.

In fifty-seven cases the bronchial arteriogram seemed to be complete, and in fourty-seven of these this was virtually certain.

There were therefore twenty cases with incomplete arteriograms. In eleven of these the vascularization of a small part of the lungs was missing and in the remaining nine only the bronchial vascularization of the right lung could be demonstrated. In nine patients, therefore, no left bronchial arteries could be catheterized, whereas there was no case in which only left bronchial arteries were found.

a. Normal origin

Normal anatomical situation

The situation with one intercosto-bronchial trunk and two left bronchial arteries was also the most frequent in our material (Fig. 14), but in a lower percentage than is mentioned in the literature (Table 4); depending on the classification, our values were 19.3 to 25.5 per cent (Table 11, 'NORMAL ANATOMY' I).

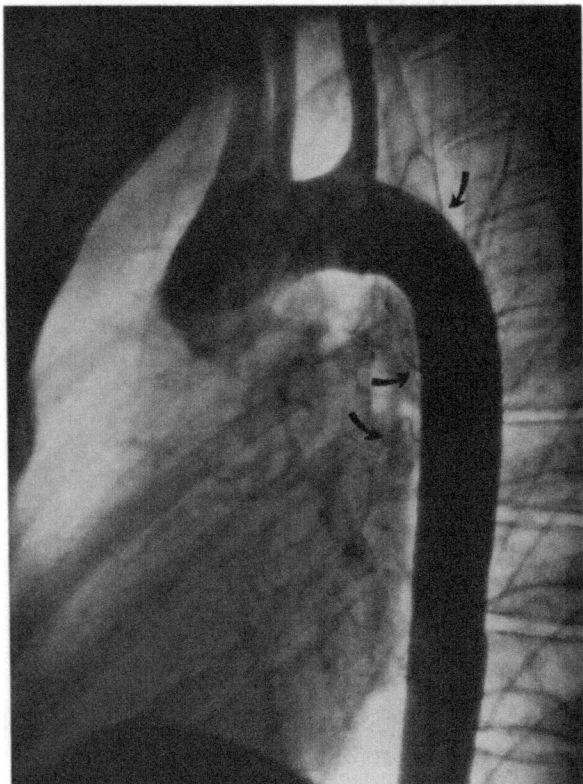

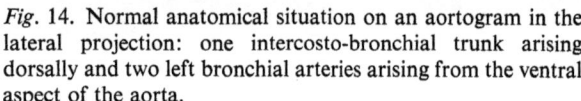

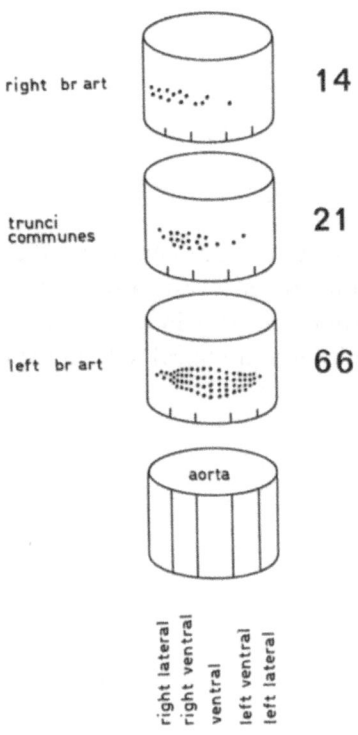

Fig. 14. Normal anatomical situation on an aortogram in the lateral projection: one intercosto-bronchial trunk arising dorsally and two left bronchial arteries arising from the ventral aspect of the aorta.

Fig. 15. Transverse spread of the sites of origin on the ventral side of the aorta for the different types of bronchial arteries. Most of these origins can also be seen in Fig. 27.

a.1. *Origin from the descending aorta*

Most of the bronchial arteries arose from the descending aorta. The part of the aortic wall from which they arose, the level, and range of the distribution of the origins will be discussed separately.

Dorsal-ventral

All the bronchial arteries in our material arose from the ventral aspect of the aorta. The site of origin could be accurately determined for 14 right bronchial arteries, 21 trunci communes, and 66 left bronchial arteries (Table 7). Disregarding their level of origin, these arteries were put on the ventral wall of the aorta which for that purpose as shown in fig. 15 was subdivided into five equal longitudinal bands to facilitate the visual representation of the distribution of the origin sites per type of bronchial artery in the transverse direction (see also fig. 27).

Discussion

The origin of right bronchial arteries is almost entirely restricted to the right side of the ventral part of the aortic wall. Only one artery (7 per cent) arose from the left side.

Most of the trunci communes also arise from the right ventral side but on the average the location is slightly more central. In 14 per cent of the cases they took origin from the left ventral side.

Left bronchial arteries arise on the average much further to the left. Although their origin shows a slight predilection for the right side, the distribution over the anterior wall of the aorta is nevertheless almost proportional. An origin on the left ventral side of the aorta was seen in 44 per cent of the cases.

The scanty data on this point in the literature are shown in table 1. There is some agreement between our findings and those of CAULDWELL ET AL. Although GIORDANI AND PINNA give percentages, these are not based on the number of ostia. CAULDWELL ET AL. saw one case in which a left bronchial artery arose from the dorsal aspect of the aorta.

Conclusions

Bronchial arteries originating from the aorta must be sought on the ventral aspect of this vessel. Right bronchial arteries and trunci communes are most likely to be found on the right ventral side, although on the average the latter arise slightly more centrally. Left bronchial arteries must be sought over the entire ventral part, but most of them have a central site of origin.

Cranial – caudal

Most of the bronchial arteries arose between the levels of T5 and T6. The level and distribution range of the origins will be discussed in detail below (page 57-65), where the origin of intercosto-bronchial trunks and bronchial arteries from the aortic arch can be included in the discussion.

a.2. *Origin from intercostal arteries*

An intercosto-bronchial trunk is easy to find for catheterization because this artery has a fixed location and a relatively large caliber. Therefore, our entire material is representative for the study and discussion of the intercosto-bronchial trunks, (even though a complete selective bronchial arteriogram was not obtained in all cases). The data are tabulated in table 8. Identification of the intercostal spaces supplied by intercostal arteries of intercosto-bronchial trunks was done in a separate study (Table 9).

Discussion

Bronchial arteries: A single intercosto-bronchial trunk was present in 81.8 per cent of the cases, which agrees with NAKAMURA's percentage (Table 2).

Two intercosto-bronchial trunks (Fig. 16) were seen in only two cases (2.6 per cent), which is fewer than mentioned in the literature (Table 2). This may mean that a second intercosto-bronchial trunk was not always found, although CAULDWELL ET AL. also report a low percentage (3.3) for this situation. In both of our cases one of the two bronchial arteries was much smaller, and with it the caliber of one of the intercosto-bronchial trunks (Fig. 16*b*). This difference in size may make it easier to overlook a second intercosto-bronchial trunk.

A total of 65 intercosto-bronchial trunks were seen, which is 30.1 or 31.4 per cent of all bronchial arteries (with or without aberrant arteries). This percentage agrees well with the data in the literature (Table 2).

In our material no left bronchial arteries arising from intercostal arteries were seen, although this situation is reported in both the anatomical (Table 2) and the radiological literature (e.g. VIAMONTE ET AL., 1965). We are unable to explain this discrepancy.

Intercostal arteries: These proved able to supply one or two intercostal spaces. Two-thirds (66.1 per cent) of the intercostal arteries supplied either both the 2nd and 3rd intercostal spaces or only the 3rd.

Comparison can be made with the data of CAULDWELL ET AL. and LAUWERIJNS. There is reasonably good agreement with the former, except with respect to the supply of the 2nd and the combined supply of the 2nd and 3rd intercostal spaces. The percentages for arteries supplying the 2nd and 3rd intercostal spaces (both separately and combined) show, however, very close agreement: 79.0 per cent in our material and 79.5 per cent for CAULDWELL ET AL. LAUWERIJNS's data are much less differentiated; 90 per cent of the intercostal arteries are reported to have supplied the 2nd and 3rd intercostal spaces.

Only in two cases (2.6 per cent) was an intercostal artery found which arose from the aorta cranial to the intercosto-bronchial trunk. Although NAKAMURA gives almost the same percentage (Table 2, III), this number is probably too small because it is based on a selective study and it is difficult or impossible to determine on an aortogram, whether there is any aortic intercostal above the intercosto-bronchial trunk.

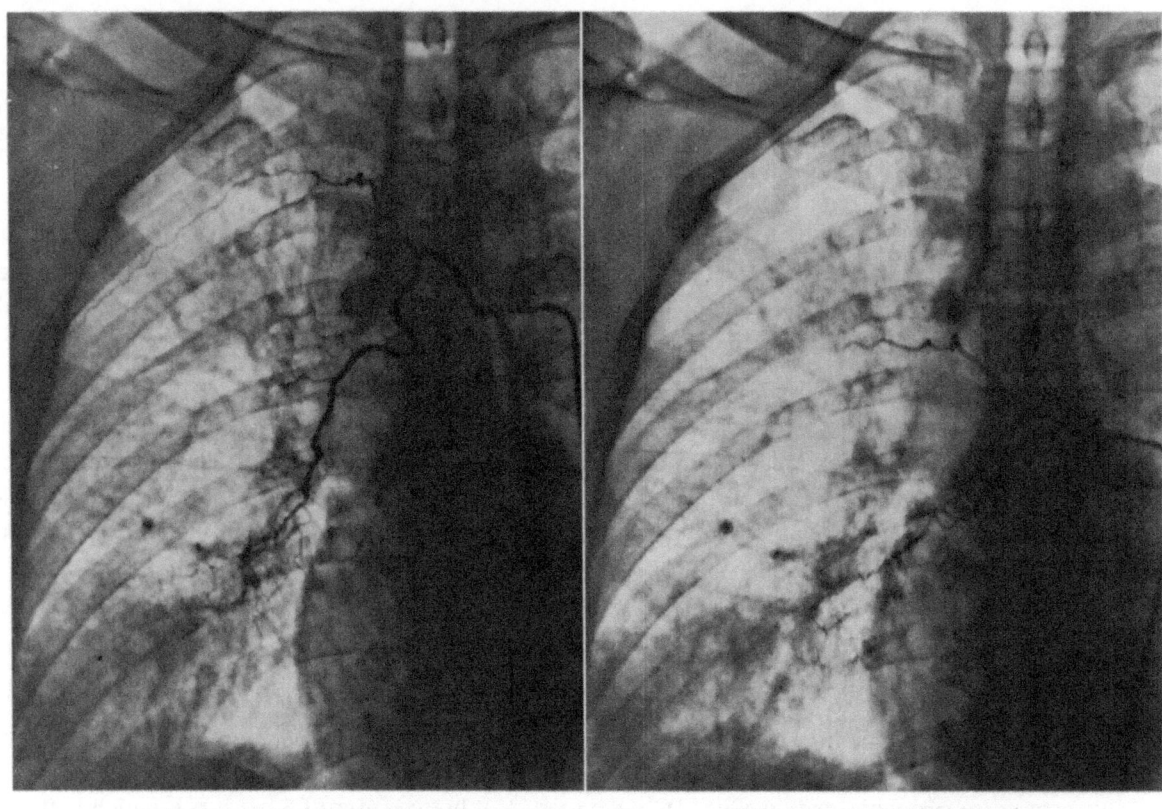

3rd intercosto-bronchial trunk
a

5th intercosto-bronchial trunk
b

Fig. 16. Two intercosto-bronchial trunks in a patient with a pulmonary neoplasm in the right lower lobe. The intercostal arteries supply the 3rd and 5th intercostal spaces. Both bronchial arteries take part in the supply of the tumor.

Conclusions

An intercosto-bronchial trunk is present in four out of five cases. Because of its well-defined location and relatively large caliber, the artery need not be missed. When, however, a second intercosto-bronchial trunk is present, it may not always be found.

A deliberate effort should be made to find the arteries supplying the 2nd and 3rd intercostal spaces, since almost four out of five intercosto-bronchial trunks supply these spaces.

The occurrence of trunci communes

A truncus communis with important branches to both lungs has a larger caliber than independent bronchial arteries and will therefore seldom be missed. Our entire material may therefore be considered representative for the study of this type of artery. The data are shown in table 10 under classification I.

To permit comparison of our data with those of LIEBOW, a second classification was made with inclusion among the trunci communes of bronchial arteries with a very small twig to the contralateral hilus or lung (Table 10, classification II). For these arteries our material is not entirely representative, because they do not necessarily have a larger caliber than independent bronchial arteries. Therefore, only the 57 cases with probably complete bronchial arteriograms are used for this second classification.

Discussion

Classification I: In 29.9 per cent of the cases, a truncus communis was found. This percentage agrees with that of CAULDWELL ET AL. (Table 3). A complete truncus communis was seen more rarely than would be expected from reports in the literature, especially LIEBOW's, although our percentage and that of CAULDWELL ET AL. differ only slightly. It cannot be assumed, however, that such a large bronchial artery was missed. In our opinion, therefore, a complete truncus communis is a rare bronchial artery and occurs less frequently than LIEBOW in particular believed. This is unfortunate for the selective investigation, because the chance of obtaining a complete bronchial arteriogram is greatest in such cases.

Classification II: Although LIEBOW's percentages still lie one and a half to two times higher, the comparative analysis supports our impression that LIEBOW defined the truncus communis much more broadly than the other authors. We reserve the term truncus communis for bronchial arteries with important branches to both lungs.

Conclusions

Less than a third of the cases show bronchial arteries with distinct branches to the lungs (trunci communes).

Because of their greater caliber, trunci communes are easier to find during catheterization than independent right and left bronchial arteries. The schematic representations in figs. 15 and 26 are intended to provide orientational information for catheterization.

Cases with a complete truncus communis, i.e. with one bronchial artery, unfortunately proved to be even more rare than the anatomical literature suggests.

Other anatomical situations

For the discussion of the anatomical variants, reference must be restricted to cases in which the probability that the bronchial arteriogram was complete is very great. The relevant data are shown in table 11, in which under *I* the origin from intercostal arteries is disregarded; this is taken into consideration under *II*. The formations were studied in four groups. Group A comprises the 47 almost certainly 'complete' cases, and groups B, C, and D the 57 probably 'complete' cases. In group A, only normal bronchial arteries with a normal origin are included; groups B, C, and D comprise the accessory bronchial arteries from the aorta as well, and group D also comprises the aberrant bronchial arteries. Group C is the same as classification II in table 10, in which the common trunk for right and left bronchial arteries is defined in the widest sense.

For classification I, the tabulation of the number of possible combinations is done in the same sequence as that applied for table 4. Four combinations did not occur in our material (7, 17, 18, 20), but six new combinations could be added (21–26).

If the origin from intercostal arteries is taken into consideration (classification II), the number of possible combinations increases appreciably, in group B from 13 to 18 and in group D from 16 to 22.

The normal anatomical situation (Table 11, under 'NORMAL ANATOMY' I) has already been discussed (see page 45). More importance must be assigned, however, to the percentage of the combined situations in which one intercosto-bronchial trunk and one or two bronchial arteries arising ventrally from the aorta are present (Table 11, under 'NORMAL ANATOMY' II).

Discussion

Classification I, group A: The arteries included in this group can be reached selectively. In addition, they are unmistakably bronchial arteries supplying variably larger areas of the bronchial tree. These are the arteries of paramount importance for selective bronchial arteriography.

Ten combinations of bronchial arteries occurred among these fourty-seven cases. The percentages agree with those of CAULDWELL ET AL. (Table 4). If it is also considered that our series and even that of CAULDWELL ET AL. are actually very small for this type of analysis, the agreement is even striking, and also constitutes an indication that the bronchial arteriograms in our fourty-seven patients were indeed complete. The three arrangements occurring most frequently in their and our material are: one right bronchial artery with two left bronchial arteries; one right and one left bronchial artery; and a truncus communis with one right and one left bronchial artery (Fig. 17). CAULDWELL ET AL. found these three combinations in exactly 70 per cent of their cases and we in 61.7 per cent of ours.

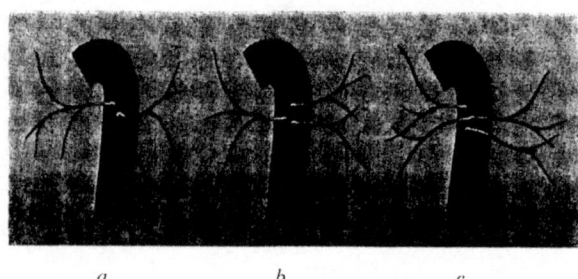

a   *b*   *c*

Fig. 17. Schematic representation of the three combinations of bronchial arteries occuring most frequently. In these situations all the arteries arise from the descending aorta or from high right intercostals.

The agreement with the other authors is limited, which supports our assumption that the study of CAULDWELL ET AL. is the most reliable.

Classification I, groups B, C, and D; and classification II: This part of table 11 serves only to illustrate the large number of possible combinations and the wide range of the variations. For this small series, little value may be attached to the percentages. If for classification II the intercostal spaces supplied by the intercosto-bronchial trunks are also taken into consideration, thirty-six combinations are observed. Therefore, 63 per cent of the cases show a divergent anatomical situation, which certainly demonstrates the irregular anatomical pattern of the bronchial arteries.

'NORMAL ANATOMY' II: These combined arrangements were found in virtual independence of the form of classification in two out of three cases. Our analysis of the data in the literature yielded a slightly higher percentage (Table 4).

Conclusions

The number of anatomical variations among the bronchial arteries appears to be very great, and many combinations occur. However, two conclusions of use for selective arteriography can be drawn.

1. If the bronchial arteries having minor importance for arteriography are not included, one of the following arrangements will be found in almost two of the three cases (Fig. 17 and table 11, I A, 1, 2, and 3):
   a. One right bronchial artery and two left bronchial arteries.
   b. One right bronchial artery and one left bronchial artery.
   c. One truncus communis and one right and one left bronchial artery.
2. The combination of one intercosto-bronchial trunk and one or two bronchial arteries from the aorta is, regardless of whether accessory and aberrant bronchial arteries are included, also found in two out of three cases.

Numbers of bronchial arteries

For the discussion of this point we may again refer only to those cases for which there is some certainty that the bronchial arteriogram was complete. Table 12 therefore concerns the same groups of patients as those used in table 11 for the anatomical variants. The data in table 12 are thus derivable from those in table 11. To groups A-D, a group E is added in table 12 comprising all the bronchial arteries in our material and therefore incomplete cases. The data belonging to group A have the most value for practical purposes. The analysis of the total numbers of bronchial arteries in these five groups was done both with (classification II) and without (classification I) differentiation of an origin from intercostal arteries.

The analysis of the numbers of bronchial arteries per individual in groups A-D was performed for all bronchial arteries, for left bronchial arteries, and for right bronchial arteries. The numbers of left and right bronchial arteries per individual were determined in two ways: in the first (I), the trunci communes were counted as one right and one left bronchial artery, and in the second (II), the cases with a truncus communis were excluded.

Discussion

Total numbers of bronchial arteries: The percentages show the greatest agreement with those of CAULDWELL ET AL. (Table 5). The number of left bronchial arteries and intercosto-bronchial trunks in group B also agrees well with NAKAMURA's classification A. In our material too, more left than right bronchial arteries were seen, although the difference is smaller than in the literature.

In group A, the average number of bronchial arteries per individual is 2.81, which is higher than the value calculated for the data in the literature (Table 5). In groups B and D the number ranges from an average of 3 to 3.16 per individual[1], depending on the number of arteries counted. According to the literature, an average of 2.70[2] was found by others authors. This implies that in our study per two patients on the average about one additional bronchial artery was seen. Since it is hardly likely that our accuracy was that much higher, we think that the difference must lie in the presence in our material of a number of cases with congenital or long-standing anomalies. In such cases an above-average number of bronchial arteries is usually found, as will be discussed in the next chapter. This would also explain the comparatively smaller percentage of normal anatomical variations (Table 11, 'NORMAL ANATOMY' I and II).

Total numbers of bronchial arteries per individual: These data too correspond with those of CAULDWELL ET AL. (especially the percentages for group A). As generalization it may be said that in half of the cases there are three bronchial arteries, and in a fourth two bronchial arteries. In one out of six or seven cases there are four bronchial arteries. In sporadic cases, one or five bronchial arteries occur. Five or more bronchial arteries were usually limited to cases with long-standing or congenital anomalies.

Distribution of left and right bronchial arteries per individual: When the trunci communes are counted as left and right bronchial arteries about half of the cases had two left bronchial arteries and more than one-third of the cases *one* left bronchial artery, whereas on the right *one* bronchial artery occurred most frequently (also in about half of the cases). Only group C, in which the increase in the number of trunci communes led to a marked increase in the number of bronchial arteries, has more cases with *two* right bronchial arteries than with one. In comparison with the data from the literature shown in table 5, CAULDWELL ET AL. found a higher percentage of cases with two left bronchial arteries but fewer with two right bronchial arteries than we, but our data agree better with those of GIORDANI AND

---

[1] If dubious aberrant bronchial arteries are also included, the average number of bronchial arteries per individual amounts to 3.26.
[2] See under Literature, Numbers of Bronchial Arteries (page 18).

PINNA. In particular we did not find the specific distribution of CAULDWELL ET AL., with two times as many cases with two left bronchial arteries as with one, and conversely with twice as many cases with one right bronchial artery as two.

If the cases with a truncus communis are excluded, the numbers of left and right bronchial arteries per person drop, especially the right ones. Under these circumstances there are twice as many cases with one bronchial on the right as with two, but on the left the ratio shows only a small change.

Some cases show three bronchial arteries on one side. For both modes of calculation, this occurred in our material less frequently on the right than on the left side. If all accessory and aberrant arteries are admitted, this situation is no longer rare on the left side (15.8 or 21.1 per cent). In the sporadic cases with more than three bronchial arteries on one side, long-standing or congenital anomalies were usually present.

Conclusions

According to our analysis, man possesses on the average more than three bronchial arteries. This value is distinctly higher than the literature indicates. Since our degree of accuracy cannot have been so much higher, we assume that our material included more cases with a higher than average number of bronchial arteries. This was encountered in cases with long-standing or congenital anomalies.

The number of bronchial arteries in our material amounted per individual to three in half of the cases, to two in a fourth of the cases, and to four once in six to seven cases. Cases with one or with more than four bronchial arteries were exceptional.

More bronchial arteries go to supply the left lung than to the right lung. The number of left bronchial arteries per person amounted in half of the cases to two and in more than one-third to one. The number of right bronchial arteries occurring most frequently per person was one. When cases with trunci communes are excluded, there are even twice as many cases with one right bronchial artery than with two. As compared with our results, CAULDWELL ET AL. found on the average more cases with two left bronchial arteries and fewer cases with two right bronchial arteries. Otherwise, there is good agreement between their data and ours.

The occurrence of three bronchial arteries is rare on the right side but less so on the left side.

b. Abnormal origin

b.1. *Origin from the aortic arch*

Bronchial arteries arising from the aortic arch were demonstrated in fourteen cases. One artery was filled selectively by chance, the others were filled collaterally (Fig. 11a) or were visible on the aortogram. Only one artery arose from the convex segment of the arch (Fig. 18). Of the fourteen arteries, six were left and five right; in the remaining three determination being impossible, because they were demonstrated on a lateral aortogram. The vessels were in general accessory bronchial arteries. Only three had a diameter of more than 1 mm, one of these supplying the entire right lung.

Discussion

The bronchial arteries mentioned so far can be catheretized selectively, but this does not hold generally for those arising from the aortic arch. For the boundary between the descending aorta and the aortic arch we chose the horizontal tangent plane with the concave segment of the aortic arch, because bronchial arteries arising at higher levels cannot be selectively catheterized via the groin. We are aware that this is not the anatomical boundary, but as the discussion of the anatomical literature showed, this boundary was not localized exactly in any of the investigations, and the widely varying percentages (see table 6) show that it differed from one investigation to another. Consequently, exact comparison with our data is not possible. Our percentages indicate, however, that we saw these bronchial arteries as frequently as did CAULDWELL ET AL. and GIORDANI AND PINNA.

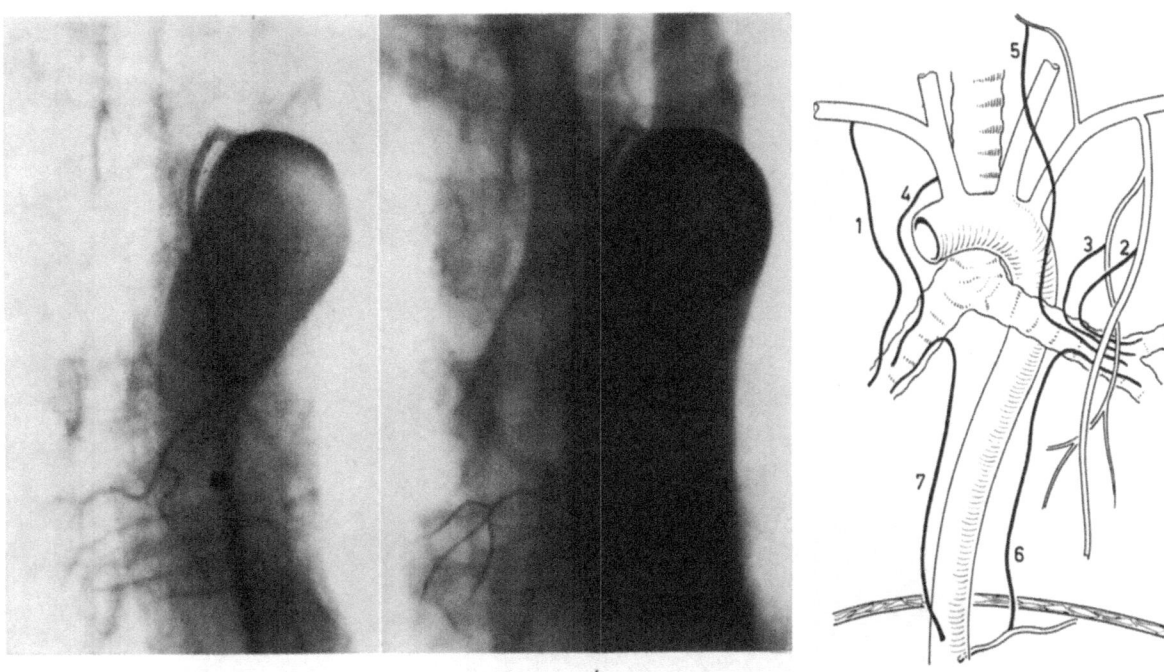

Fig. 18. Origin of a bronchial artery from the upper side of the aortic arch. Exposures made one-third of a second (*a*) and two-thirds of a second (*b*) after the beginning of the injection of contrast medium into the aorta.

Fig. 19. Usual forms of aberrant origin of the bronchial arteries from the subclavian (1), the internal mammary (2), the pericardiacophrenic (3), the innominate (4), the thyreocervical (5), the inferior phrenic (6) arteries, and the abdominal aorta (7).

Conclusion

Bronchial arteries arising from the aortic arch cannot be reached selectively via the groin. Their occurrence is, however, rare, and then they are usually of the accessory type. In very rare cases a normal bronchial artery takes its origin from the aortic arch, in which case it can be made visible aortographically or collaterally.

b.2. *Aberrant origin*

In eighteen cases (23.4 per cent) there were thirty aberrant bronchial arteries, seventeen of them demonstrated unequivocally. Ten were right and twenty were left bronchial arteries. Six were directly involved in the vascularization of a pathological process. Only one artery contributed important information to the achievement of a complete diagnostic picture. With one exception, all were accessory bronchial arteries, whether of the normal or pathological type. Only four had a caliber greater than 1 mm. The most common forms of aberrant origin are shown in fig. 19. The first six possibilities were encountered in our material. In order of decreasing frequency, these arteries arose from:

internal mammary artery . .	10	(Fig. 20)
pericardiacophrenic artery. .	7	(Fig. 21)
inferior phrenic artery . . .	5	(Fig. 22)
thyreocervical artery	4	(Fig. 23)
left subclavian artery	3	(Fig. 24)
innominate artery	1	

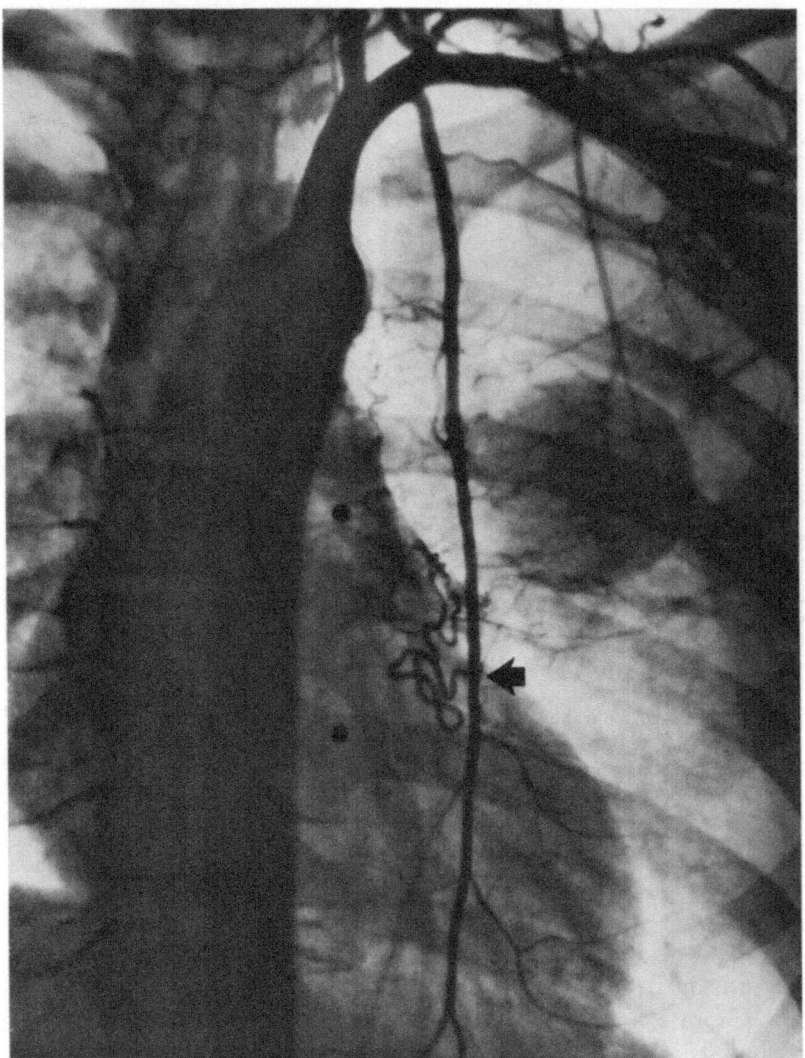

Fig 20. Aberrant origin of an accessory left bronchial artery from the left internal
mammary.

Fig. 24 is also an example of the only normal bronchial artery with an aberrant origin in our material.
This was a case with three bronchial arteries on the left side, the most cranial arising from the left
subclavian artery.

Fig. 23. Injection of contrast medium at the level of the bifurcation of the innominate artery. Heavy dilatation of the first
part of the right subclavian, the right thyreocervical, and inferior thyroid arteries. Through the shadow of the thyreocervical
the right vertebral artery is visible. The inferior thyroid continues, directly and without reduction in caliber, as a much dilated
and aberrantly originating bronchial artery with a centrally located tortuous anastomosis (black arrows) with the pulmonary
artery of the right upper lobe. As a result of retrograde flow, the contrast medium reaches the right pulmonary trunk (white
arrows) (later investigated patient excluded from the present material).

Fig. 24. Aberrantly originating bronchial artery from the left subclavian.

a: Start of the injection of the contrast medium. The arrow indicates the origin of the bronchial artery. After a short distance
     the course of the artery is projected over the shadow of the aorta, remaining just barely visible (up to the white arrow).

b: Later phase of the aortogram, in which the contrast medium has already disappeared from the aortic arch. From the point,
     indicated by the white arrow in *a*, the further course of the aberrant bronchial artery is visualized (arrows).

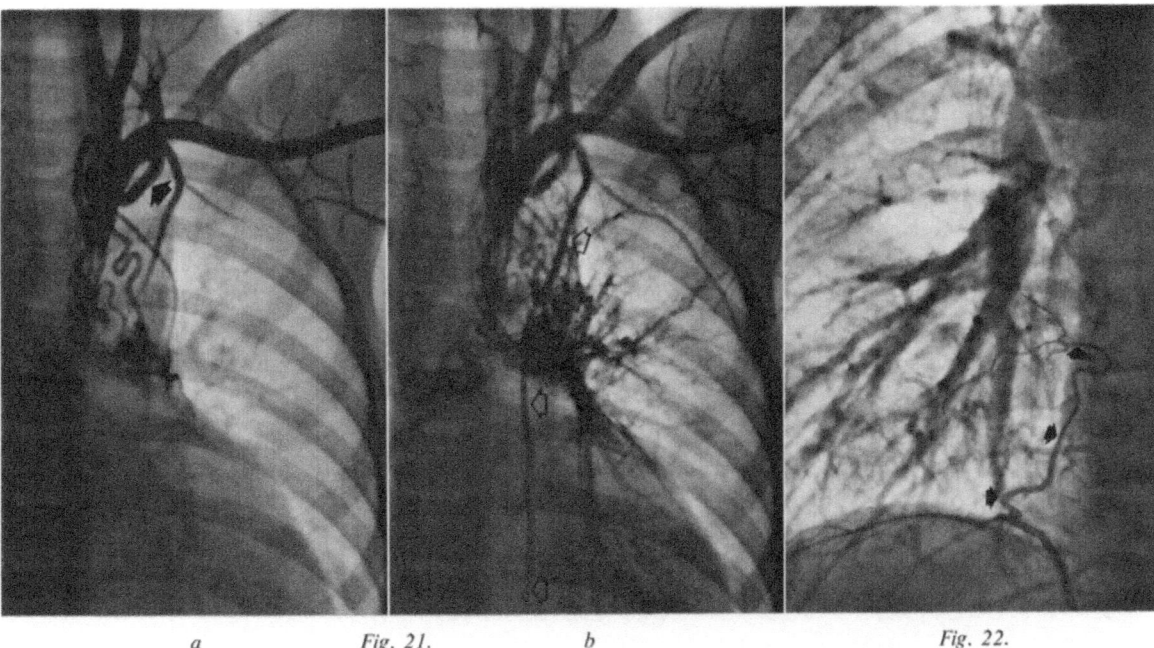

a   *Fig. 21.*   b   *Fig. 22.*

Fig. 21. Left bronchial arteries with aberrant origin from a strongly dilated left pericardiacophrenic artery (arrow in *a*). In *b* the further course of the left internal mammary artery is indicated by the arrows; this picture also shows contrast medium in branches of the pulmonary artery in the presence of central broncho-pulmonary anastomoses (previously investigated patient excluded from the present material).

Fig. 22. Aberrantly originating bronchial artery from the phrenic artery (arrows). The artery reaches the lung via the pulmonary ligament.

a

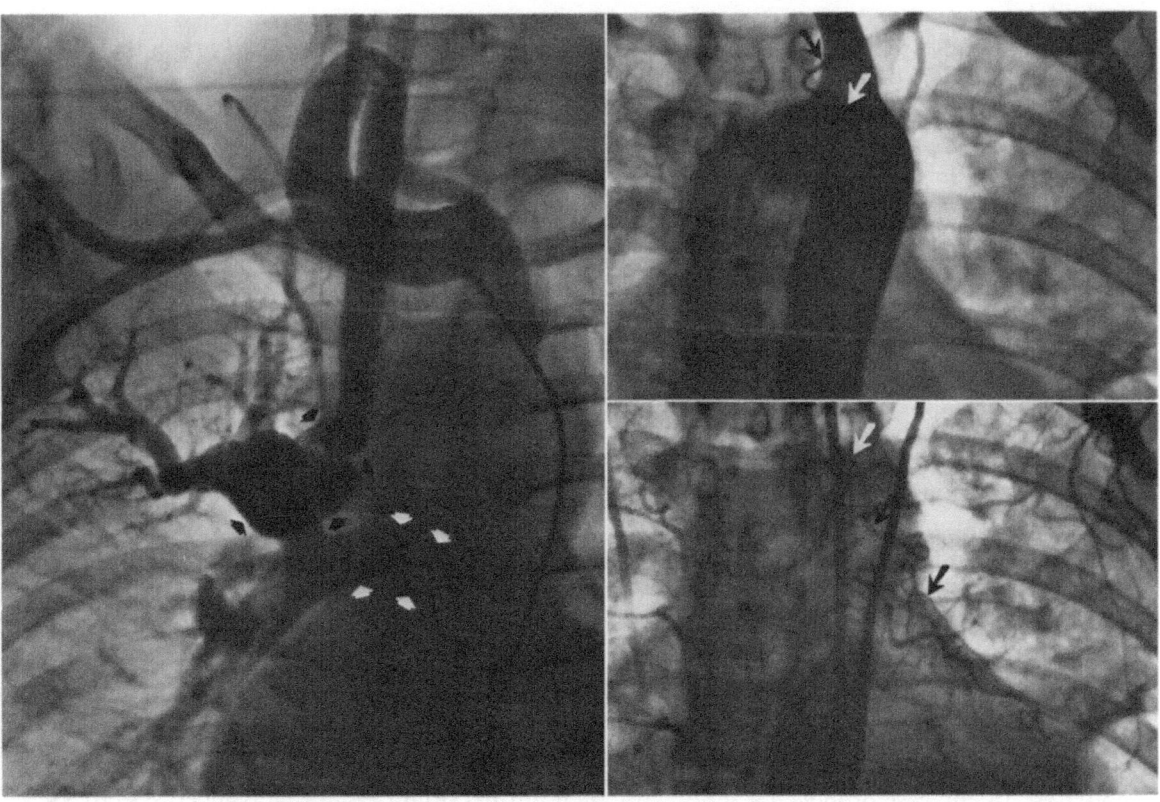

Fig. 23.   b   *Fig. 24.*

Discussion

Our total number of arteries with an aberrant origin is higher than any found in the literature, which confirms LIEBOW's opinion that the currently used preparation techniques probably only permit demonstration of a minimal number of these arteries. In our material it is also unlikely that all the 'aberrant' bronchial arteries were seen. Our high percentage is explained in the first place by a certain selection in our study with respect to this type of origin. Two of our patients, for instance, had congenital anomalies, together accounting for eight aberrant arteries. But even if the patients with long-standing or congenital anomalies are excluded, the percentage of cases with 'aberrant' bronchial arteries is still much higher than those found in the literature. A second explanation for our high numbers may be that 43 per cent of these arteries were filled collaterally and therefore became visible coincidentally on a selective arteriogram of a bronchial artery with a normal origin.

Conclusion

Bronchial arteries with an aberrant origin are considerably less rare than the percentages in the literature suggest. Fortunately for the selective investigation they are, like the other group of arteries with an abnormal origin, almost all accessory bronchial arteries. A number of these were found to be of the pathological type involved in the vascularization of a pathological process, but with one exception they were of minor importance for the diagnosis.

Accessory bronchial arteries and anastomoses

Accessory bronchial arteries of normal origin were found by chance due to selective catheterization or collateral filling. A total of twenty-eight such arteries were visualized, which represents 15 per cent of all bronchial arteries with a normal origin. All arteries were derived from the aorta, none from the intercostals.

We have already seen in the discussion of bronchial arteries with an *abnormal* origin that the great majority of these (90.9 per cent) are of the accessory type.

Pulmonary sequestrations do not occur in our material.

Discussion

Of the accessory bronchial arteries arising from the aorta, five served mainly for the vascularization of the esophagus and four mainly for the vascularization of the aorta. These nine arteries can also be classified under the bronchial arteries of aberrant origin, since it is difficult to determine whether they are accessory bronchial arteries with rami to the esophagus and aorta or esophageal arteries and vasa aortae with bronchial derivatives to the lung.

The presence of anastomoses is confirmed by the high number (43 per cent) of collaterally filled aberrantly originating bronchial arteries described above. An example of this type is shown in fig. 25 (small arrows).

In the discussion of the numbers of bronchial arteries it was noted that in cases of long-standing or congenital anomalies many bronchial arteries are present (sometimes as many as seven). Most of these were found to be large pathological accessory bronchial arteries or dilated anastomoses.

Conclusion

Of the bronchial arteries with a *normal* origin 15 per cent are of the accessory type, and of those with an *abnormal* origin 91 per cent are accessories. This distribution is not unfavorable for selective bronchial arteriography, since accessory bronchial arteries make a subordinate contribution to the bronchial vascularization and proved to be relatively unimportant for the diagnosis of pulmonary anomalies. In any case bronchial arteries with an abnormal origin cannot be reached selectively.

In our material, both normal and pathological accessory bronchial arteries were present.

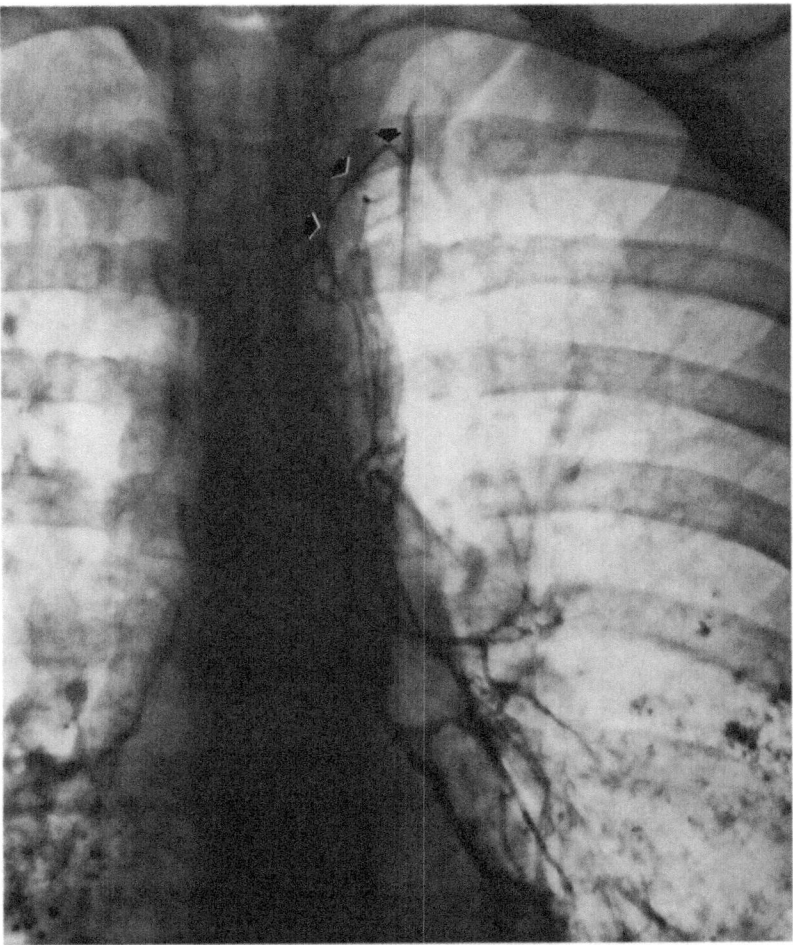

Fig. 25. Aberrantly originating accessory bronchial artery (arrows) from the left internal mammary artery, these vessels being collaterally filled through vasa aortae (see also Fig. 53). A similar artery is visible in Fig. 11*a*.

Level of origin of the bronchial arteries

The level of origin could be determined for 182 bronchial arteries (61 intercosto-bronchial trunks, 48 normal left bronchial arteries, 26 accessory left bronchial arteries, 16 right bronchial arteries, 22 trunci communes, and 9 bronchial arteries arising from the aortic arch). As in the literature, the site of origin was related to the vertebral levels divided for that purpose into three equal parts of the vertebral bodies and one of the intervertebral disk. The results of our study are shown in table 13 and illustrated by figs. 26 and 27. Since several of the left bronchial arteries were accessories, we used two classifications: classification A comprises only normal bronchial arteries; in classification B all left bronchial arteries are admitted.

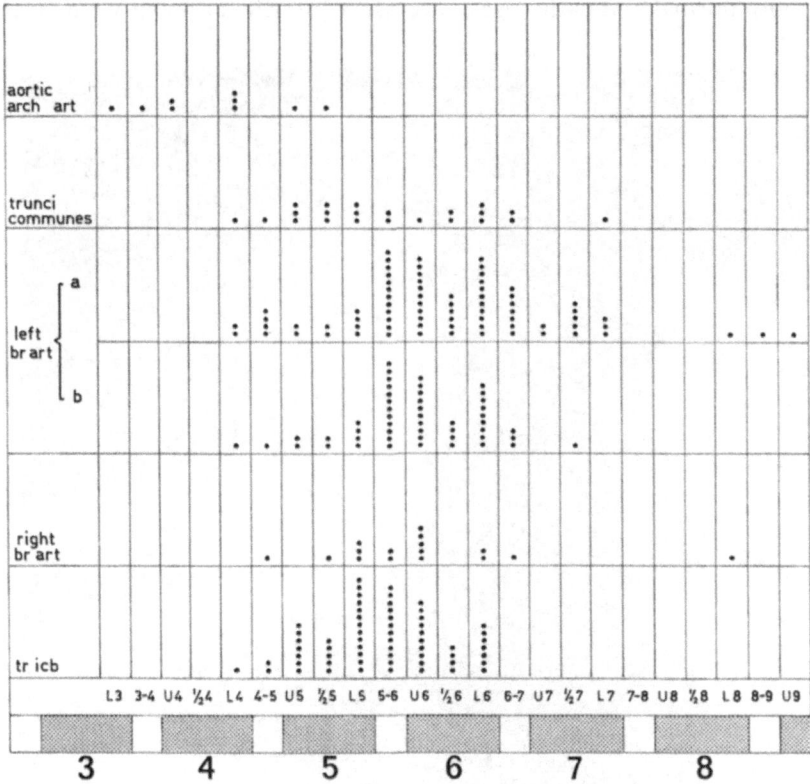

Fig. 26. Level of the origin per type of bronchial artery. As reference points serve the thoracic vertebrae, schematically represented at the bottom. The classification, abbreviations, and numbers used here are identical to those in Table 13. On the average, trunci intercosto-bronchiales and communes arise at a slightly higher level than left and right bronchial arteries.

TABLE 14.   Comparison between the data of CAULDWELL ET AL. and those of the present study with respect to the bronchial origins from the descending aorta in relation to the vertebral levels. A: Normal left bronchial arteries. B: All left bronchials (including the accessories).

	CAULDWELL ET AL.				THE PRESENT STUDY					
	Right br art	Left br art	Trunci communes	Total	Right br art	Left br art A	B	Trunci communes	Totals A	B
T4		7	2	9		1	4	1	2	5
T5	10	69	11	90	6	15	16	11	32	33
T6	29	119	2	150	9	30	38	9	48	56
T7	2	24	2	28		2	13	1	3	14
T8		1		1	1		2		1	3
T9							1			1
TOTAL	41	220	17	278	16	48	74	22	86	112

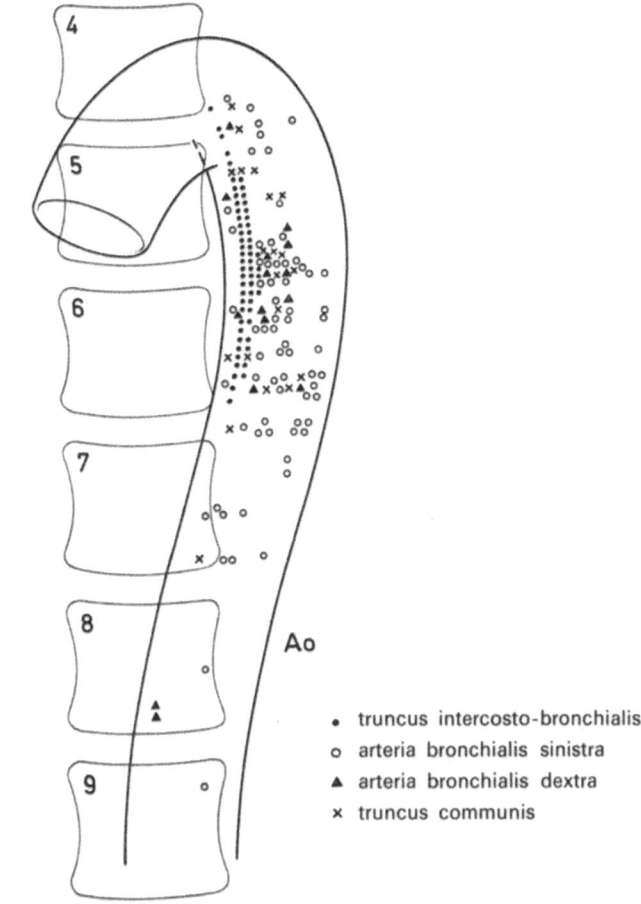

Fig. 27. Representation of all the
bronchial arteries whose level and
site of origin on the aortic wall could
be determined with certainty.

TABLE 15. Aortic origins related to the 5th and 6th thoracic vertebral levels, in proportion to the total numbers of aortic origins in Table 14. A: Normal left bronchial arteries. B: All left bronchials.

		CAULDWELL ET AL.	THE PRESENT STUDY	
			A	B
ALL[1] AORTIC BR ART	Opposite T5	32.4	37.2	29.5
	Opposite T6	53.9	55.8	50.
	Opposite T5 and T6	86.3	93.0	79.5
LEFT BR ART	Opposite T5	31.3	31.3	21.6
	Opposite T6	54.1	62.5	51.4
	Opposite T5 and T6	85.4	93.8	73.0
RIGHT BR ART	Opposite T5	24.4	37.5	
	Opposite T6	70.7	56.3	
	Opposite T5 and T6	95.1	93.8	

[1] Exclusive of bronchial arteries from the aortic arch.

The level of origin of the bronchial arteries was also investigated by CAULDWELL ET AL. and VIA-MONTE ET AL. (Table 1). In tables 14 and 15 our data can be compared with those of CAULDWELL ET AL.[1] For purposes of this comparison, in our material half of adjacent disks were included with the vertebral bodies, since CAULDWELL ET AL. refer only to the bodies.

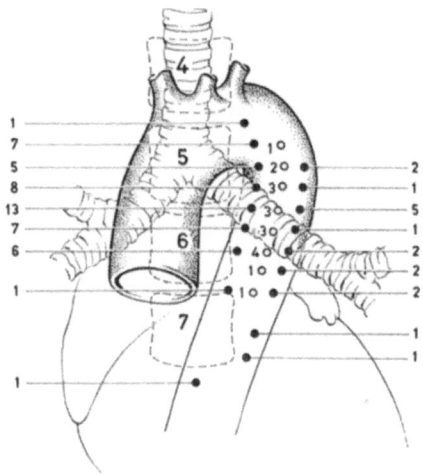

art. bronch. dextra   : 49
art. bronch. sinistra : 17
truncus communis   : 18
total   : 84

Fig. 28. Level of the origin of right and left bronchials and trunci communes (central circles) according to VIAMONTE ET AL. (1965) (after their Fig. 1).

TABLE 16.   Relation to vertebral levels of the origins of the bronchial arteries catheterized by VIAMONTE ET AL. (1965), according to their data. The vertebral levels are divided into four equal parts comprising three of the bodies (upper third: U; middle third: $\frac{1}{2}$; lower third: L) and one representing the intervertebral disk (4–5).

	RIGHT BR ART*	LEFT BR ART	TRUNCI COMMUNES	TOTAL
4–5	1			1
U5	7		1	8
$\frac{1}{2}$5	5	2	2	9
L5	8	1	3	12
5–6	13	5	3	21
U6	7	1	3	11
$\frac{1}{2}$6	6	2	4	12
L6		2	1	3
6–7	1	2	1	4
U7				
$\frac{1}{2}$7		1		1
L7		1		1
7–8	1			1
TOTAL	49	17	18	84

* As appears from the publication of VIAMONTE ET AL. almost all these arteries are intercosto-bronchial trunks.

[1] Table IV B of the publication of CAULDWELL ET AL. shows the level of origin of left and right bronchial arteries from the aorta, and comprises the trunci communes as left and right bronchial arteries as well as the bronchial arteries from the aortic arch. To permit comparison, some conversion was necessary. After comparison with their table IV A, the bronchial arteries arising from the aortic arch could be removed from table IV B. The trunci communes, specified for table IV B, were subtracted from the left and right bronchial arteries and listed separately. The result which is shown in our table 14, must be regarded with some reserve. According to CAULDWELL ET AL.'s table IV B, 17 trunci communes would arise from the descending aorta, but elsewhere they give a figure of 36 (e.g. in Table III). This seems to imply that only half of their trunci communes were included in table IV B or mentioned in the legend.

TABLE 17. Comparison between the data of VIAMONTE ET AL. and those of the present study with respect to the level of points of origin of the bronchial arteries. According to VIAMONTE ET AL. the bronchial arteries originate somewhat more cranially than according to our findings. A: Normal left bronchial arteries. B: All left bronchials.

	VIAMONTE ET AL.								THE PRESENT STUDY											
	Right br art[1]		Left br art		Trunci communes		Total		Right br art[2]		Left br art				Trunci communes		Totals			
											A		B				A		B	
	No.	%	No.	%	No.	%	No.	%	No.	%	No.	%	No.	%	No.	%	No.	%	No.	%
OPPOSITE T5	20	41	3	18	6	33	29	35	29	38	8	17	8	11	9	41	46	31	46	27
OPPOSITE DISK T5–T6	13	27	5	29	3	17	21	25	14	18	12	25	12	16	2	9	28	19	28	16
OPPOSITE T6	13	27	5	29	8	44	26	31	28	36	22	46	28	38	6	27	56	42	62	36
OPPOSITE T5 AND T6	46	94	13	77	17	94	76	91	71	92	88	88	48	65	17	77	130	93	136	79

1 Almost exclusively intercosto-bronchial trunks.
2 Trunci intercosto-bronchiales and independent right bronchial arteries.

The data of table 16 are based on fig. 1 of VIAMONTE ET AL. (1965) (see our fig. 28). The right bronchial arteries in this table are almost all intercosto-bronchial trunks. VIAMONTE ET AL. did not distinguish between intercosto-bronchial trunks and right bronchial arteries, so that we added up these vessels in our material (Table 13) to permit comparison. The results being shown in table 17.

Discussion

The site of origin of the bronchial arteries arising from the aortic arch varied from the lower margin of T3 to the middle of T5 (Table 13, Fig. 26). It appears, therefore, that as reference points for the site of origin from the descending aorta, the thoracic vertebrae are not entirely reliable. We have, however, made use of them in our investigation because they are clearly visible fluoroscopically.

The outer limits of the origins from the descending aorta in our material (including intercosto-bronchial trunks) were the lower margin of T4 and the upper margin of T9; if the accessory left bronchial arteries are left out of consideration, these limits are the lower margins of T4 and T7 (Figs. 26 and 27, Table 13). The left bronchial arteries and the trunci communes showed the widest range. The level of origin of the intercosto-bronchial trunks was, despite their large number (61), of course the most constant.

The majority of the arteries arose at the level of T5 and T6. If the accessory left bronchial arteries are excluded, 92.5 per cent of the normal sites of origin were situated in the aortic segment opposite T5 and T6, but if they are included this value is 78.6 per cent. The greatest number of origins was located opposite the disk between T5 and T6 (Table 13). About twice as many left and right bronchial arteries arose opposite T6 as opposite T5. Conversely, trunci intercosto-bronchiales and communes arose slightly more often opposite T5 than opposite T6.

Generally speaking, most of the sites of origin of the normally arising bronchial arteries were situated opposite T6.

With respect to the level of origin per type of artery, fig. 26 shows that independent right and left bronchial arteries arose at about the same level, and on the average both trunci intercosto-bronchiales and communes arose slightly higher. The latter fact deserves attention, because trunci communes and isolated left and right bronchial arteries all arise from the ventral wall of the aorta. This also emerged from our analysis of the data of CAULDWELL ET AL. (Table 14), although it is not explicitly stated by them.

Comparison with the data of CAULDWELL ET AL.: The percentages for the total number and the number of left bronchial arteries from the descending aorta show good agreement (Table 15). For the right bronchial arteries the agreement is not as good, but our number of right bronchial arteries is small.

CAULDWELL ET AL. state that in general right bronchial arteries arise lower in the aorta than left bronchial arteries because there is usually an intercosto-bronchial trunk arising at the same level as the latter. This is not confirmed by our material, as shown above. Our main left bronchial arteries, however, were found to arise slightly higher than the intercosto-bronchial trunks, and a second artery with a ventral origin one-half to one vertebra lower.

Comparison with the data of VIAMONTE ET AL.: We found a lower percentage of arteries opposite T5 and T6, but they found a narrower distribution, i.e. from the disk between T4 and T5 to the disk between T7 and T8. They also found a much lower number of bronchial arteries per individual (1.18), which implies that those with an unusual location were probably missed relatively more frequently. In their material the bronchial arteries arise slightly more cranially with as many arteries opposite T5 as opposite T6, possibly because of the inclusion of the relatively high number of intercosto-bronchial trunks, which, as our material shows, on the average have a higher origin.

Conclusions

Although the origin of the bronchial arteries is usually related to the thoracic vertebrae, the varying levels of origin of the bronchial arteries from the aortic arch indicates that these reference points are not ideal. No better ones are available, however.

Accessory bronchial arteries showed a wider spread of their points of origin than normal bronchial arteries. Although the maximum spread amounted to almost six vertebral levels, 8 to 9 out of 10 bronchial arteries arose opposite the 5th and 6th thoracic vertebrae and most of them opposite the intervertebral disk in between. Almost twice as many right and left bronchial arteries arose opposite T6 as T5, but intercosto-bronchial trunks and trunci communes arose more often opposite T5. The average truncus communis, therefore, appears to arise somewhat higher from the ventral aortic wall than the average left and right bronchial arteries.

The level of origin was understandably the most constant for the intercosto-bronchial trunks and the least constant for the left bronchial arteries.

The correlation between our data and those of CAULDWELL ET AL. is good, but that with the results of VIAMONTE ET AL. is poorer. The reasons for this have been discussed.

Range of the distribution of the bronchial origins per case

Under this range is understood the portion of the aorta between the most cranial and caudal levels of origin of the bronchial arteries in a single case. The length of this segment provides, for each individual an impression of the distribution of the bronchial origins.

In 57 probably complete bronchial arteriographies, the origin of all bronchial arteries could be accurately localized. The results are shown in table 18. In group A only those with a normal origin are listed; in group B also those from the aortic arch. Eleven cases showed an accessory artery with an aberrant origin.

TABLE 18.   Range of the points of origin of all bronchial arteries, per case. In the cases shown in the first top row, all bronchial arteries originated within a segment of the aorta opposite one-third of a vertebral body (indicated by v). The second row shows the cases with all bronchial arteries within a aortic segment opposite two-thirds of a vertebral body (the disk being counted as one-third of a vertebra).

In group A only bronchial arteries of normal origin are included, in group B also the bronchial arteries from the aortic arch.

RANGE OF THE ORIGINS PER CASE	CASES (NUMBERS) A	B
$\frac{1}{3}$v	12	12
$\frac{2}{3}$v	6	6
1v	6	6
1$\frac{1}{3}$v	10	7
1$\frac{2}{3}$v	8	8
2v	4	5
2$\frac{1}{3}$v	2	2
2$\frac{2}{3}$v	1	1
3v		1
3$\frac{1}{3}$v	1	2
3$\frac{2}{3}$v	1	1
TOTAL	51	51

To obtain an impression of the significance of the data in table 18, the percentage of cases in which all bronchial arteries arose opposite $\frac{1}{3}$, 1 and $1\frac{2}{3}$ of a vertebra were calculated (Table 19, Fig. 29). For $1\frac{2}{3}$ of a vertebra one should visualize a verbebra plus the adjacent disks.

TABLE 19. Range of the points of origin of the bronchial arteries, per case, in proportion (round figures) to the total number of analysed cases (51). Under A, only bronchial arteries of normal origin are considered; under B, also the ones from the aortic arch.

ORIGINS OF THE BR ART OPPOSITE	CASES (PERCENTAGES)	
	A	B
$\frac{1}{3}$ VERTEBRA	24	24
1 VERTEBRA	47	47
$1\frac{2}{3}$ VERTEBRA	82	76

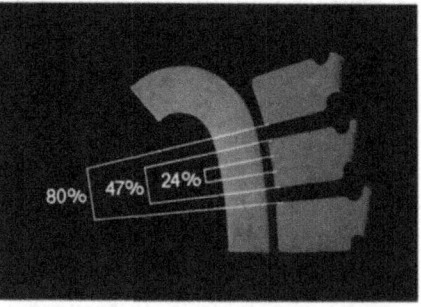

Fig. 29. Spread in the cranio-caudal direction of the points of origin of the bronchial arteries per case in proportion to the total number of analysed cases (51). The percentage of cases in which the bronchial arteries arose opposite one vertebra with the adjacent disks has been rounded off to 80.

CAULDWELL ET AL. determined the number of cases in which the bronchial arteries arose opposite one, two, or three vertebrae, restricting their counts to those originating from the descending aorta. Since they did not include the disks, we equated, for purposes of comparison, $1\frac{1}{3}$ of a vertebra in our material with one vertebra in their material (Table 20). We also excluded the arteries arising from the aortic arch but not the intercosto-bronchial trunks, since the latter rarely increase the range in question.

TABLE 20. Pro rata comparison between the data of CAULDWELL ET AL. and those of the present study with respect to the range of the points of origin of the bronchial arteries, per case, measured as vertebral heights (v). For the cases of CAULDWELL ET AL. only the bronchial arteries from the descending aorta are taken into account; in ours also the intercosto-bronchial trunks.

RANGE OF THE ORIGINS PER CASE	CASES (PERCENTAGES)	
	CAULDWELL ET AL.	THE PRESENT STUDY
1v	38	67
2v	57	29
3v	5	4
TOTAL	100	100

Discussion

For group A, which comprises the bronchial arteries relevant for arteriography, the following may be said:

About one in four cases shows a very limited spread of the origin levels amounting to one-third of the height of a vertebra. In almost half of the cases the bronchial arteries arise opposite a single thoracic vertebra, and in more than four out of five cases all the bronchial arteries arise opposite a single vertebra with the adjacent disks. The percentages in group B show little variation.

There is a divergence in our material from the data of CAULDWELL ET AL. (Table 20). In two out of three of our cases the bronchial arteries arise opposite a single thoracic vertebra (with its disk), but in their cases this holds for only slightly more than one out of three. In more than half of their cases the segment of the aorta in which the bronchial arteries originated represented the height of two vertebrae (with disks), but in ours this was seen in less than one-third of the cases. The number of cases with the greatest spread, i.e. three vertebrae, however, was about equally small. We are unable to explain these differences.

Conclusion

The bronchial arteries per case usually arise from only a small segment of the aorta. In about a quarter of the cases this segment is only as long as a third of a vertebra, in half of the cases one vertebra, and in about four out of five cases one vertebra with its adjacent disks.

CAULDWELL ET AL. found a greater spread of the sites of origin of the bronchial arteries per case than we saw.

IV.1.1.2. CENTRAL COURSE OF THE BRONCHIAL ARTERIES

We did not perform a special study of this point, because the X-ray picture does not lend itself for this purpose. In a few of our cases an arched course indicated passage on the ventral side of the left main bronchus or the trachea. Great importance must be attached to the central anastomoses between bronchial arteries, which permit the collateral filling already referred to (Fig. 11). One patient with carcinoma of the lung and glandular metastases, and two patients with bronchiectasis and probably infected hilar glands showed centrally located constrictions of the bronchial arteries probably caused by pathological lymph glands (Figs. 30 and 94). The central segment of the bronchial arteries is highly mobile, as shown by comparison of exposures made during inspiration and expiration (Fig. 31). When the left bronchial arteries ramify, caudal or inferior branches often appear first and cranial branches last.

IV.1.1.3. INTRAPULMONARY COURSE OF THE BRONCHIAL ARTERIES

The bronchial arteries were found to follow the bronchi. In some cases a small bronchus accompanied by two bronchial arteries was clearly visible (Fig. 32). Three instances were seen in which a branch closely followed the interlobium (Fig. 33), apparently an interlobar pleural artery.[1]

---

[1] Mentioned in the literature by LATARJET (1956) and CUDKOWICZ AND ARMSTRONG (1952).

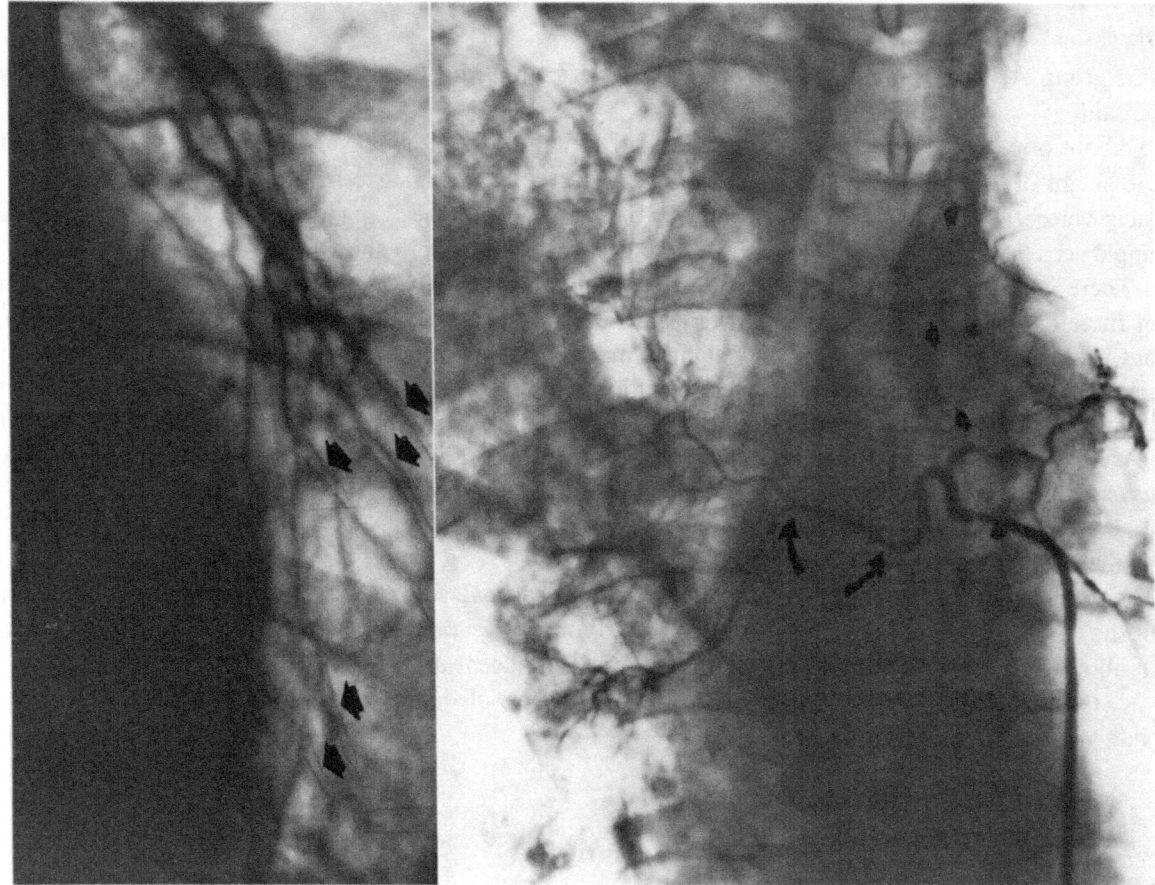

Fig. 32.   *Fig. 30.*

Fig. 32. Arteriogram of the left bronchial artery. In the paracardiac region a few small bronchi are visualized (arrows), because they are paralleled by twigs of the bronchial artery on either side.
Fig. 30. Centrally located constriction (large arrows) of the right branch of a truncus communis in a case of extensive glandular
metastases at the level of the carina and the right hilus. A small artery for the vascularization of the left main bronchus and
the trachea (small arrows) is derived from the left branch.

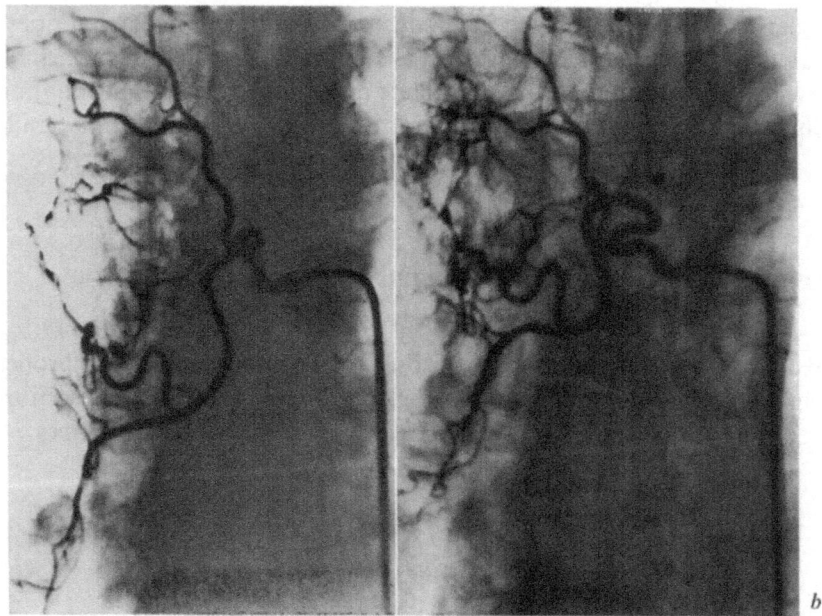

Fig 31. Exposures made during inspiration (*a*) and expiration (*b*) showing the mobility
of the central segment of the bronchial artery.

IV.1.1.4. FUNCTION OF THE BRONCHIAL ARTERIES

a. Bronchi

In some cases a kind of bronchogram could be seen on the last of a series of arteriograms, usually when excessive pressure had occurred at injection. One case showed coating of the wall of the right main bronchus (Fig. 34).

b. Esophagus

Almost all the patients complained not only of irritation leading to coughing which was caused by the contrast medium in the bronchial vessels, but also of a hot feeling in the throat. Often this hot, sometimes painful sensation was much stronger than the coughing stimulus. In agreement with the general opinion in the literature we initially took this sensation of heat in the throat as an indication that a bronchial artery had been catheterized, even wehn the smallness of this artery prevented its being seen on the monitor of the image amplifier–television circuit, and on the X-rays the presence of

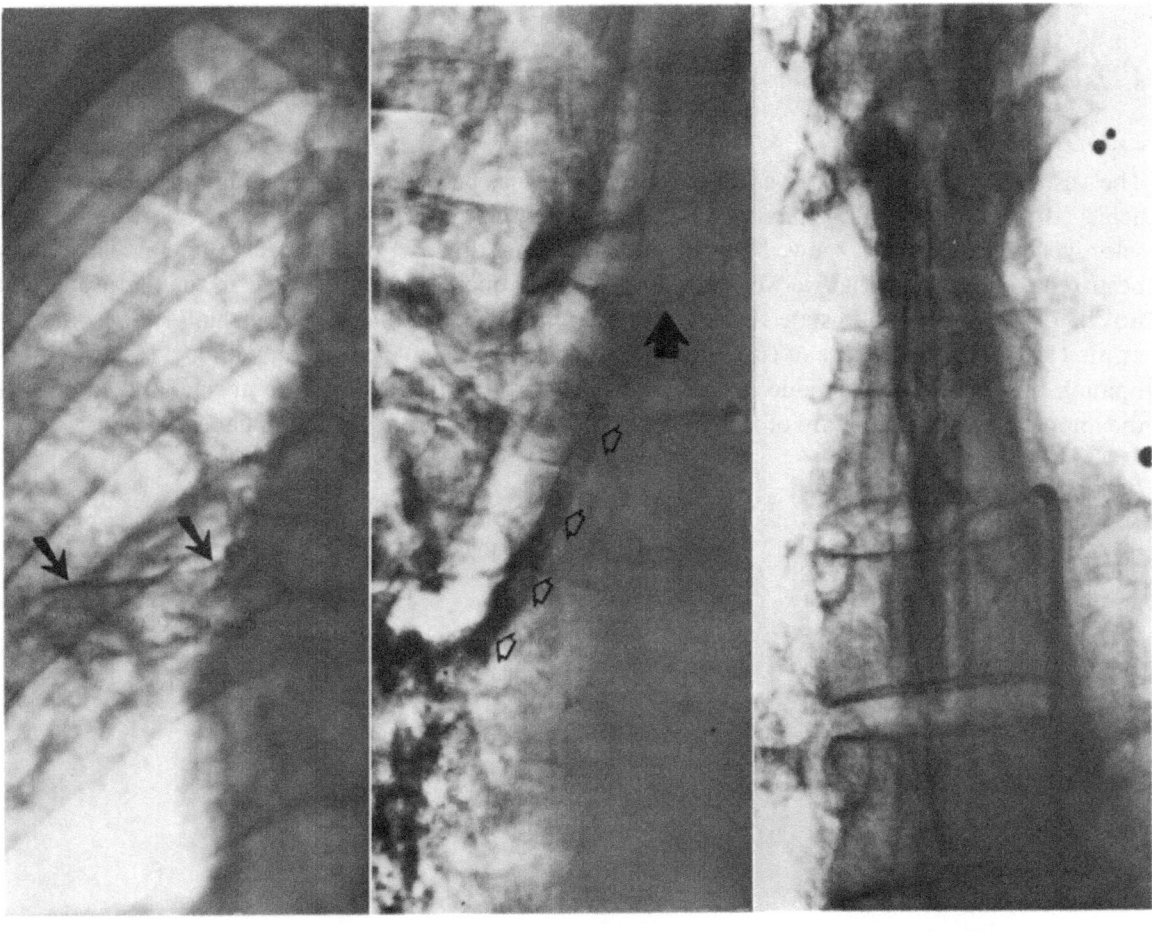

Fig. 33.   Fig. 34.   Fig. 35.

Fig. 33. The vascularization of the interlobar pleura is provided by the bronchial arteries, as demonstrated by this bronchial arteriogram showing an interlobar artery between the middle and lower lobes (arrows).
Fig. 34. Coating of the wall of the right main bronchus in the capillary phase of a bronchial arteriogram (arrows). The carina is marked by a large arrow.
Fig. 35. Capillary phase of a bronchial arteriogram. The vertical streaky shadows in the median line are caused by contrast medium in the wall of the esophagus.

a bronchial artery was indeed confirmed. Later, however, we realized that the rami to the esophagus were responsible for this sensation of heat. Some cases showed in the mid-line, vague vertical streaky shadows representing the contrast medium in the wall of the esophagus (Fig. 35). This was especially clear during the selective injection of five arteries, which led to an intense burning sensation in the throat, predominating over the coughing-stimulus. On the relevant arteriograms only a very small branch was found running to the hilus or the lung, so that probably the five catheterized arteries[1] were primary esophageal arteries with bronchial derivatives (accessory bronchial arteries of aberrant origin) or anastomoses with the bronchial circulation. All of them arose caudally and ventrally from the descending aorta.

Conclusion

The sensation of heat and sometimes of painful burning in the throat, interpreted in the literature as an indication that a bronchial artery has been injected, actually demonstrates the presence of contrast medium in esophageal arteries. Since this sensation almost always occurs during bronchial arteriography, it can be deduced conversely that branches to the esophagus are almost always present. This is in agreement with the findings reported in the literature.[2]

c. Vasa vasorum

c.1. *Vascularization of the aorta*

The vascularization of the aortic arch and the proximal part of the descending aorta is apparently achieved primarily by the left bronchial artery. Every left superior bronchial artery, whether filled selectively or collaterally, showed a branch vascularizing this part of the aorta (Fig. 36). This finding occurred so constantly that we were surprised to find almost no mention of it in the literature. Only HOVELACQUE ET AL. (1936) state that the aortic arch can be supplied by bronchial arteries. STECKEL ET AL. (1967) reported a case of rupture of the aorta after selective perfusion with a cytostatic. In our opinion this must have been due to damage to the aortic wall via these vasa aortae, and emphasizes the importance of being aware of the existence of these branches of the bronchial arteries.

---

[1] See also under the anatomical section of the present study 'Accessory Bronchial Arteries' (page 56).
[2] See under Literature, 'Function Bronchial Arteries' (page 23).

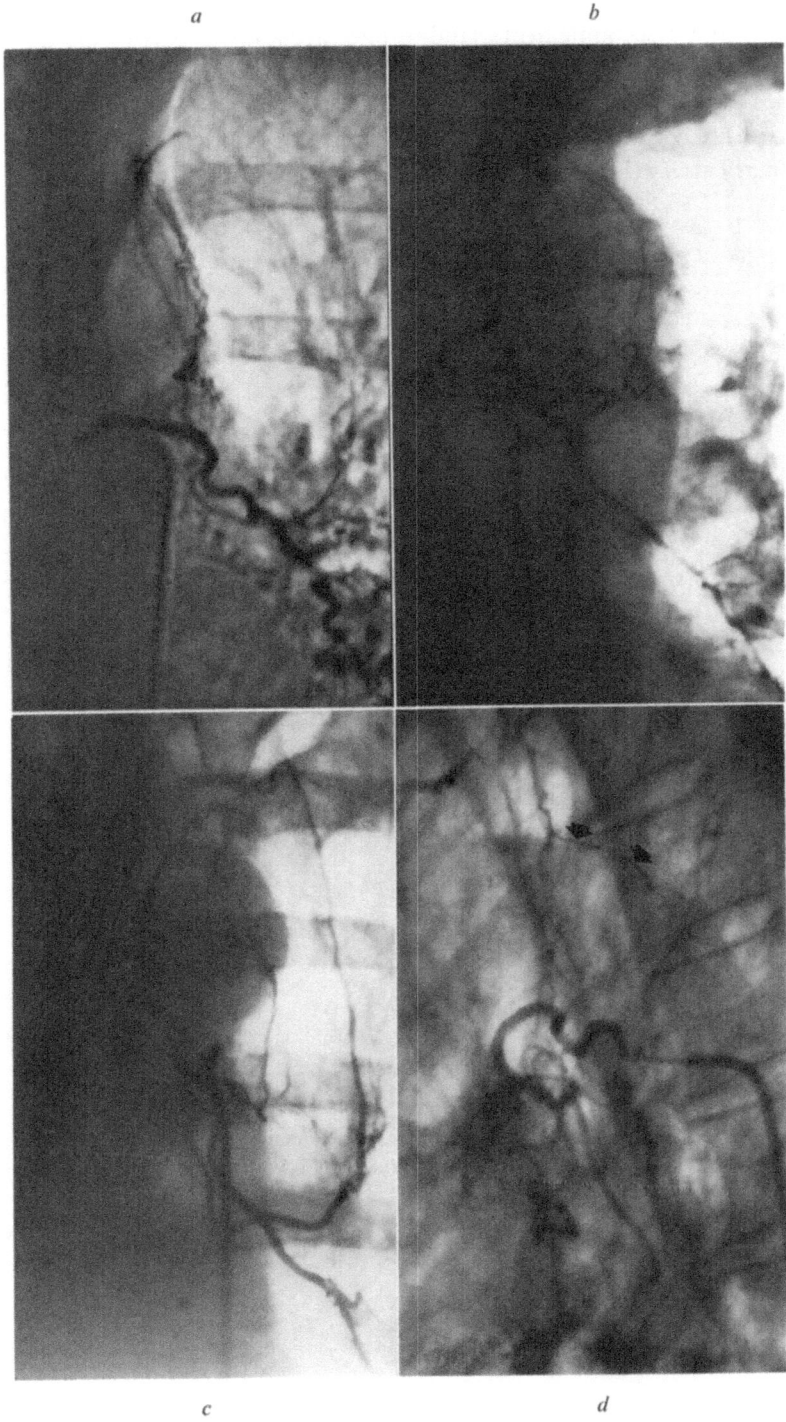

Fig. 36. The vascularization of the aortic arch and the proximal part of the wall of the descending aorta appears to be effected by branches of the left bronchial artery.

a: vasa aortae deriving from the left bronchial artery.

b: Vasa aortae from the left branch of a truncus communis.

c and *d*: Left-sided bronchial arteriogram with vasa aortae in anteroposterior (*c*) and in lateral (*d*) projection. In the lateral view a small branch follows the contour of the aortic arch (arrows).

Two cases showed small branches arising from the left inferior bronchial artery to supply the proximal segment of the descending aorta, and in one case a lower part of the descending aorta was vascularized by a branch of the left inferior bronchial artery. In two cases the right bronchial artery provided branches for the ascending aorta.

Via these vasa aortae connections with the thyreocervical arteries (Figs. 37, 38a, and 50) and the left internal mammary artery (Figs. 11a, 25, and 53a) sometimes run through the anterior mediastinum.

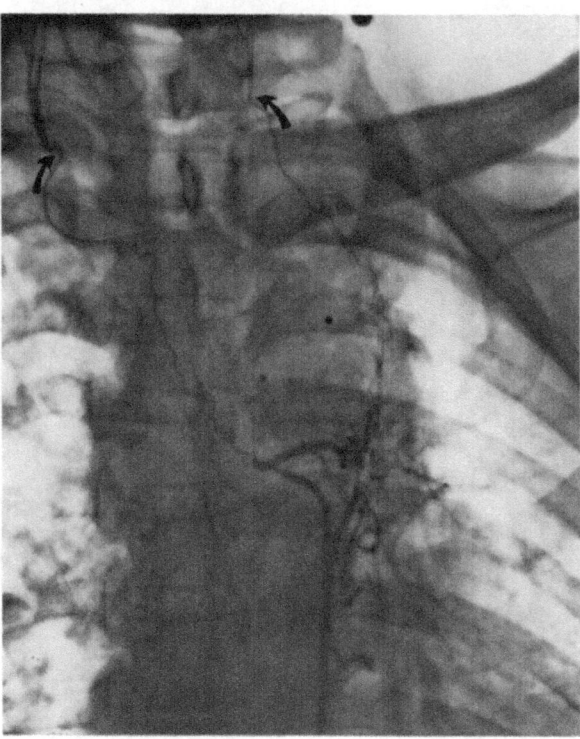

Fig. 37. Via vasa aortae there are sometimes connections between the bronchial and the thyreocervical arteries (arrows). These intercommunicating vessels run through the anterior mediastinum.

In four cases[1] a vas aortae was selectively catheterized, two of them supplying the aortic arch (Fig. 38a) and two the descending aorta (Fig. 38b). In these cases the arteriograms showed bronchial branches or anastomoses with the bronchial circulation. One patient developed severe unexplained retro-sternally located pain during the injection of contrast medium into a vas aortae (aorta descendens). In two patients the vas aortae was distinctly enlarged due to its contribution to the collateral circulation supplying the lung.

---

[1] See also under the anatomical section of the present study 'Accessory Bronchial Arteries' (page 56).

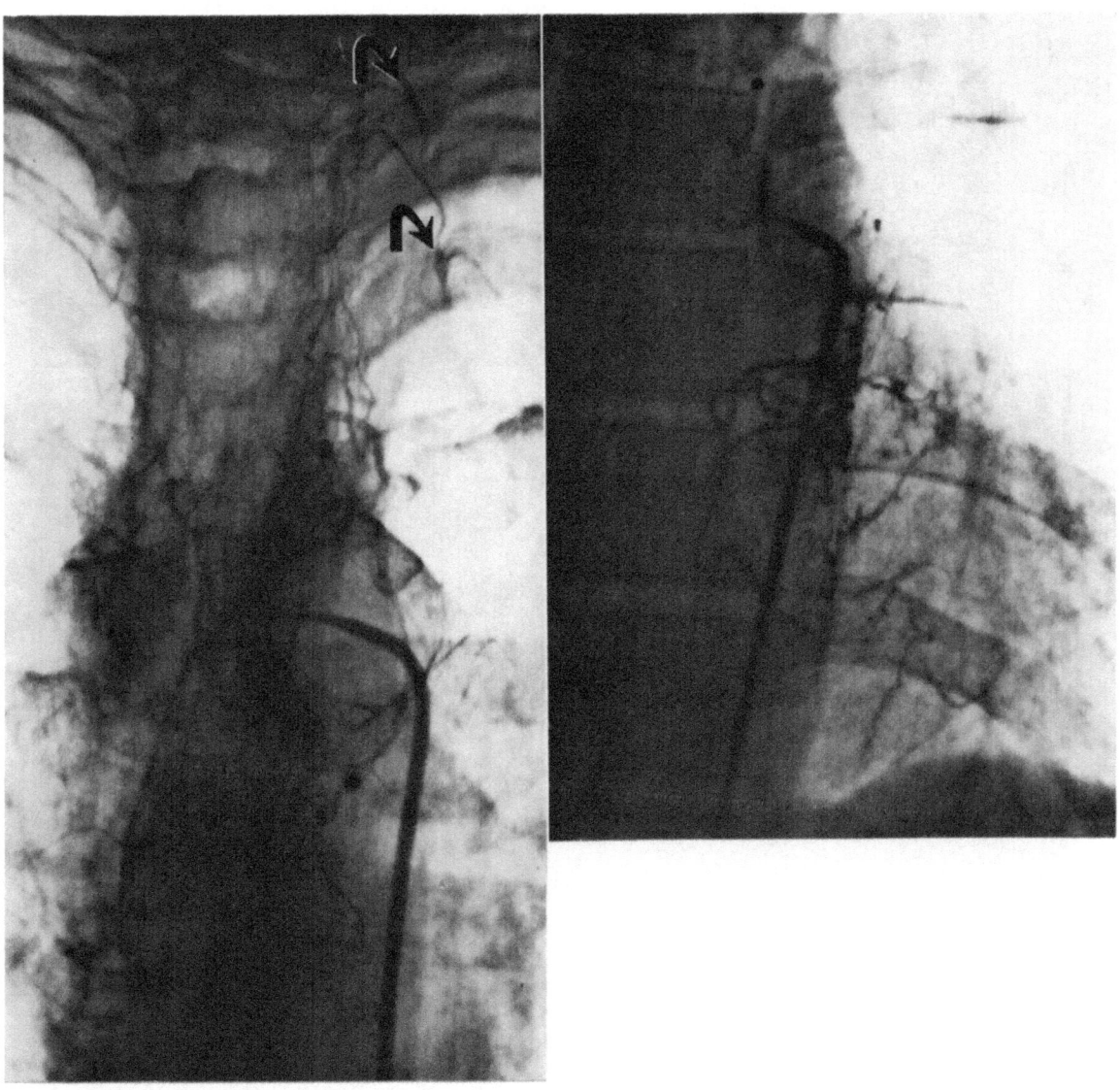

a   *b*

Fig. 38. Selectively catheterized vasa aortae.
a: Vas for the aortic arch. A few fine arteries (projected left paravertebrally) run in the cranial direction and form connections with two thyreocervical arteries (arrows).
b: Vas for the descending aorta with ramifications closely following the lateral contour of the aorta and several accessory bronchial arteries penetrating into the parenchyma of the lung.

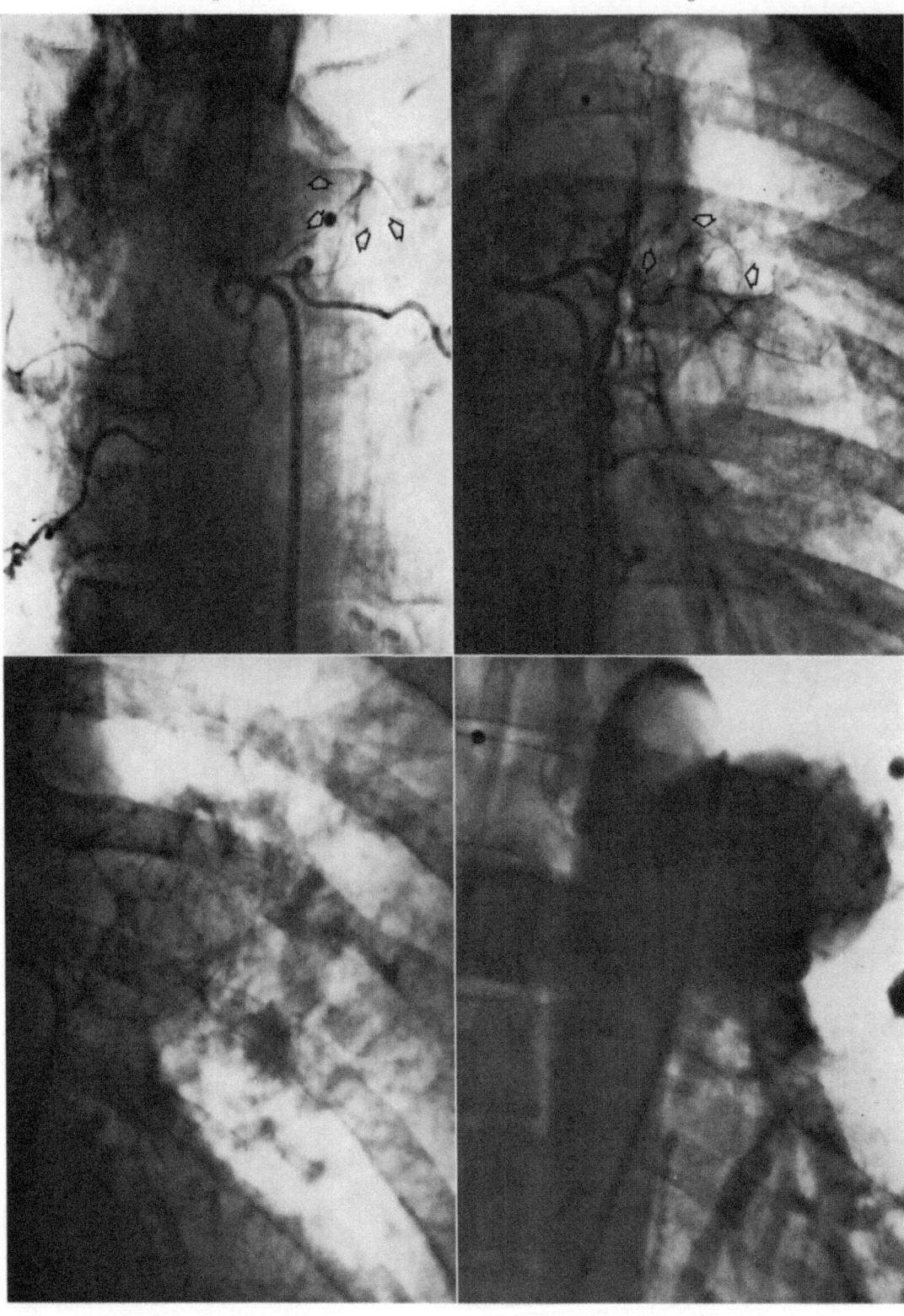

a   *b*

c   *d*

Fig. 39. Three cases showing vasa pulmonalis on bronchial arteriograms.
a and *b*: The fine rami for the vascularization of the pulmonary trunk and the left main branch are indicated by the arrows.
c and *d*: Patient with a heavily dilated pulmonary artery as a result of a POTT operation. The vascularized area on the bronchial arteriogram (*c*) corresponds with the region of the pulmonary trunk and the left branch on the aorto-gram (*d*).

c.2. *Vascularization of the pulmonary artery*

In five cases vasa pulmonalis were derived from the bronchial artery (Fig. 39). Two dubious cases of similar derivation were also seen. In one patient treated with a POTT operation for tetralogy of FALLOT there was marked vascularization of the heavily dilated main pulmonary trunk (Fig. 39c and d). This possibility must be kept in mind if re-operation is considered.

d. Hilar glands

In a few cases (seven probable and seven dubious), vascularization of usually pathological hilar glands was visible on the bronchial arteriogram (Figs. 40 and 93).

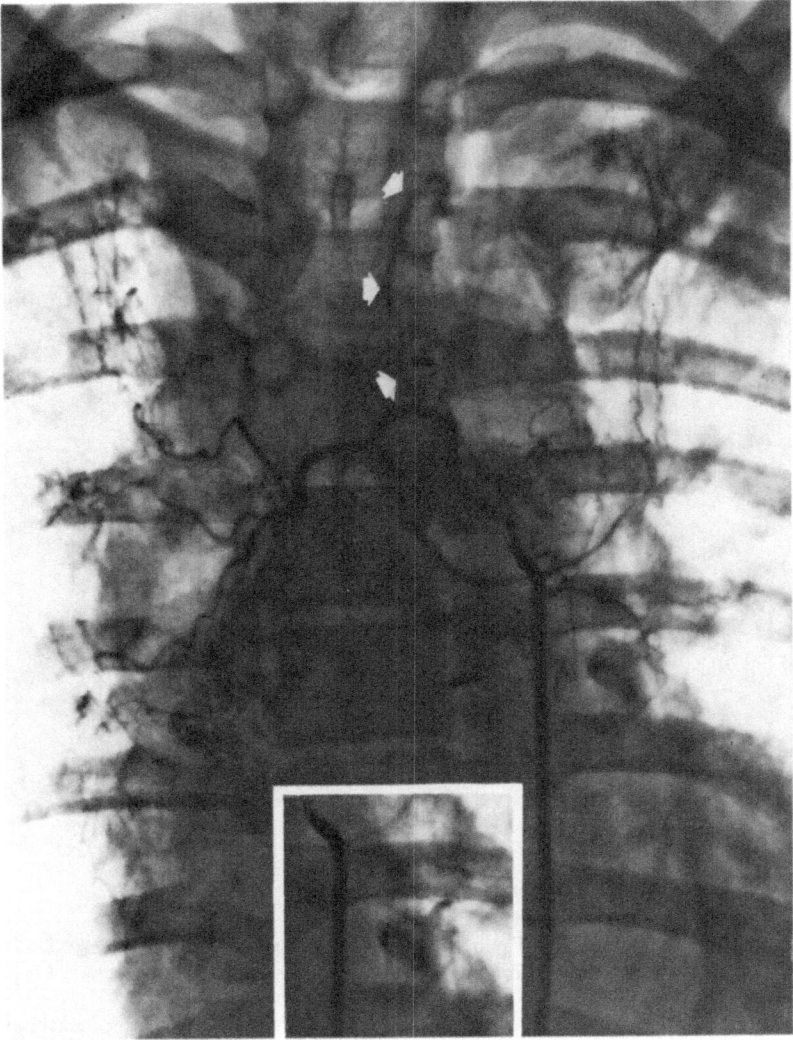

Fig. 40. Vascularization of a gland in the lower pole of the left hilus in a patient with tuberculous lesions in the upper lobes. In the capillary phase the amount of contrast medium in the gland is augmented (inset). The white arrows indicate the rapid drainage of part of the contrast medium via a bronchial vein to the superior hemiazygos vein.

e. Trachea

Vascularization of the trachea was seen in three cases (e.g. Fig. 30).

IV.1.2. Bronchial veins

In the discussion of the anatomical data in the literature a simplified schematic representation was given of the two pathways of venous drainage of the bronchial circulation (Fig. 2). Fig. 41 shows these two pathways *in vivo*.

In four cases with richly vascularized intrapulmonary pathological processes the draining pulmonary veins were visible on the arteriogram (Fig. 41*a*). In thirty-two cases (41.6 per cent) veins were visible on the antero-posterior view running on both sides in a paravertebral zone most often in the vicinity of the pulmonary hili. Most of these were bronchial veins of the collecting type, since visualization of the venae bronchiales anteriores and posteriores cannot be expected because of their small caliber. In view of the straight, vertical course of some veins, we think that in some cases it was not the small bronchial veins themselves that were seen but rather the common drainage via azygos and hemiazygos veins. Left bronchial veins were visualized in twenty-three cases and right bronchial veins in seventeen cases.

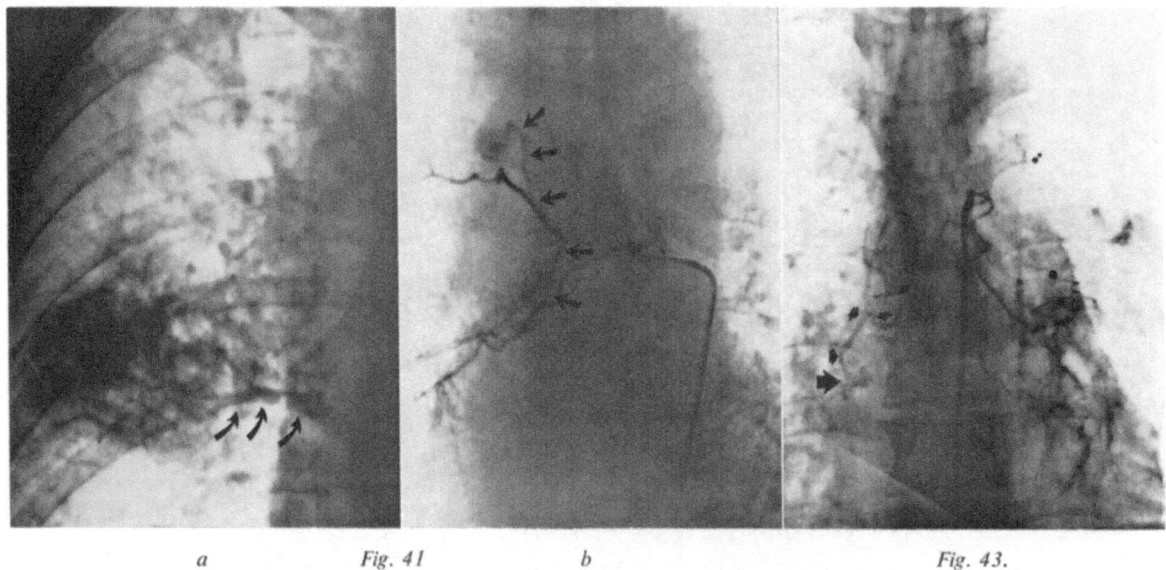

a   *Fig. 41*   *b*   *Fig. 43.*

Fig. 41. The two different modes of venous drainage *in vivo*.

a: The blood derived from this richly vascularized pulmonary tumor is drained via the pulmonary vein, which can be followed to its termination in the left atrium (arrows) during the venous phase of a bronchial arteriogram. Fig. 12*b* shows the arterial phase of this arteriogram.

b: This bronchial vein (arrows) already became visible during the arterial phase of the series, indicating rapid passage of the contrast medium through the capillaries in the region of the hilus. At the upper aspect of the right main bronchus the entry into the superior caval vein or even just into the azygos vein can be discerned as a vague spot of contrast medium.

Fig. 43. Example of a bronchial vein (small arrows) entering the central portion of the pulmonary vein or directly into the left atrium (large arrow).

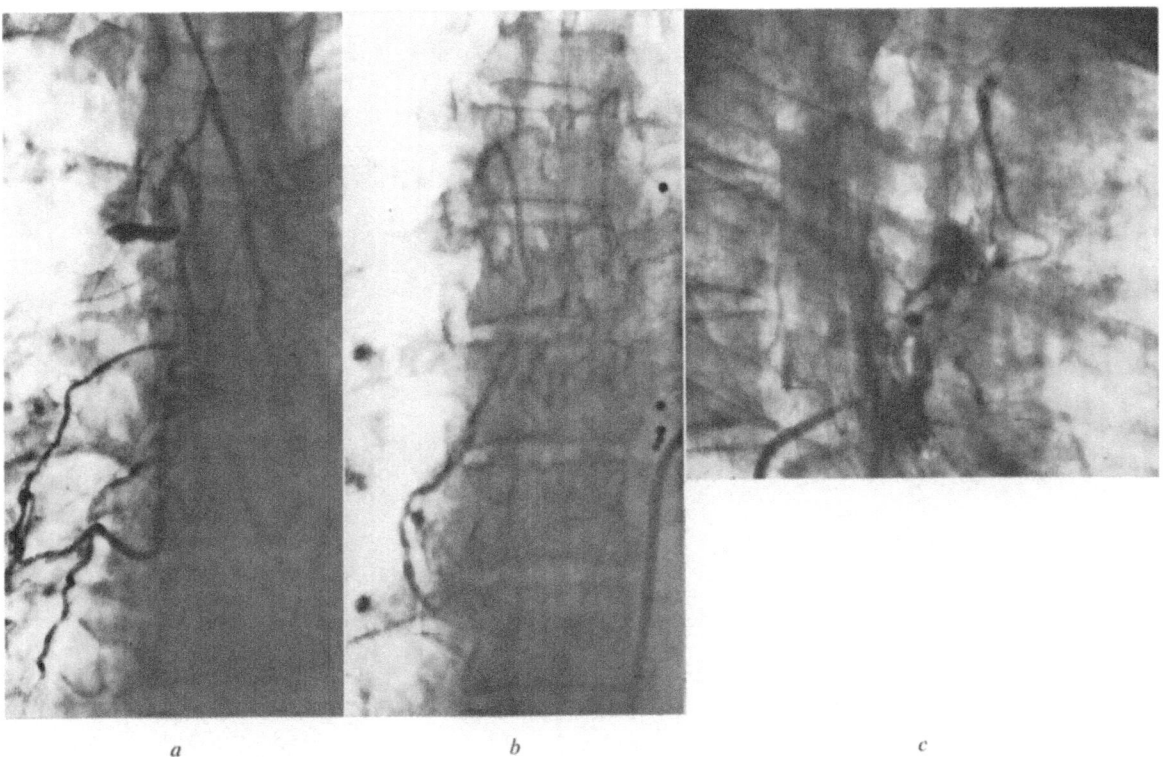

a *b* *c*

Fig. 42. Bronchial veins with drainage in the azygos vein just before the latter enters the superior caval vein, or directly into the latter. The wide vein in *a* may be the azygos vein. The bronchial vein in *b* is also present – in the lateral view – in *c*.

Discussion

Drainage via the azygos vein was visible on the right side in six cases. The entry was usually at a high level; in three cases, as described by MARCHAND ET AL. (1950), just before the termination of the azygos vein in the superior caval vein or directly into the latter (Figs. 41*b* and 42). In one case a vein seemed to empty into a central pulmonary vein or directly into the left atrium (Fig. 43), probably representing one of the central connecting veins between the bronchial and pulmonary venous systems, e.g. described by ZUCKERKANDL (1881).

On the left side drainage into the inferior hemiazygos, superior hemiazygos (Fig. 40), left innominate, and left subclavian veins was seen. In sixteen cases one of the draining veins closely parallelled the contour of the aorta (Figs. 44*a* and 44*b*). This vein was seen particularly in cases in which a distinct arterial branch vascularizing the aorta was present. We thought that this vein served for the drainage of the aortic wall, and termed this vessel vena aortae. In six cases, on the left side only this vein was visible. Probably, thus, this vein serves at the same time for drainage of the bronchial blood, since according to SCHOENMACKERS (1960) extensive anastomoses exist between bronchial and aortic veins.

In one case the broncho-pulmonary veins of LE FORT (1859), also termed the deep bronchial veins of MARCHAND ET AL. (1950), were clearly visible (Fig. 44c).

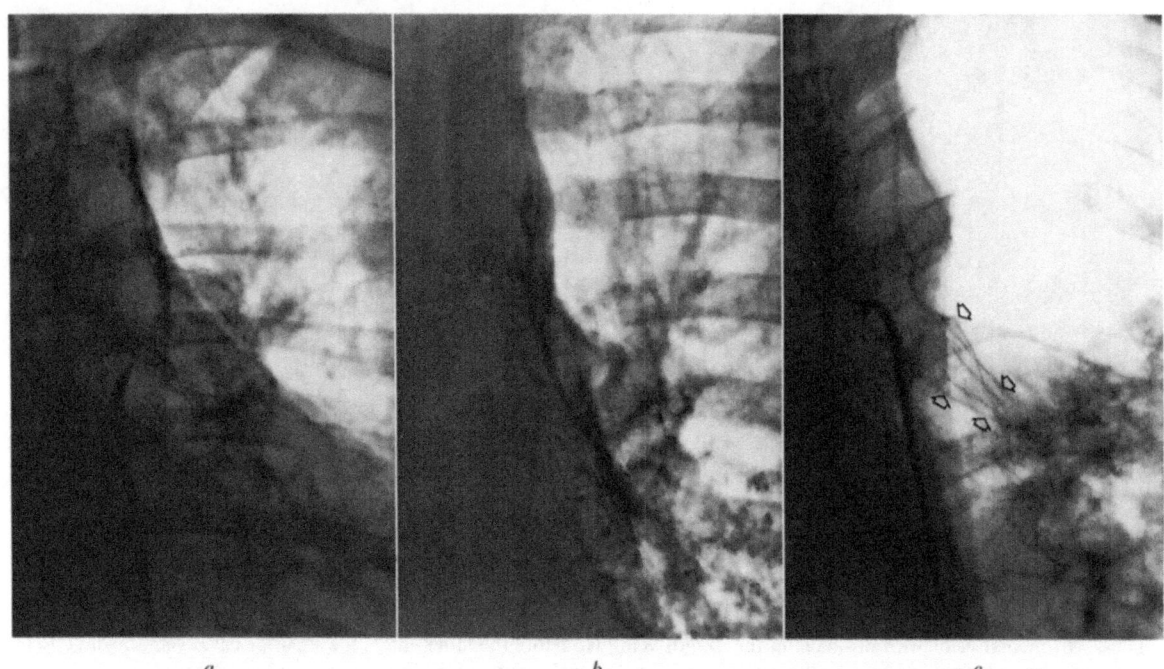

a   *b*   *c*

Fig. 44. Bronchial veins.
a and *b*: Venous phases of the arteriograms shown in Figs. 11 *a* and 25, respectively. On the left side most of the draining veins closely parallel the contour of the aorta. The latter observation was consistently made in cases with a distinct arterial branch for the vascularization of the aorta.
c: The 'broncho-pulmonary' veins of LE FORT, also termed the 'deep bronchial veins' of MARCHAND ET AL. (arrows).

We wondered whether there was a reason for the visualization of the bronchial veins. At first, there seemed to be a connexion with the presence of pathological hilar glands, but this could not be confirmed later. There proved to be a relationship between the injection pressure and the location of the point of the catheter: bronchial veins were visualized more rapidly and with greater intensity when the injection pressure was too high and the point of the catheter occluded the vessel.

Conclusions

Our findings concerning the venous drainage of the blood from the bronchial circulation are in agreement with data in the literature. In addition, the drainage of the central supply region on the left side was found to occur frequently via venae aortae (the draining veins of the wall of the aorta).

No diagnostic value could be assigned to the visualization of the bronchial veins.

IV.1.3. Intercostal arteries

A total of 120 selective arteriograms were made of intercostal arteries originating from the aorta. The most important anatomical data obtained from a study of this material can be summarized as follows.

Normal origin and course
The intercostal arteries arise in pairs from the dorsal aspect of the aorta, the origin of the right intercostal arteries being situated right dorsally and right dorso-laterally and that of the left strictly dorsally or left dorsally. In older patients this asymmetry with respect to the sagittal plane increases, as though the descending aorta had a tendency to turn to the right. This is probably the result of unrolling.

The varying oblique cranial course has already been discussed in the chapter on the technique (page 30).

After a brief course over the vertebral column, the intercostal arteries turn aside to insinuate themselves at about the middle of the intercostal spaces, where after 2 to 8 cm (Fig. 48a) – average 2.5 cm – the artery divides itself into one usually larger cranial and one (sometimes two) usually smaller caudal branches (Fig. 45). Often, proximal to this division a large muscular branch arises, most frequently at the entry into the intercostal space (Fig. 45a). The cranial branch runs 2 to 8 mm under the cranial rib, the caudal branch along the middle or the upper part of the inner aspect of the next rib. In younger individuals these branches are straight, but in older individuals they show increasing tortuosity (Fig. 45b).

Variants
Many variants occur. The intercostal artery sometimes shows a tortuous course, touching first one and then another rib (Fig. 48c). The variation increases from the cranial to the caudal direction. In our material we also found more variations of left than of right intercostal arteries. Frequently, we saw intercostal arteries for the supply of two adjacent intercostal arteries, seldom for three or four.

Anastomoses
Almost all cases showed collateral shunts to adjacent intercostal arteries (Fig. 46). In 8 instances (6.7 per cent) contralateral intercostal arteries were filled via prevertebral muscular branches (Fig. 46). An anastomosis with the phrenic artery was seen once (Fig. 47). Anastomoses with the pulmonary artery will be discussed under 'Pathology' (page 100–105).

78

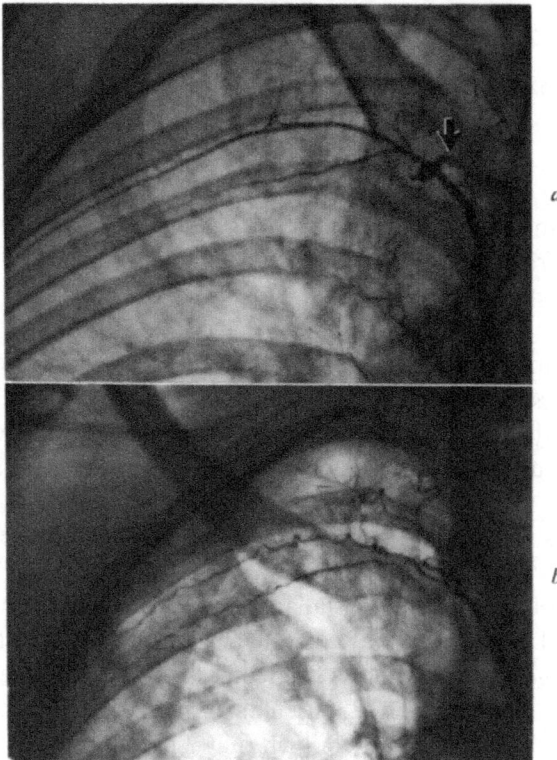

a

b

Fig. 45. Normal course of the intercostal arteries.

After an average distance of 2.5 cm in the intercostal space the artery divides into a cranial branch (below the correspondent rib) and a generally smaller caudal branch (on the inner side of the next rib). Before this bifurcation, a large muscular branch often arises (arrow in *a*). Initially, the intercostal branches show a straight course, but with advancing age they become increasingly more tortuous.

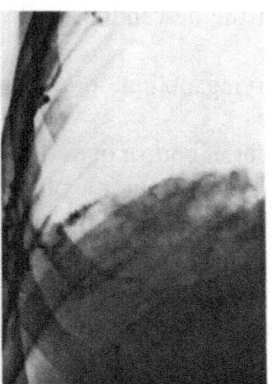

*Fig.*47. Anastomosis between an intercostal and a phrenic ⟶ artery.

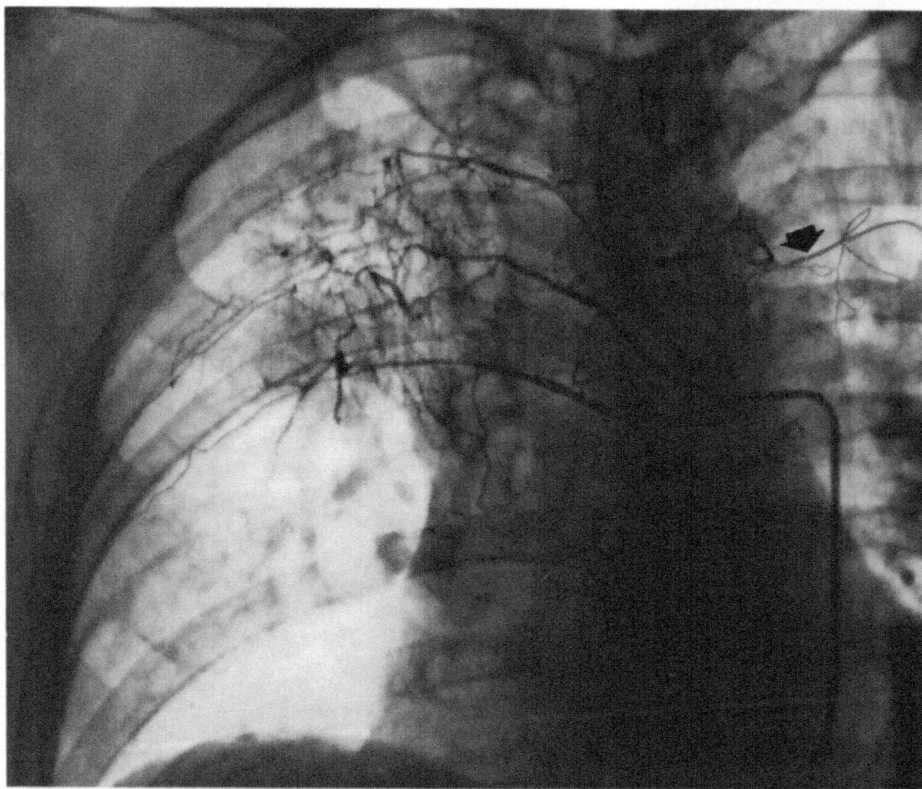

Fig. 46. Arteriogram of the 4th right intercostal artery. Visualization of the 3rd and 5th right intercostals via colleteral anastomoses and also of the 4th left intercostal artery (arrow) via contralateral anastomoses through prevertebral muscular branches.

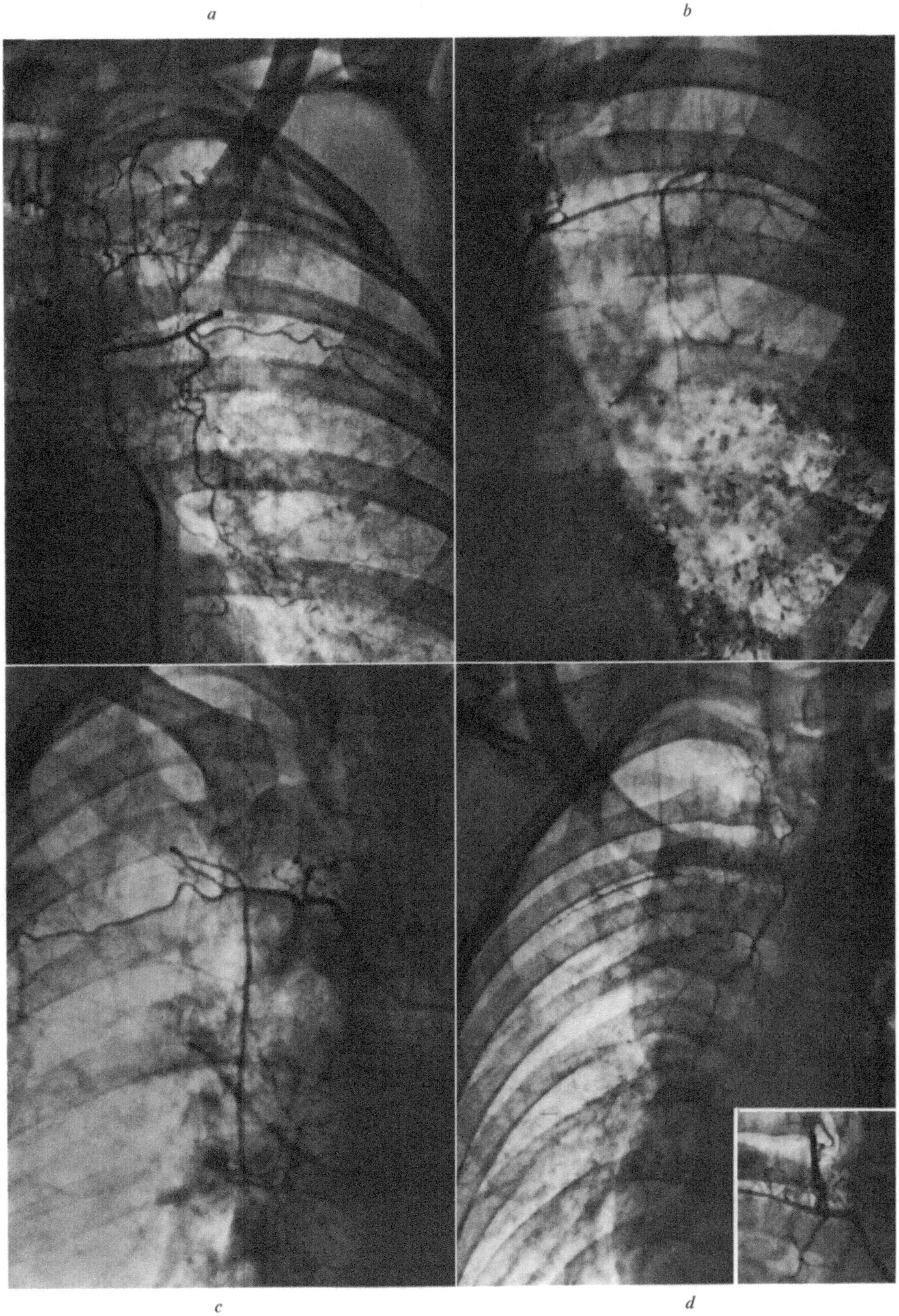

Fig. 48. Examples of intercostal arteries with large dorsal muscular branches projected over the lung field: no bronchial arteries. The intercostal artery in *a* shows a late bifurcation i.e. after a distance of 8 cm, and further shows 3 cranially localized loop-shaped derivatives possibly related to the tuberculous lesions located apically in the left upper lobe. Two muscular branches from a single intercostal are shown in *c*. The inset in *d* shows the central segment, since the contrast medium has already left this segment in *d*. None of the intercostal arteries shows the 'normal' course.

Anterior spinal artery
This artery was visualized in eight cases, as will be discussed under 'Complications' (page 170).

Discussion

According to standard works on anatomy the intercostal arteries run initially in the costal groove and then enter the intercostal spaces.[1] This is certainly not in accordance with the actual anatomical situation. In addition, the cranial and caudal branches do not run along the lower side of the cranial rib and the upper side of the caudal rib, respectively: the cranial branch often runs quite far below the cranial rib (sometimes in the middle of the intercostal space), and as a rule the caudal branch runs on the inner side of the caudal rib.

Under pathological conditions the intercostal arteries may become dilated and concomitantly tortuous, sometimes filling the entire intercostal space.

An extreme case is shown in fig. 73*a*. This tortuosity is also seen in older individuals. When an intercostal artery winds more than the neighboring or contra-lateral intercostal arteries, however, a pathological condition is to be suspected. We shall return to this point in the section on intercostopulmonary anastomoses.

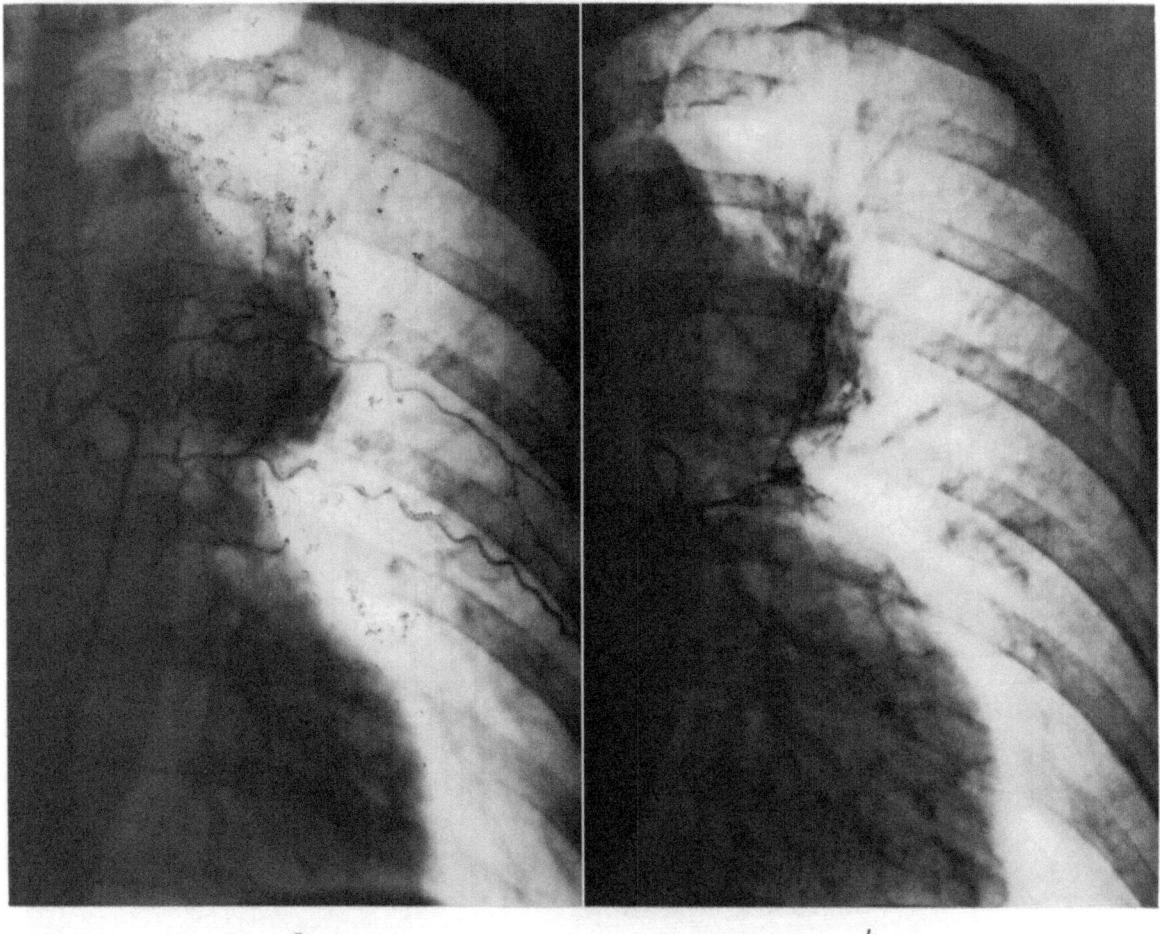

a   *b*

Fig. 49.
a: Fifth and 6th intercostal arteriogram on the left side. The para-aortal process seems to be vascularized by branches of the intercostal arteries, but this is due to superposition.
b: Bronchial arteriogram showing, for purpose of comparison, the actual vascularization of the process.

[1] See under Literature, 'Intercostal Arteries' (page 26).

The dorsal muscular branch, which usually arises from the proximal segment, may be very large and be projected over an entire lung field in the antero-posterior view, thus suggesting the presence of a bronchial artery (Fig. 48). In the radiology literature this has led to many errors, these intercostal muscular branches being mistaken for bronchial arteries (e.g. in VIAMONTE ET AL. (1965); NORDEN-STRÖM, 1966; E COSTA, 1967; MILNE, 1967). Fig. 49 shows an example from our material in a case of a para-aortal process. The process seems to be vascularized by the artery for the fifth and sixth inter-costal spaces (Fig. 49a), but is actually supplied by the bronchial artery (Fig. 49b). On the lateral view these branches can be seen running in the dorsal muscles (Fig. 50). Consequently, in doubtful cases a lateral X-ray should be made. Nevertheless when only one arteriogram is available errors can be avoided because the ramification of these muscular branches is very different from that of the bronchial arteries, being more irregular and of course not following the bronchial tree.

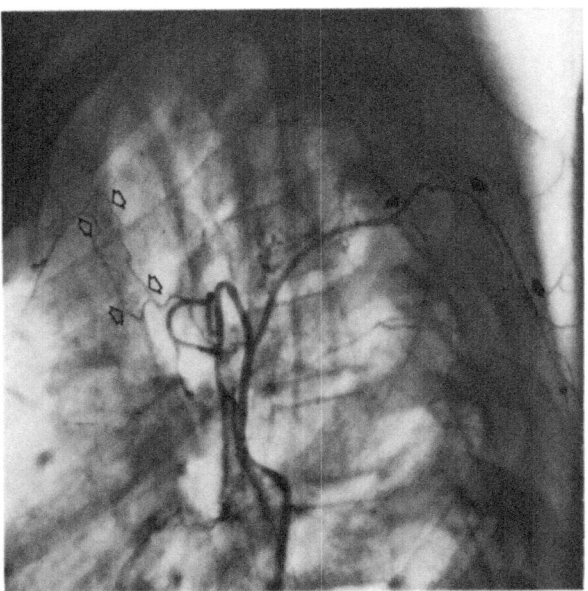

Fig. 50. Arteriogram of an intercosto-bronchial trunk, showing a dorsal muscular branch provided by the intercostal artery (solid arrows). Thin arterial branches (open arrows) run through the anterior mediastinum connecting the bronchial artery with the thyreocervicals via vasa aortae (ascendens).

Conclusions

The results of our study show considerable divergence from the situation described in standard works, especially with respect to the course of the intercostal arteries in the intercostal spaces.

In addition to the normal course, in which the intercostal artery divides to form a large cranial branch running under the cranial rib and a small caudal branch running on the inner side of the next rib, many variants occur. The variants increase from cranial to caudal, and may be more numerous on the left side.

Fine anatomoses occur between the unilateral and contralateral intercostal arteries. An intercostal artery seldom gives rise to an anterior spinal artery.

Tortuosity of intercostal arteries occurs with increasing age and also under pathological conditions. Differentiation can be made by comparison with the other intercostal arteries.

IV.1.4. Intercostal veins

The intercostal veins are not relevant to the present subject. They appeared on five intercostal arteriograms in the venous phase.

IV.2. PART II – PATHOLOGY

The following anomalies were investigated by means of bronchial arteriography:

Primary lung tumors	: 23	Diffuse small focal lesions	: 2
Tuberculosis		Bronchoplasty	: 2
Focal lesions	: 18	Hamartoma	: 2
Cavities	: 4	Aspergillosis	: 2
Tuberculoma	: 2	Hemoptysis of unknown cause	: 2
Bronchiectasis	: 11	Pleural tumor (benign)	: 2
Emphysema	: 11	Bronchogenic cyst	: 1
FALLOT's tetralogy	: 4	Suppurative pneumonia	: 1
Chronic infiltration	: 4	Histiocytosis X	: 1
Metastases	: 4	Subphrenic abscess	: 1
Chronic asthmatic bronchitis	: 4	Esophageal carcinoma	: 1
Infected cavities	: 3	HODGKIN's disease[1]	: 1

The number of anomalies is higher than the number of patients in whom bronchial arteriography was successful (77). There are two reasons for this discrepancy. In the first place, several of the patients suffered from more than one disease; for instance, a case with old tuberculous lesions in the upper lobes, localized bronchiectatic changes, and a peripherally located pulmonary tumor. In the second place, a few patients, examined later, were added to the original series.

In the order of the list given above, the anomalies will be discussed under 'Bronchial Vascularization in Pulmonary Diseases' with the exception of the tetralogy of FALLOT, for which the cases will be discussed separately under 'Bronchial Circulation in Heart Disease'. The cases of subphrenic abscess and esophageal carcinoma will be dealt with after the discussion of the pulmonary anomalies.

For the proper interpretation and understanding of the radiological picture, attention must be paid to certain forms of arterial anastomoses prior to the discussion of the bronchial circulation in the various anomalies.

---

[1] This patient will not be discussed, since he was treated in several ways for HODGKIN's disease and the arteriographical findings therefore cannot be considered typical with respect to the type of vascularization of HODGKIN glands.

IV.2.1. Anastomoses

In this section four forms of arterial anastomoses playing a part in the vascularization under pathological circumstances will be discussed. Fig. 51 shows a schematic representation of all these forms. Two types also occur under normal circumstances: intercommunicating anastomoses between the bronchial arteries (1) and anastomoses between bronchial and pulmonary arteries (2). The anastomoses between intercostal and pulmonary arteries (3) only occur under pathological circumstances; this probably also holds for the anastomoses between intercostal and bronchial arteries (4). There are also intercommunicating anastomoses between intercostal arteries[1] playing no role, however, in pathological conditions. Intercommunicating anastomoses between pulmonary arteries are denied in the literature, e.g. by LAUWERIJNS (1962).

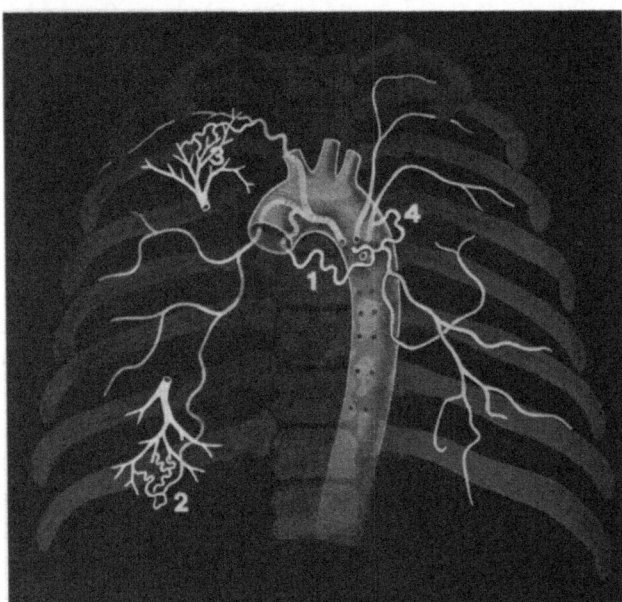

Fig. 51. Schematic representation of the different forms of arterial anastomoses between the bronchial arteries, other arteries of the systemic circulation, and the pulmonary artery.

1: Broncho-bronchial anastomoses
2: Broncho-pulmonary anastomoses
3: Intercosto-pulmonary anastomoses
4: Intercosto-bronchial anastomoses

IV.2.1.1. BRONCHO-BRONCHIAL ANASTOMOSES

Under broncho-bronchial anastomoses is understood fine and constantly present connections between the bronchial arteries in the region of the hilus.[2]

---

[1] See the anatomical section of the present study, 'Intercostal Arteries' (page 77).
[2] See under Literature, 'Central Course Bronchial Arteries' (page 22).

LITERATURE

The literature on both anatomy and pathology contains several descriptions of these anastomoses, but they are neglected in the radiology literature.

FINDINGS IN ARTERIOGRAPHY

Broncho-bronchial anastomoses were demonstrated in 31 patients (40.3 per cent). Of the total number of 216 bronchial arteries, 63 (29.2 per cent) were filled collaterally, and of these 17 could also be reached selectively and 7 were also visible on a aortogram. Therefore, 39 bronchial arteries (18.1 per cent) *only* became visible as a result of collateral filling and 46 collaterally filled bronchials could not be reached selectively.

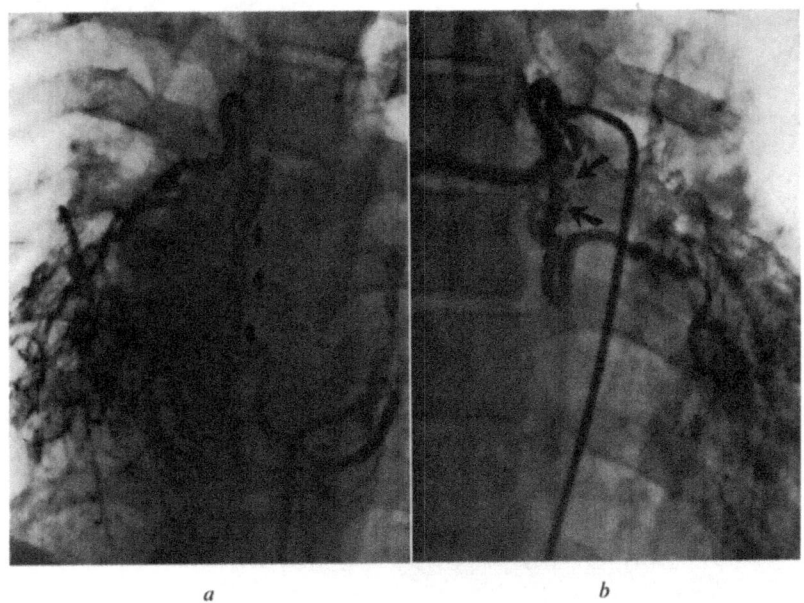

a   *b*

Fig. 52. Enlarged broncho-bronchial anastomoses
a: Enlarged anastomosis (arrows) in tetralogy of FALLOT.
b: Greatly enlarged left-sided anastomosis (arrows) in tetralogy of FALLOT.

Normal broncho-bronchial anastomoses are barely visible on the X-ray (Figs. 11, 13*b*, 56, and 102). In twelve cases, however, the anastomoses were enlarged (Fig. 52), mainly in bronchiectasis and congenital cardiac diseases. In most of the cases the anastomoses were all found on one side (Fig. 52*b*), most frequently between the left superior and inferior bronchial arteries (Fig. 53). Fig. 54 shows an example of a distended anastomosis running via the mediastinum to a contralateral bronchial artery. The anastomotic canals were often long (Figs. 53 and 54). The anastomoses are usually situated centrally but may also occur in the region of the hilus (Fig. 57).

New broncho-bronchial anastomoses can also be formed. In one patient with a probably thrombotic bronchial artery we observed a by-pass consisting of small bridging collaterals (Fig. 55). In two patients who had undergone bronchoplastic surgery similar pictures were seen (Figs. 98 and 99), obviously as a result of ligation of the bronchial artery.

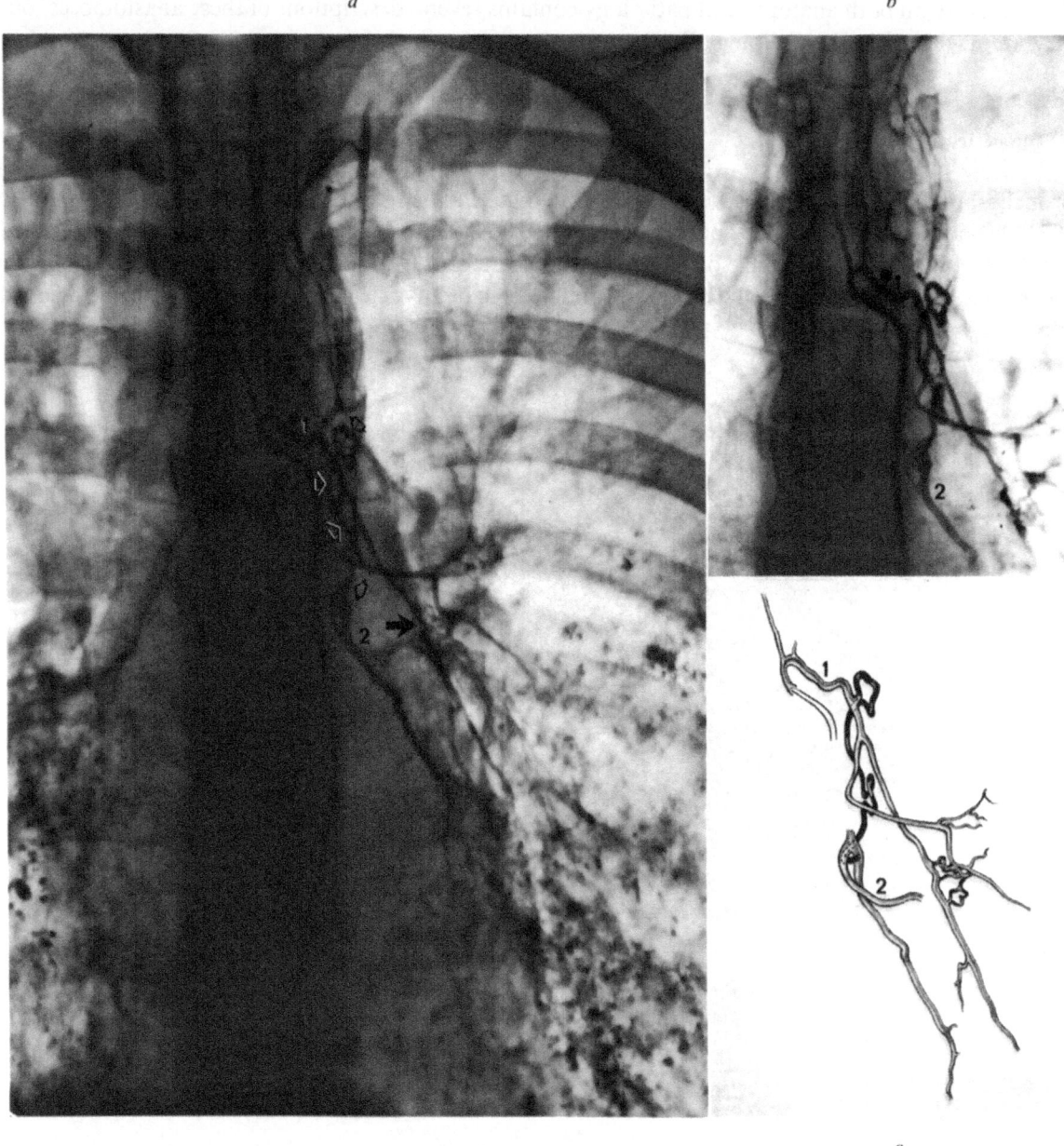

Fig. 53. Enlarged broncho-bronchial anastomoses between the left superior (1) and inferior (2) bronchial arteries in a patient with bronchiectasis in the left lower lobe and lingula.

a: Catheter in the left superior bronchial artery. The centrally localized, long, and tortuous anastomotic canal between the left superior (1) and inferior (2) bronchial arteries is indicated by small open arrows. The large arrow indicates a second area with anastomoses near the lower pole of the left hilus. Via vasa aortae and an aberrantly originating accessory bronchial artery, the contrast medium reaches the internal mammary artery (see also Fig. 25).

b: Detail of the central anastomotic canal.

c: Schematic representation. The darkest vessels are the anastomoses.

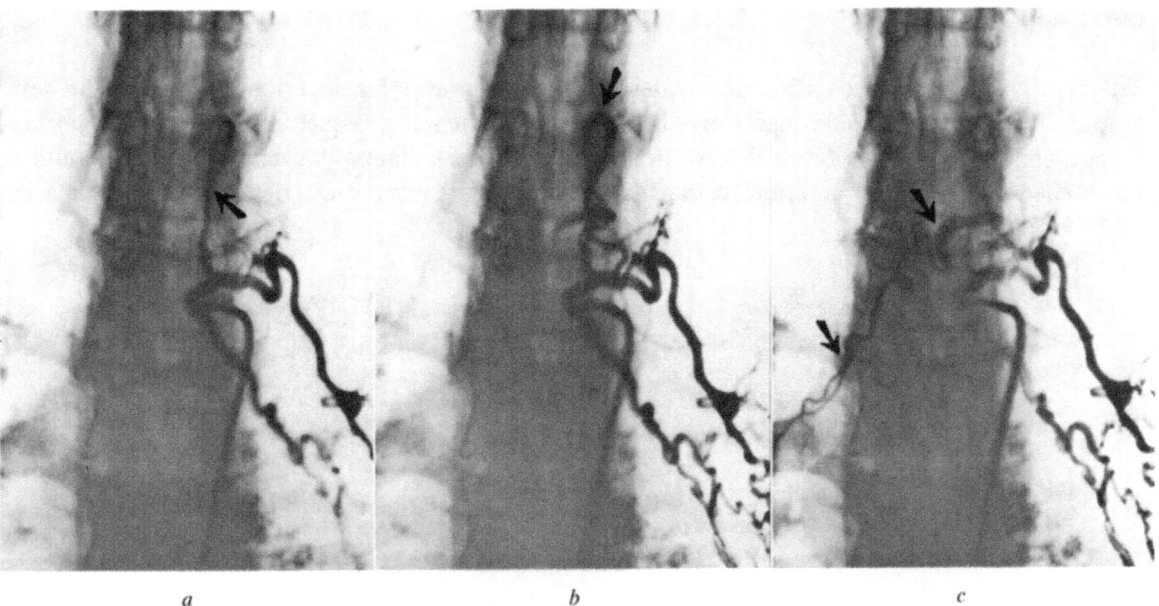

a   b   c

Fig. 54. Enlarged transmediastinally intercommunicating broncho-bronchial anastomosis in successive arterial phases (*a*, *b*, and *c*). Bronchiectasis in both lungs.

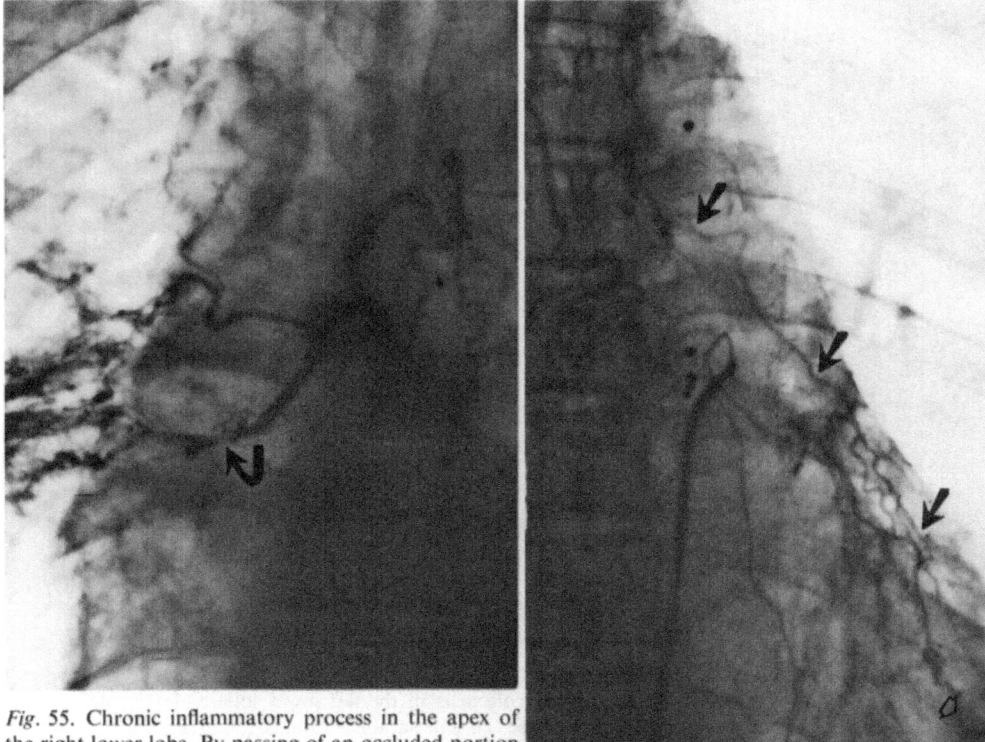

Fig. 55. Chronic inflammatory process in the apex of the right lower lobe. By-passing of an occluded portion of the bronchial artery (arrow) by collaterals. The bronchial artery is probably thrombosed.

Fig. 56. Patient with a tumor in the left lower lobe (small arrows). The tumor is poorly vascularized by branches of the left superior bronchial artery. The catheter is located in the left inferior bronchial artery. The superior bronchial artery (large arrows) could not be catheteirzed but has filled collaterally.

DISCUSSION

The quality of the representation of collaterally filled arteries is far superior to those of the aorto-graphically filled vessels and roughly equals the quality of the selective pictures. Of special importance here, therefore, are the 46 bronchial arteries that were filled collaterally even though they could not be reached selectively. In addition to the 143 selectively catheterized arteries, this represents a gain of 32.3 per cent.

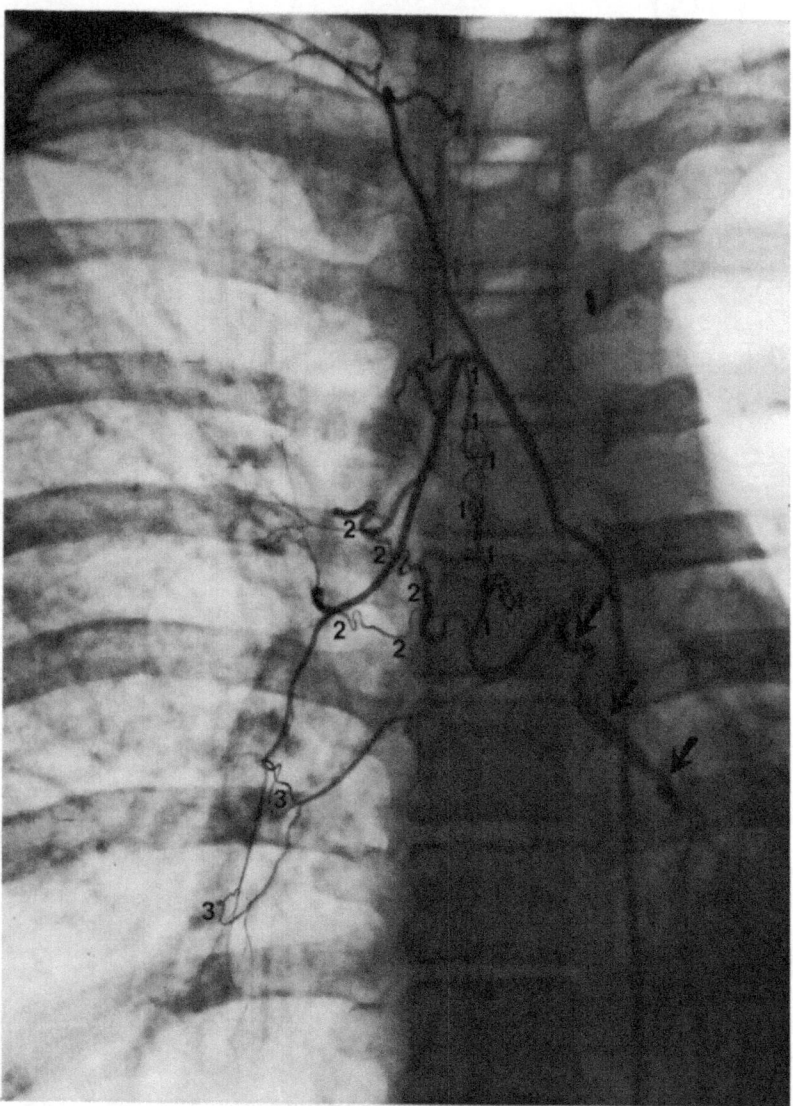

Fig. 57. Multiple wide broncho-bronchial anastomoses to the left inferior bronchial artery (arrows) in a patient with serious bronchiectasis in the left lower lobe and lingula (see Fig. 92B). There are central (1), hilar (2), and parahilar (3) anastomoses.

In this way we succeeded in some cases in obtaining a picture of the bronchial vascularization of certain parts of the lung equalling the results of the selective study even when the bronchial artery in question had not been found. In one patient, for example, the artery supplying a tumor could only be filled collaterally (Fig. 56). The neglect of these anastomoses in the radiology literature is not justified, since they greatly increase the chances of performing a complete investigation.

The anastomoses proved to be wider the longer the anomaly with an increased bronchial blood supply had been present. Conversely, it may be said that wide broncho-bronchial shunts, such as shown in figs. 52, 53, 54, and 57, indicate long-term and probably congenital anomalies with an increased bronchial circulation. In patients with localized pulmonary lesions and an increased bronchial circulation, e.g. bronchiectasis in one segment or lobe, this dilatation can easily be accounted for: the anastomoses come into active use due to the increased bronchial flow (Fig. 57). In generalized changes with an increased bronchial circulation, e.g. in the presence of a pulmonary stenosis or atresia, the explanation is more difficult. In these cases, however, there are always parts of the lung requiring a still larger supply of blood.

CONCLUSIONS

1. The presence of broncho-bronchial anastomoses considerably increases the chance of a complete and successful arteriographic investigation.
2. The demonstration of wide broncho-bronchial anastomoses has diagnostic value. They indicate long-term or congenital anomalies accompanied by an increased bronchial blood supply.
3. Broncho-bronchial anastomoses are always present, although the contrast medium does not always pass them (in 2 out of 5 cases in our material). Newly formed broncho-bronchial anastomoses can be seen when a bronchial artery is occluded.

IV.2.1.2. BRONCHO-PULMONARY ANASTOMOSES

Under broncho-pulmonary anastomoses is understood arterial connections between the bronchial and pulmonary circulations. The anatomical and pathological literature on these anastomoses is abundant. All the investigators agree that capillary communications between bronchial and pulmonary arteries occur. The occurrence of precapillary shunts or broncho-pulmonary anastomoses in the normal lung, however, has long been a controversial problem which, according to some authors, has not yet been solved. These anastomoses have a special importance because they mean that a circulatory tract with oxygenated blood and a relatively high pressure is in communication with a tract with a relatively low pressure and desoxygenated blood.

LITERATURE

a. In normal lungs

Although broncho-pulmonary anastomoses have been known since 1721 (RUYSCH), their presence in normal lungs has been authoritatively denied since the end of the last century by MILLER (1906, 1947). MILLER's opinion, however, was primarily based on observations in dogs. Nevertheless, his view has been supported by many other investigators, including GHOREYEB AND KARSNER (1913), BERRY (1935), CUDKOWICZ AND ARMSTRONG (1951), HARRIS AND HEATH (1962), and SMITH (1964).

These anastomoses were unequivocally demonstrated in normal lungs by VON HAYEK (1940, 1953b & c, 1954) and by the well-known detailed study by VERLOOP (1948). Since then, they have been seen by TOBIN (1952), LAUWERIJNS (1962), PUMP (1963), and OUDET ET AL. (1967), the excellent investigation of LAUWERIJNS deserving special mention.

They have also been seen in the lungs of normal neonates by BRUNI (1954) and WAGENVOORT (1966).

According to VERLOOP (1948), VON HAYEK (1954), and LAUWERIJNS (1962), the anastomoses are localized both peribronchially and subpleurally but, according to OUDET ET AL. (1967), only peribronchially. Subpleural anastomoses were also demonstrated by MILNE (1967). TOBIN (1952) distinguishes two kinds of probably intrapulmonary anastomoses: long (10–40 mm) and short (1–2 mm). PUMP (1963) in particular states that the number of these anastomoses increases from the centre toward the periphery.

Through the communications between the bronchial and pulmonary circulations, blood from the left ventricle flows via the lesser circulation into the left atrium. The precapillary broncho-pulmonary flow has been measured in normal lungs by a number of investigators (LEVINSON ET AL., 1959; CUDKOWICZ ET AL., 1960, 1962; FRITTS ET AL., 1961; RYAN AND ABELMANN, 1961; CUDKOWICZ, 1962; MANDELBAUM AND GIAMMONA, 1966). According to the results of physiological studies by BERRY AND DALY (1931), DALY (1936), BRUNER AND SCHMIDT (1947), STATE ET AL. (1957), HORISBERGER AND RODBARD (1960), and GOETZ ET AL. (1965) in dogs and the study in man by HALLER ET AL. (1966), this bronchopulmonary flow can be influenced pharmacologically but is primarily determined mechanically by the difference in pressure between the lesser and the greater circulations. On the question of a possible nervous, vasomotoric influence there is no agreement. According to ARAMENDIA ET AL. (1962a), the flow is regulated by contraction of bronchial veins. In animal experiments not only a bronchopulmonary flow but also a pulmo-bronchial flow was demonstrated (SCHOEDEL AND BALTZER, 1962; ARAMENDIA ET AL., 1967b).

b. In pathological conditions

There is general agreement that broncho-pulmonary anastomoses can occur under pathological conditions. Depending on the anomaly, these anastomoses can be very wide. Although the various investigators found anastomoses in all anomalies, the largest shunts were seen in congenital cardiopathies with pulmonic stenosis or atresia, bronchiectasis, tuberculosis, and chronic inflammatory processes. The authors who deny the existence of these anastomoses in normal lungs attribute their genesis to the enlargement of capillary connections and to neoformation. The following theories are put forward in the literature.

1. Enlargement of the capillary shunts: LIEBOW ET AL. (1949–1950), SMITH ET AL. (1964), ORELL AND HULTGREN (1966).
2. Dilatation of pre-existing broncho-pulmonary anastomoses: this view is maintained by the investigators who have demonstrated these anastomoses in normal lungs. According to TOBIN (1952) and DONKERS (1968), the central anastomoses they observed in certain pathological conditions were remnants from the fetal period.
3. Recanalization of thrombotic pulmonary arteries by vasa vasorum: since the vascularization of the pulmonary artery is provided by bronchial arteries, a shunt can develop in this way. The chief advocate of this theory is CUDKOWICZ, who believes that such shunts can develop in all anomalies. TURNER-WARWICK (1963a), SMITH ET AL. (1964), and ORELL AND HULTGREN (1966) saw similar recanalization in their material.
4. Proliferation of vascular endothelial buds of pulmonary and bronchial arteries in granulation tissue. This hypothesis is strongly supported by LIEBOW ET AL. (e.g. 1949, 1949–1950, 1958, 1962), but DELARUE ET AL. (1952), TURNER-WARWICK (1963a), and SMITH ET AL. (1964) also found these newly formed anastomoses in their material.

In animal experiments, wide broncho-pulmonary anastomoses developed after ligation of the pulmonary artery in one lung (BLOOMER ET AL., 1949; COCKETT AND VASS, 1951; MAKSIMUK, 1962), and very wide anastomoses when an infection was present at the same time (MATHES ET AL., 1931). Measurement of the broncho-pulmonary flow (LIEBOW ET AL., 1950; ARAMENDIA ET AL. 1962b; AVERILL ET AL., 1962) showed that after the ligation it could become 40 times greater and reach a volume of 1 l/min. Behind the ligature the pulmonary artery remains patent (e.g. LIEBOW ET AL., 1950), although OSIPOV

ET AL. (1965) sometimes observed the formation of small clots. After removal of the ligature the bloodflow soon normalizes (ALLEY ET AL., 1961), according to GAHAGAN ET AL. (1966) even within a few hours.

The very heavy broncho-pulmonary flow obtained after experimental ligation or in the presence of stenosis or atresia of the pulmonary artery in one lung puts an extra load on the left ventricle, since a shorter pathway has been formed to the left atrium via the bronchial arteries. According to most of the authors this explains the long misunderstood left-ventricle hypertrophy seen in chronic lung diseases, in which very wide anastomoses are often present. FISHMAN (1961), however, thinks that no hypertrophy of the left ventricle can develop in this way, because the largest broncho-pulmonary flow is by far inferior to the left-right shunts in cardiac defects.

These wide anastomoses bring the systemic blood pressure into contact with the pressure in the pulmonary circulation. The pressure and oxygen saturation are increased on the diseased side (ROOSEN-BURG AND DEENSTRA, 1954; TROCMÉ AND CHÉDAL, 1958), sometimes with reflux of saturated blood to the pulmonary artery of the healthy side (GILROY ET AL., 1951). The 'amputation' of the pulmonary artery on a pulmonary arteriogram often proved to be a pseudo-amputation (LIEBOW ET AL., 1949–1950; HERTZOG ET AL., 1952; KOURILSKY AND DECROIX, 1960; WILLIAMS ET AL., 1963; NEYAZAKI, 1964; MASSUMI ET AL., 1965a & b; BENNET ET AL., 1966; PADOVANI ET AL., 1966, SOSSAI, 1966), for during catheterization the 'amputated' artery proved to be normal and patent.

The earlier investigators attributed the pulmonary hypertension seen in many lung diseases to this high pressure in the pulmonary artery (e.g. WOOD AND MILLER, 1938). Although GARDÈRE (1953) connects primary pulmonary hypertension with broncho-pulmonary shunts, most modern authors are of the opinion that there is no direct relationship between broncho-pulmonary anastomoses and pulmonary hypertension. Furthermore, normal lung tissue has such a great capacity for adaptation that a third or a fourth of it can cope with the entire pulmonary circulation without an increase in pressure (COURNAND, 1947; FROMANT ET AL., 1954; ARNOULD ET AL., 1957; DAUSSY AND DAUMET, 1960; ELBERT ET AL., 1967). In the presence of narrowing or occlusion of the pulmonary artery or its branches, however, there appeared to be a relationship between the site and the degree of this stenosis, the development of pulmonary hypertension, and the development of broncho-pulmonary anastomoses, but between the last two in inverse proportion (FALKENBACH ET AL., 1959; HEIMBURG, 1964).

In acquired pathological conditions the anastomoses are mainly found peripherally in the lungs (LIEBOW ET AL., 1950) ,but in congenital anomalies centrally localized anastomoses are also seen (e.g. HALES AND LIEBOW, 1948). According to TURNER-WARWICK (1963a), all broncho-pulmonary anastomoses, with the exception of a few acquired forms, are end-to-end anastomoses.

What stimulus leads to the genesis of these connections? Almost all investigators have sought an explanation in which the following factors might play a role.

1. Mechanical factors: generally considered to be important.
2. Nervous factors (CUDKOWICZ AND WRAITH, 1957).
3. Chemical factors: made plausible by the results of studies by VIDONE AND LIEBOW (1957) and WEIBEL (1960).
4. Hormonal factors: demonstrated by animal experiments of LIEBOW (1962).

According to LATARJET (1956), broncho-pulmonary anastomoses develop as a reaction to an in-flammatory process. CUDKOWICZ AND ARMSTRONG (1953c), FISHMAN ET AL. (1958), and TURNER-WARWICK (1963b) associated finger clubbing with broncho-pulmonary anastomoses.

No data are available on the developmental course of the broncho-pulmonary anastomoses. ABEL-ANET (1961) surmises, on the basis of data obtained by catheterization, that the broncho-pulmonary flow changes in the course of time. According to GASTAING ET AL. (1961) this change could be the result on the one hand of stricture or dilatation of contractile anastomosing arteries – found by DELARUE ET AL. (1952) around extatic bronchi – or, on the other hand of variations in the inflammatory process.

The radiological literature contains reports of the visualization and identification of broncho-pulmonary anastomoses in the region of the hilus but not of peripheral anastomoses.

c. Discussion of the data in the literature

After studying the literature we have come to the following conclusions. In normal lungs there are subpleural and intrapulmonary precapillary broncho-pulmonary anastomoses that can become wider under pathological conditions. Connections between bronchial and pulmonary arteries can also be *formed:* by recanalization of a thrombotic pulmonary artery as well as in granulation tissue in an inflammatory process. Fig. 58 gives examples of all these possibilities.

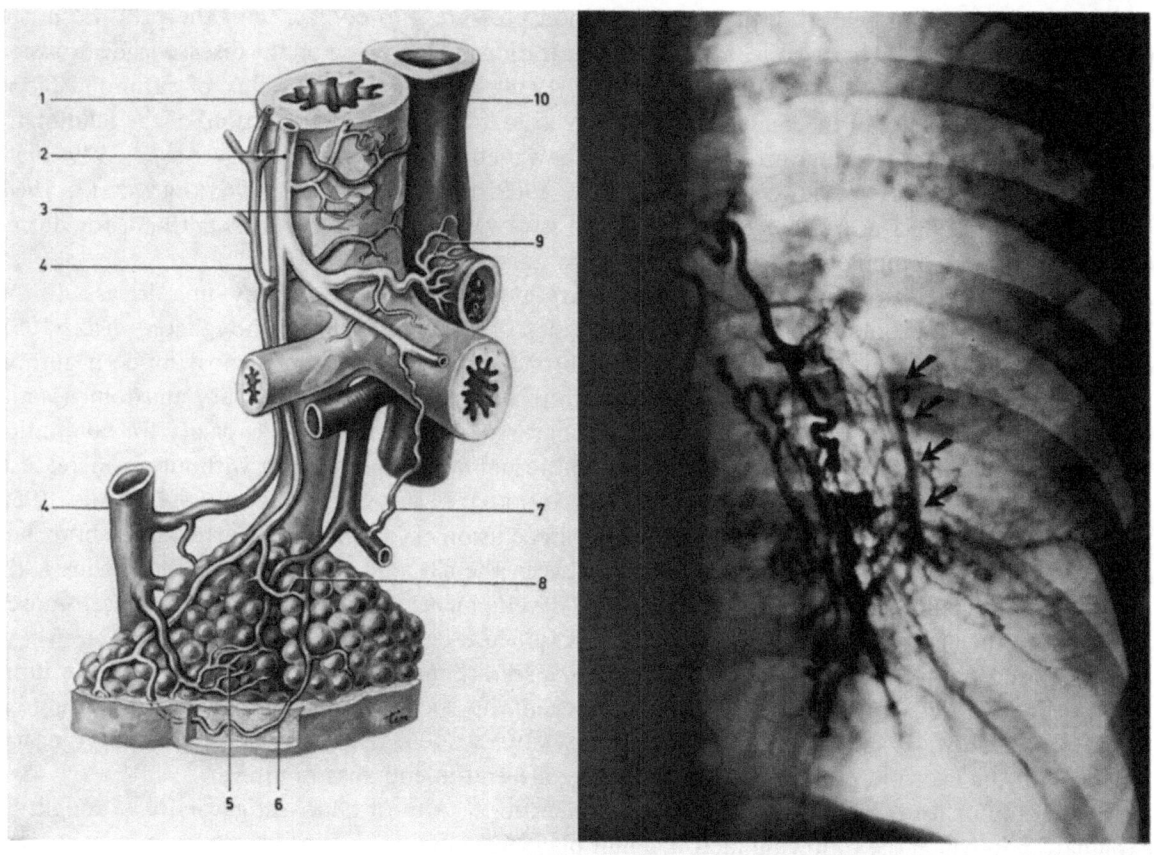

Fig. 58   *Fig. 59*

Fig. 58. Various types of broncho-pulmonary shunts (after TOBIN, 1952). (1) Bronchus. (2) Bronchial artery. (3) Enlarged capillary broncho-pulmonary connection. (4) Pulmonary vein. (5) Capillary bed of the pulmonary circulation. (6) Pleural broncho-pulmonary anastomosis. (7) Long intrapulmonary broncho-pulmonary anastomosis, developed by enlargement or neoformation. (8) Short intrapulmonary broncho-pulmonary anastomosis. (9) Enlarged vasa vasorum: recanalization of a thrombotic branch of the pulmonary artery. (10) Pulmonary artery.

Fig. 59. Marked enlargement of the left bronchial artery. Multiple parahilary broncho-pulmonary anastomoses. Intensive filling of the pulmonary artery. Note tortuous course of the bronchial arteries and fern-like pattern of branches of the pulmonary artery. Arrows: retrograde filling of pulmonary artery.

According to results obtained by WOOD AND MILLER (1938), NAKAMURA ET AL. (1961), and TURNER-WARWICK (1963a), the anastomoses can occur in all anomalies; therefore, broncho-pulmonary anastomoses are not specific.

What is the reason for the occurrence or widening of these shunts? Mechanical, or rather hemodynamic, factors are certainly important in this respect, since the anastomoses are widest in the presence of a ligated or congenitally stenosed or occluded pulmonary artery. The anastomoses around and in inflammatory processes, and especially the sometimes very wide broncho-pulmonary shunts associated with bronchiectasis, cannot be entirely explained in this way, however. Hormonal and probably also nervous and chemical factors can influence the development of anastomoses. Various investigators have attempted to find a common cause for the genesis of these shunts. ROOSENBURG AND DEENSTRA (1954), LIEBOW (1962), and MORAND ET AL. (1963) are among those who have seen this development as a protective mechanism preventing desaturation of the peripheral blood. In an inflammatory process the gas exchange is hampered, especially in cases in which the process leads to atelectasis. This is usually associated with a decrease in the pulmonary circulation, but the still appreciable amount of pulmonary blood cannot take up enough oxygen, if any. If oxygenated bronchial blood can be supplied precapillarily, the danger of desaturation of the peripheral blood is avoided. This hypothesis is reasonable, but it does not explain why ligation of the pulmonary artery leads to the development of such large shunts, since in this situation there is no danger of desaturation.

The only phenomenon shared by all these anomalies is, in our opinion, hypoxia of alveolar and peripheral interstitial lung tissue normally supplied by the already well-oxygenated blood of the pulmonary capillaries. It is clear that this could be a result of either reduced gas exchange or reduced flow. This is where, in our opinion, the *primary* cause must be sought for the development of wide broncho-pulmonary shunts, whereas *secondarily*, hemodynamic factors are of great importance. HEIMBURG (1964) is the only author to point in this direction, since he says that hypoxia of interstitial tissue of the alveolar walls might form a chemical stimulus for the genesis of a collateral broncho-pulmonary circulation.

FINDINGS IN ARTERIOGRAPHY

The question of whether broncho-pulmonary shunts exist in normal lungs, cannot be answered by arteriography, because there is no histological confirmation that the radiologically normal parts of the lungs are actually normal.

Under pathological conditions, broncho-pulmonary shunts proved to be extremely frequent. They were found in 66 per cent of our patients (51 cases), and even in 92 per cent of the cases in which a complete selective bronchial arteriogram was made.

a. Diagnosis

The recognition of large shunts is not difficult, because when they are present large branches of the pulmonary artery are usually filled with contrast medium (Fig. 59). More time is required to learn to recognize small peripheral shunts, but once one has become familiar with the typical, slightly tortuous course of the bronchial arteries and the fern-like branching of the pulmonary artery, the diagnosis offers no difficulties. Fig. 60 shows some clear examples of peripheral broncho-pulmonary anastomoses. The smaller branches of the pulmonary artery, however, are not usually so distinct. In evaluating the arteriograms, one must be on the lookout for small Y-shaped vessels which always represent small peripheral branches of the pulmonary artery (Fig. 61).

The bronchial artery sometimes shows a corkscrew pattern just before entering a peripheral anastomosis (Fig. 62). This picture is highly characteristic, since it is known from the literature that the bronchial artery frequently winds itself several times around the branch of the pulmonary artery with which it is about to form an anastomosis.

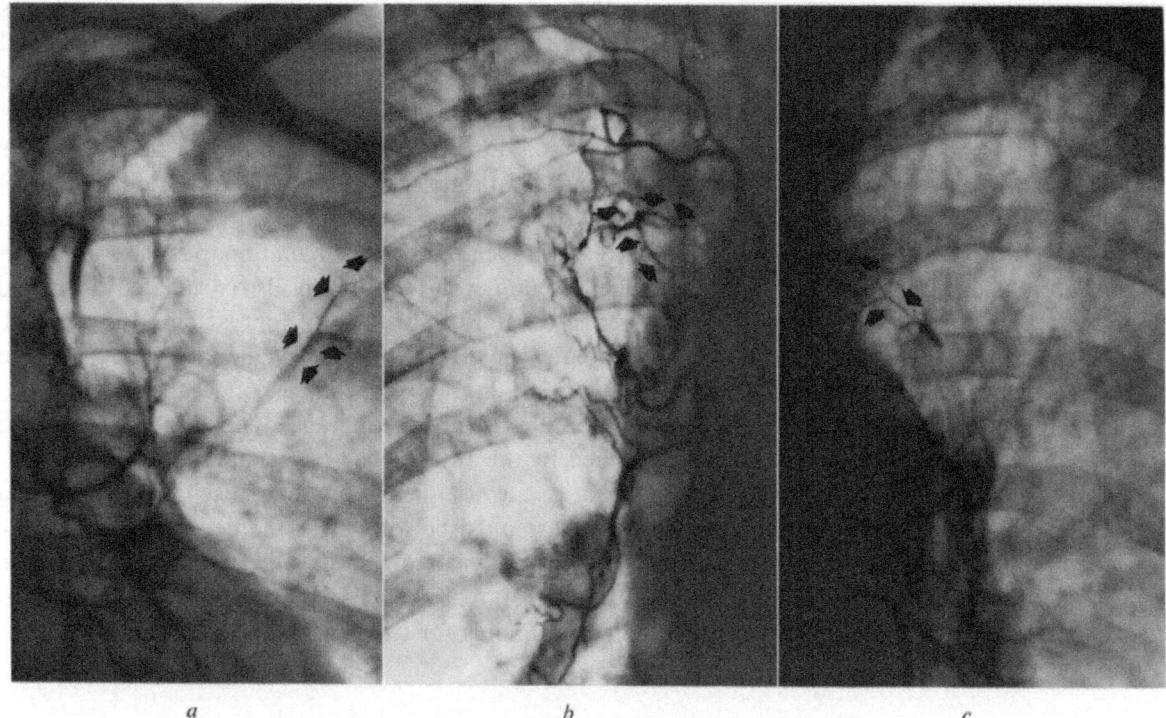

Fig. 60. Three examples of peripheral anastomoses in cases of tuberculosis (*a*), chronic asthmatic bronchitis (*b*) and radiologically normal lungs (*c*). Arrows indicate peripheral branches of the pulmonary artery.

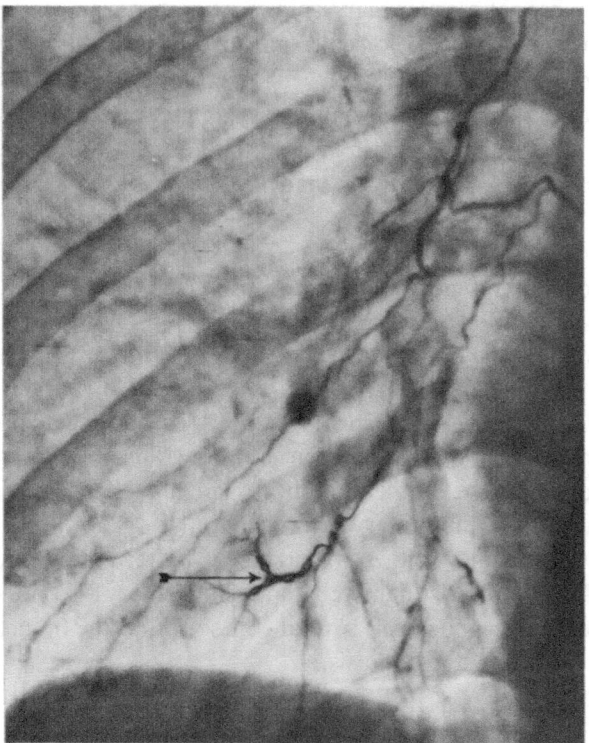

Fig. 62. Peripheral broncho-pulmonary shunt. The bronchial artery is wound several times around the branch of the pulmonary artery with which it is anastomosed (arrow).

In occasional cases – in agreement with the anatomical situation – we have seen bronchial arteries on one side of the bronchi and branches of the pulmonary artery on the other side (BOTENGA, 1969).

In a number of patients a series of exposures were made during inspiration and expiration. The broncho-pulmonary anastomoses are much less distinct on the radiograms made during expiration than on those made during inspiration (BOTENGA, 1968).

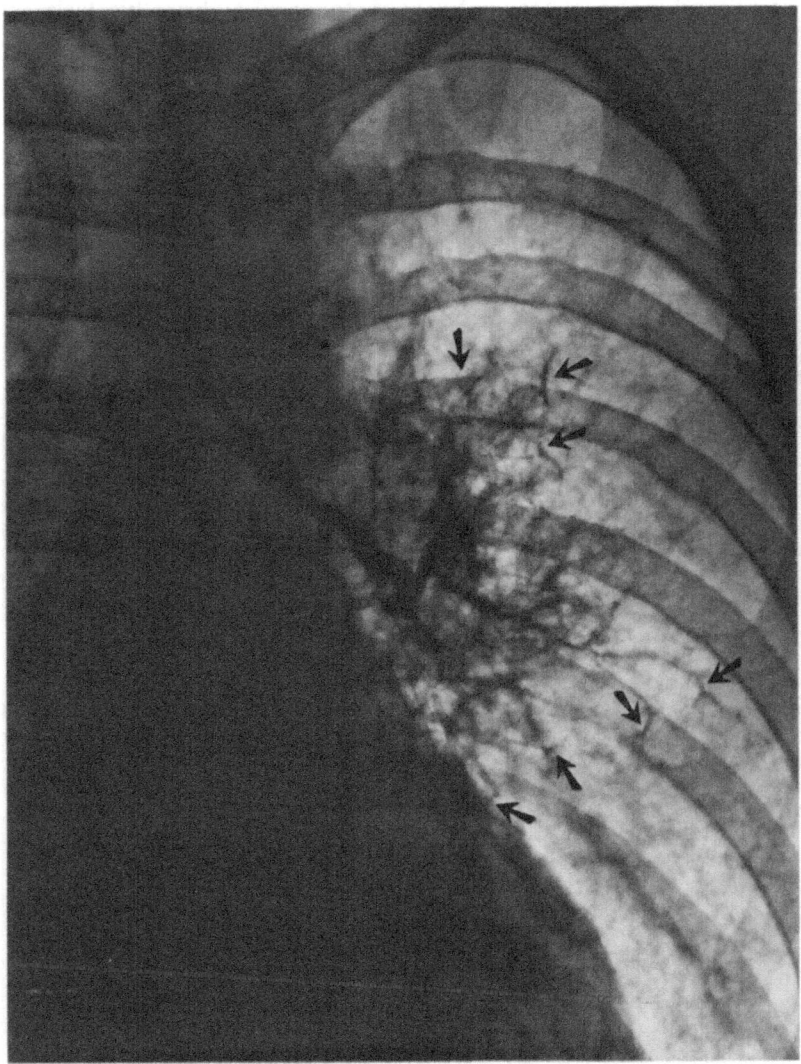

Fig. 61. Greatly enlarged left bronchial artery in tetralogy of FALLOT; multiple peripherally localized broncho-pulmonary anastomoses (arrows). Note fork-shaped configurations (see also Fig. 106a).

b. Results

Occurrence

We observed broncho-pulmonary shunts in all the anomalies we studied. They were present in all cases of the tetralogy of FALLOT and less often in patients with bronchiectasis, tuberculosis, and chronic infections, in that order. They were seen only rarely in cases of bronchial carcinoma.

Number of shunts per case

For further differentiation, we classified according to the number of shunts per case. Very high numbers were seen in the tetralogy of FALLOT and most of the cases of bronchiectasis. Many shunts were observed in most of the inflammatory processes and in the remaining cases of bronchiectasis. A few shunts were present in tuberculosis and infections; in tumors, when present, they were observed only sporadically.

Width

A similar sequence of the anomalies was found with respect to the caliber of the anastomoses. The widest shunts were found in the tetralogy of FALLOT, followed by bronchiectasis; increasingly smaller anastomoses were found in infections, tuberculosis, and bronchial carcinoma.

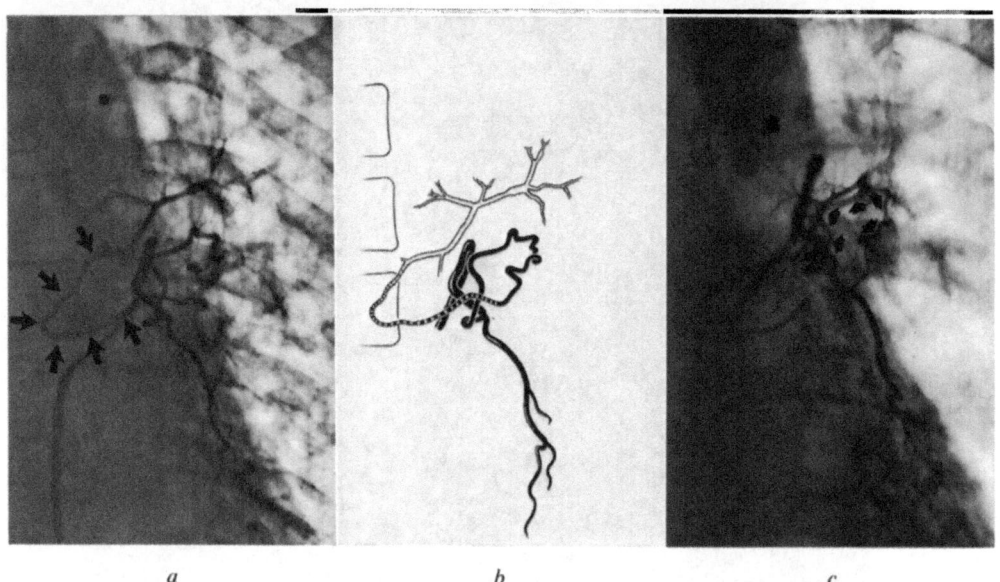

a   b   c

Fig. 63. Pleural broncho-pulmonary anastomosis.

a: Ventro-dorsal view. The bronchial artery runs dorsally and is very distinct. The anastomotic canal runs
   ventrally (arrows) and is indistinct, like the terminally filled branch of the pulmonary artery.

b: Schematic representation.

c: Dorso-ventral view. The bronchial artery is now indistinct (arrows) and the ventrally localized pleural
   anastomosis is very distinct.

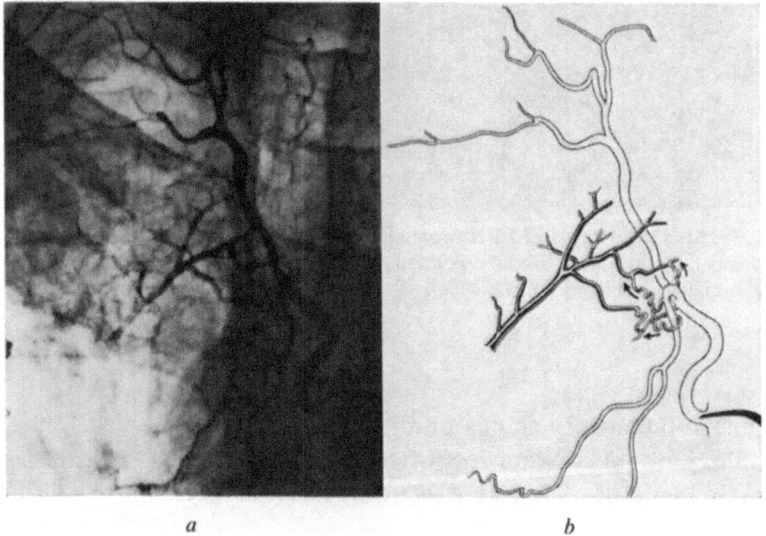

a   b

Fig. 64.

a: Broncho-pulmonary anastomosis in close vicinity of the mediastinal pleura in a
   patient with an obstruction infiltrate in the right upper lobe.

b: Schematic representation.

Localization

Pleural anastomoses were seen in two cases. In one of these patients they occurred in radiographically normal parts of the lung (Fig. 63) and in the other they occurred in an affected area (Fig. 64). The intrapulmonary anastomoses were classified according to central, parahilar, and peripheral localizations. The central shunts are the widest, the peripheral the narrowest. Central anastomoses were seen only in patients with the tetralogy of FALLOT; an extreme case of this form is shown in fig. 65 (see also figs. 21 and 23). Parahilary anastomoses were seen 13 times in association with bronchiectasis (Fig. 69a, see also figs. 59 and 66), serious infections (Fig. 89) a bronchogenic cyst (Figs. 76 and 101) and again tetralogy of FALLOT (Fig. 104, see also 107). In Figs. 69a and 104 the area of the anastomoses is marked by a dotted line. In cases with parahilary broncho-pulmonary shunts there was almost always retrograde filling of the pulmonary artery as a result of the difference in pressure between the

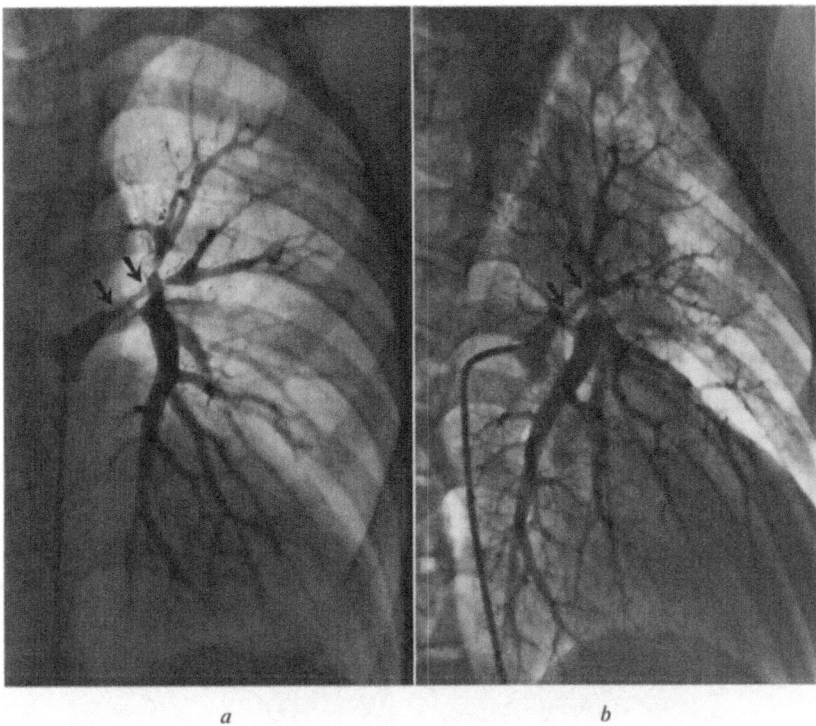

a   *b*

Fig. 65. Aneurysmatically enlarged left bronchial artery with central broncho-pulmonary anastomosis (arrows) on the stenosed left pulmonary artery. A pea-sized aneurysm is seen on the inferior wall of the bronchial artery.
a: Anteroposterior view.
b: Right oblique view.

systemic and the pulmonary circulations (Figs. 59 and 66). It is, of course, difficult to determine to what extent the injection pressure was responsible for this retrograde flow of contrast medium in the pulmonary artery. In the patient shown in fig. 66, however, this last factor could be excluded, since the wide left bronchial artery was filled via fine broncho-bronchial anastomoses with the selective injected bronchial artery. In such collaterals the injection pressure is levelled.

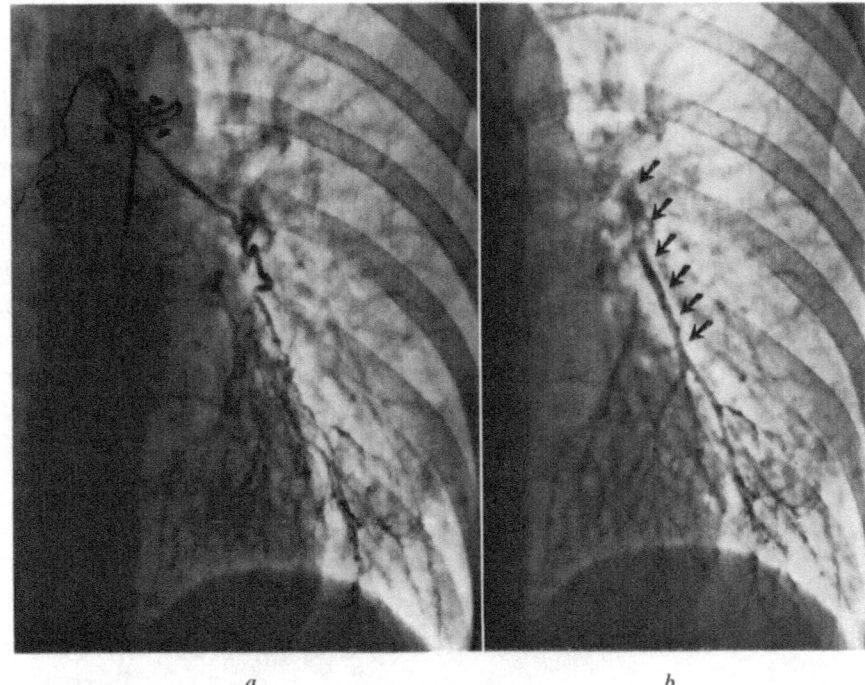

a   b

Fig. 66. Retrograde filling of the pulmonary artery via parahilary broncho-pulmonary anastomoses in a patient with bronchiectasis.

a: The catheter is located in a small right bronchial artery. The dilated left bronchial artery is filled collaterally via fine broncho-bronchial anastomoses (arrows) with the catheterized artery. Therefore, injection pressure cannot be responsible for the retrograde filling.

b: A later phase of the arteriogram shows the contrast medium in the left lower lobe branch of the pulmonary artery with retrograde flow to the region of the hilus (arrows).

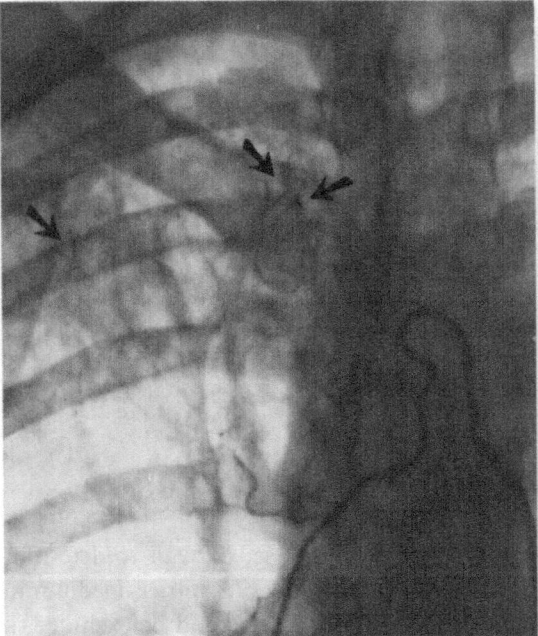

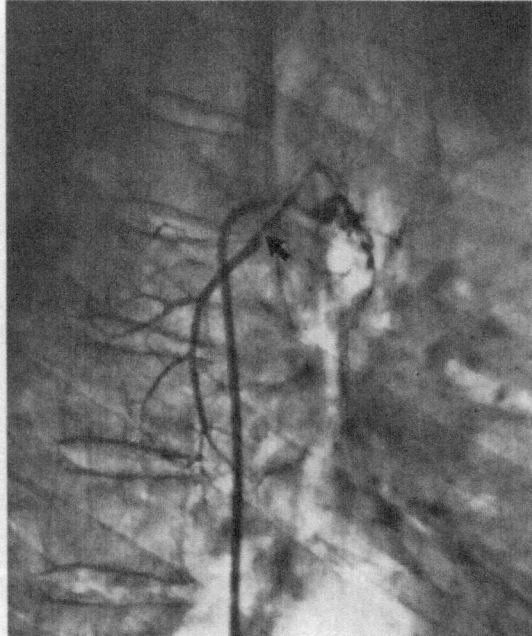

Fig. 67. Very small peripheral broncho-pulmonary shunts (arrows) in tuberculosis.

Fig. 68. Iatrogenic broncho-pulmonary anastomosis (arrow).

Peripheral shunts were found 39 times in the remaining anomalies. In tuberculosis the shunts sometimes lie extremely peripherally, which makes them difficult to recognize (Fig. 67).

In one case an artificial iatrogenic anastomosis was seen in a patient after broncho-plastic surgery (Fig. 68).

Developmental course

In two patients with bronchiectasis we performed bronchial arteriography twice with an interval of one year.

The first of these two patients was suffering from bronchiectasis in the right upper lobe, especially the anterior segment (Fig. 92A). The arteriographical examination in March, 1966 showed the pulmonary branches of the right upper lobe filled via multiple parahilar broncho-pulmonary shunts (Fig. 69a). During this period the patient had serious complaints, but these disappeared in course of time. Bronchial arteriography was performed again in March, 1967 (Fig. 69b). All the broncho-pulmonary shunts had vanished. Fig. 69a is exactly comparable to fig. 69b, both demonstrating a late arterial phase during inspiration.

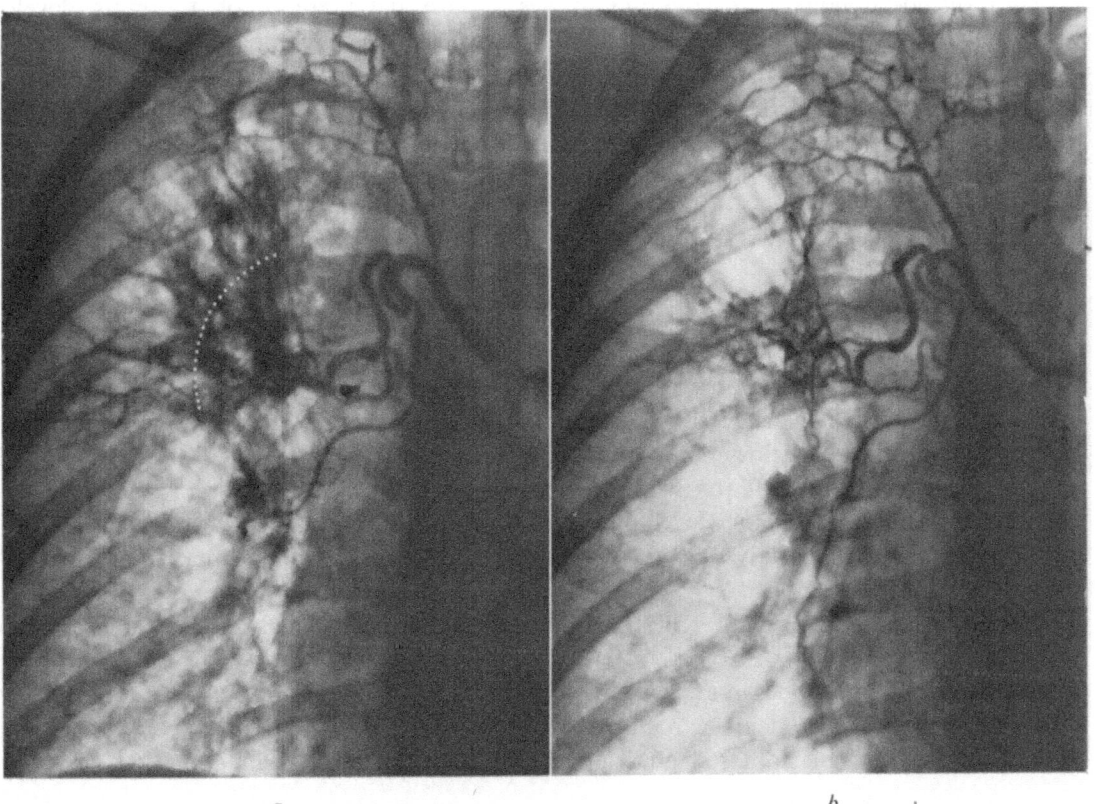

a   b

Fig. 69.
a: Bronchial arteriography in 1966. Multiple parahilary localized broncho-pulmonary anastomoses. The site of the anastomoses is indicated by a dotted line. Fig. 93 is a later phase of the same arteriogram with better visualization of the branches of the pulmonary artery.
b: Second arteriogram, 1967. The bronchial circulation is still slightly augmented but the anastomoses are no longer visible. The caliber of the bronchial artery is reduced.

The second patient was also examined for the first time in 1966 during a period of serious complaints. The arteriogram showed multiple broncho-pulmonary anastomoses. At the time of our second examination in 1967 the complaints had almost disappeared and only one anastomosis was still visible on the bronchial arteriogram (BOTENGA, 1968).

DISCUSSION

Since broncho-pulmonary shunts are not specific for a given anomaly, what is the value of identifying these structures? There is a relationship between the nature of the diseases and the frequency of occurrence, the number, the width, and the localization of these connections.

In some anomalies (tetralogy of FALLOT and bronchiectasis) many wide, parahilary shunts are always seen; others (carcinoma of the lungs) seldom show shunts, and when present they are few, small, and peripherally located. The widest anastomoses are located centrally, and the smallest shunts in the periphery. This finding confirms the hemodynamic factor in the development or enlargement of the anastomoses.

We found an increasing number of broncho-pulmonary anastomoses in lung tumors, tuberculosis, chronic infections, bronchiectasis, and tetralogy of FALLOT, in that order. In the same sequence, the duration of these diseases is usually increasingly longer. It is, therefore, tempting to suggest that *broncho-pulmonary anastomoses are more numerous, wider, and more centrally localized, the longer the patient has suffered from a disease or anomaly.* In other words, the presence of many wide, centrally localized broncho-pulmonary anastomoses argues against the presence of a rapidly developing anomaly and is, therefore, a favorable sign with respect to the differentiation between malignant and benign processes.

No data were available with respect to the developmental course of broncho-pulmonary anastomoses. In two cases the reduction in the number of broncho-pulmonary shunts was accompanied by a decrease in the inflammatory phenomena and the patient's complaints. Broncho-pulmonary anastomoses seem therefore to be a measure for the severity of the inflammatory process.

CONCLUSIONS

1. Broncho-pulmonary anastomoses are not specific. They can be present in the normal lung, but can also be newly formed. They can result from dilatation of capillary broncho-pulmonary connections, recanalization of a thrombotic pulmonary artery, or penetration by vascular endothelium of pulmonary and bronchial arteries in granulation tissue.
2. The primary stimulus for the development of wide broncho-pulmonary shunts arises, in our opinion, from hypoxia of alveolar and interstitial lung tissue, hemodynamic factors playing an important part secondarily.
3. The longer a disease has been present, the more wide and centrally localized anastomoses are to be expected.
4. The presence of many wide, more centrally localized anastomoses argues against a rapidly developing anomaly, e.g. a bronchial carcinoma.
5. Broncho-pulmonary anastomoses can disappear after treatment of the inflammatory process.

IV.2.1.3. INTERCOSTO-PULMONARY ANASTOMOSES

LITERATURE

Intercosto-pulmonary anastomoses traverse the pleural leaves and are therefore always acquired. Like the broncho-pulmonary anastomoses they represent arterial connections between the systemic and the pulmonary circulations.

Special attention was first paid to these anastomoses in the cardiovascular literature (BING ET AL., 1947; BROCK, 1949; BLALOCK, 1951). It was observed that a number of patients with tetralogy of FALLOT, in whom it proved impossible to establish a surgical anastomosis during the operation, nevertheless improved after the thoracotomy, with disappearance of the cyanosis. In these cases extensive inter-costo-pulmonary anastomoses had developed post-operatively, leading to augmentation of the pulmonary circulation. COCKETT AND VASS (1950), HURWITZ ET AL. (1954), VIDONE AND LIEBOW (1957), LIEBOW (1962), and TAKAHASHI (1963) studied the development of such anastomoses experimentally in animals.

Intercosto-pulmonary anastomoses can also be formed in chronic inflammatory processes with a pleuro-pulmonary localization (DAUSSY AND ABELANET, 1956; BRUWER, 1966; and SOSSAI, 1966). DAUSSY AND ABELANET visualized these shunts on magnification radiograms of preparations in which the intercostal arteries had been filled with contrast medium (Fig. 70). BRUWER and SOSSAI also describe anastomoses of other arteries running along the thoracic wall, e.g. branches of the axillary artery (see also LURUS ET AL., 1969).

Although these anastomoses were demonstrated arteriographically by a number of investigators (GUNTHEROTH ET AL., 1962; VAILLAUD, 1962; WILLIAMS ET AL., 1963; VACCAREZZA, 1966), they were not mentioned by most authors dealing with selective arteriography, despite the fact that they are visible on the figures illustrating their publications. BOIJSEN (1965), VIAMONTE ET AL.(1965), and E COSTA (1966) mistook such anastomoses for tumor vessels. Later, VIAMONTE (1967) inadvertently pointed to the existence of these shunts, when he thought he had demonstrated anastomoses between intercostal arteries and pulmonary veins. Since according to the anatomical and pathological data such anastomoses do not exist, the drainage VIAMONTE traced via the pulmonary veins was, in our opinion, based on the occurrence of intercosto-pulmonary anastomoses, which made it possible for the contrast medium to reach the pulmonary veins after it had passed the capillary bed of the lung.

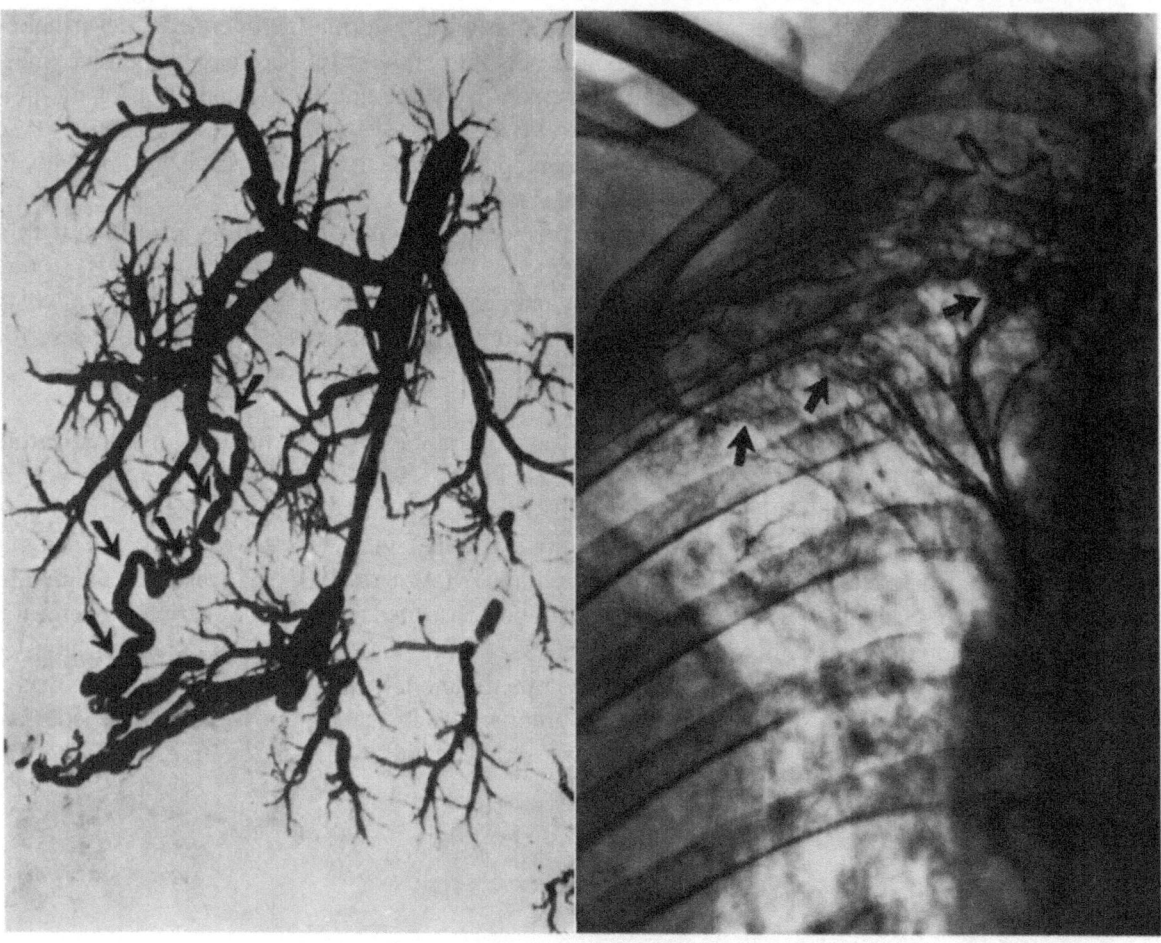

Fig. 70   *Fig. 71*

Fig. 70. Intercosto-pulmonary anastomoses in a histological preparation (DAUSSY AND ABELANET, 1956).
Fig. 71. Intercosto-pulmonary anastomoses *in vivo*. Patient with tuberculous lesions in the right upper field. The arrows indicate the areas with anastomoses.

FINDINGS IN ARTERIOGRAPHY

Intercosto-pulmonary anastomoses were found in pulmonary anomalies with pleural adhesions and also in post-operative conditions. Shunts between other arteries of the thoracic wall – mostly branches of the axillary artery – and the branches of the pulmonary artery became visible twice on aortograms.

a. Pulmonary anomalies with pleural adhesions

Anastomoses were seen most often in tuberculous apical lesions (Fig. 71), i.e. in 10 out of 15 cases (67 per cent). Sometimes they were seen in cases of tumors, bronchiectasis, and chronic infections, depending on the presence of pleural adhesions in these cases.

b. Post-operative conditions

In all surgically treated cases the anastomoses were visible upon careful examination of the intercostal arteriograms.

The anastomoses proved to be wider the longer the interval since the operation or the pleurisy, the more severe the disturbance of the gas exchange, and the greater the quantity of desoxygenated blood in the pulmonary veins. Fig. 72 gives an example of this relationship.

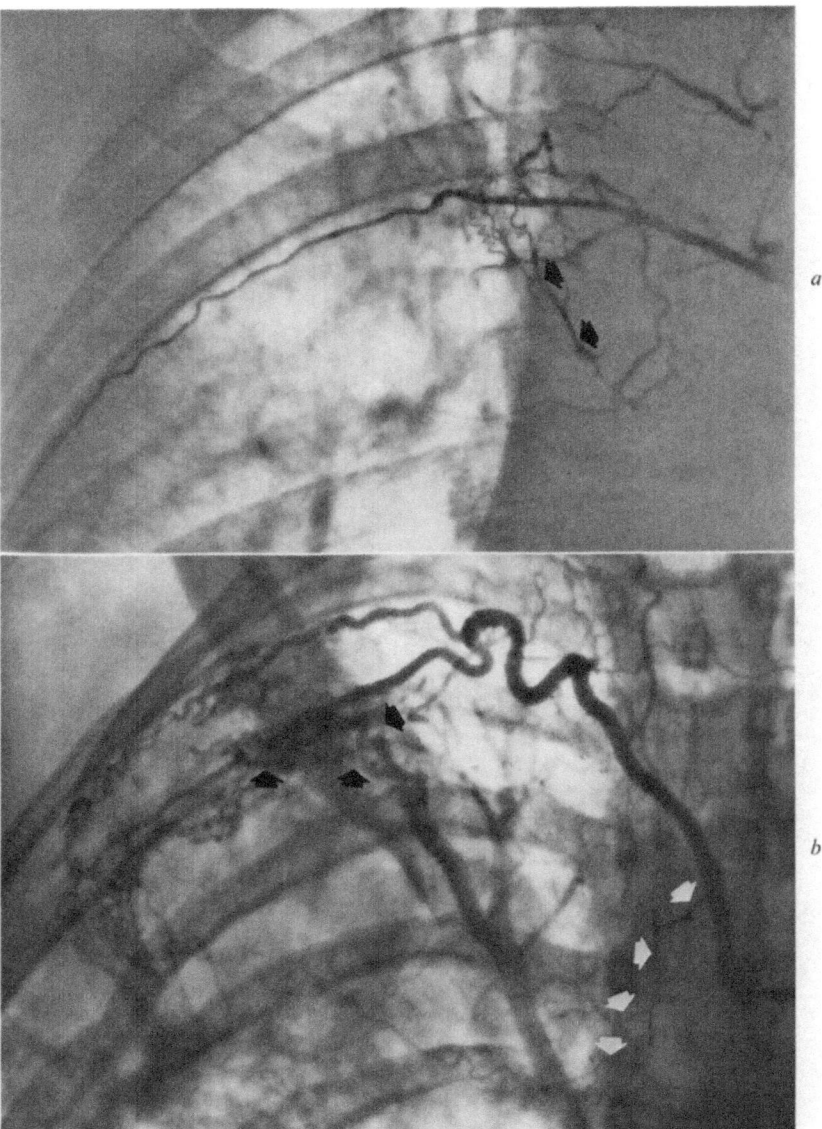

Fig. 72. Intercosto-pulmonary anastomoses become wider the older the pleural adhesions and the more the pulmonary function and oxygen saturation of the venous pulmonary blood are disturbed.

a: Fine tortuous intercosto-pulmonary anastomoses in a patient who had undergone a lobectomy 2 years earlier. The branch of the pulmonary artery is marked by arrows.

b: Wide intercosto-pulmonary anastomoses (black arrows) 4 years after thoracotomy in a patient with bullous destruction and chronic infection of the right lung. Fig. 10 shows an exposure from the same arteriogram. The catheterized artery is an inter-costo-bronchial trunk of which the very thin bronchial artery – the only right bronchial artery found in this case – is indicated by white arrows.

Concurrently the intercostal arteries become wider in the course of time. The dilatation of the intercostal arteries and the anastomoses sets in more rapidly, the greater the demand for more blood in
the pulmonary circulation, as in cases of tetralogy of FALLOT. Post-operative patients with tetralogy
of FALLOT showed the largest intercostal arteries and the heaviest intercosto-pulmonary flow.[1] Fig. 73
shows such an intercostal artery in a patient, who had been operated on 17 years earlier. The intercostal artery is strongly dilated and shows such extreme tortuosity due to elongation that the vessel
fills the entire intercostal space. In these cases notches can develop not only on the lower side but,
in contrast to the general opinion on this point, also on the upper side of the ribs (Fig. 73*b*, arrows).

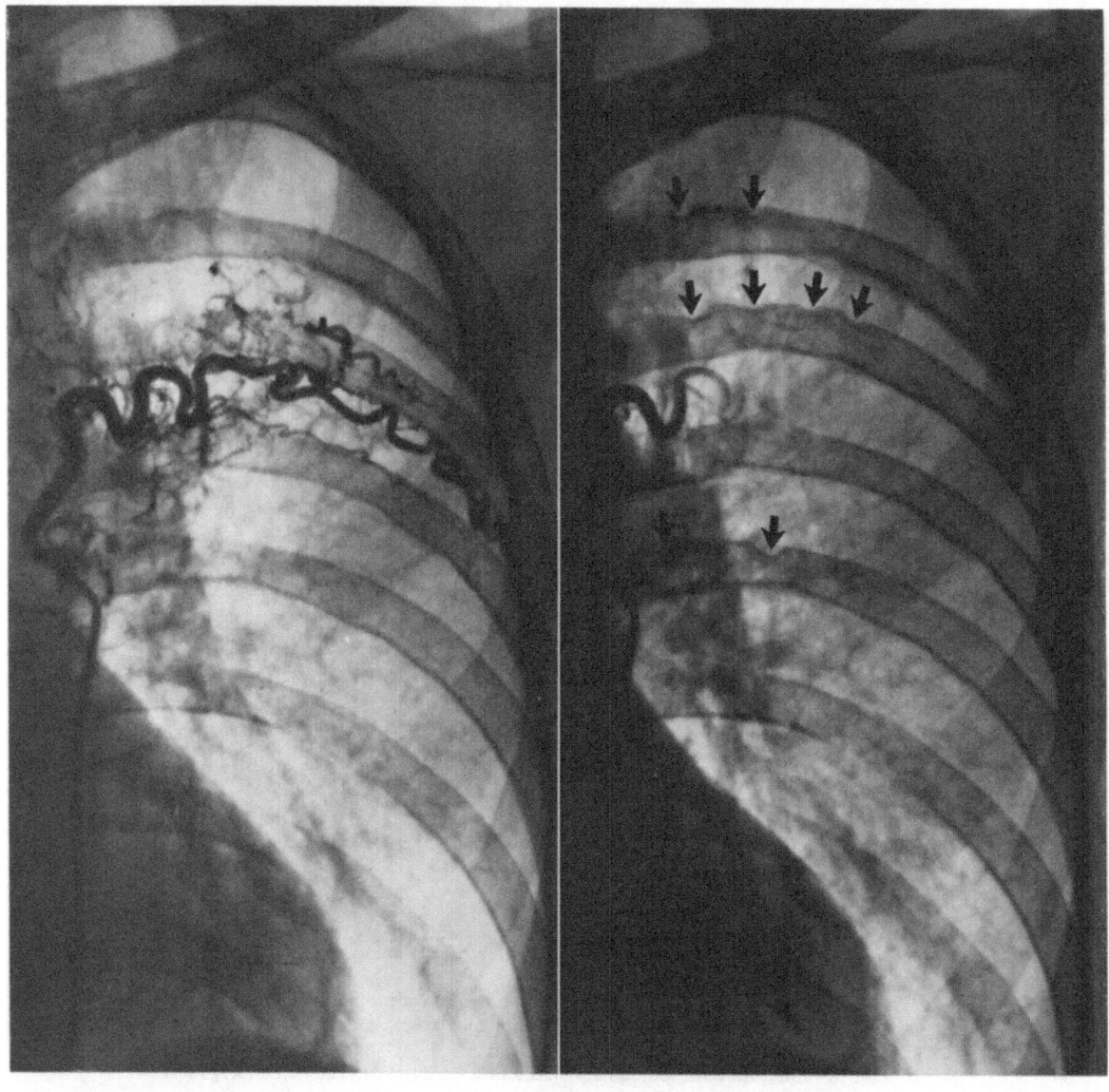

a   *b*

Fig. 73. Intercostal arteriogram in a patient treated surgically for tetralogy of FALLOT.
a: As a result of the heavy dilatation and elongation of the intercostal artery the proximal part of the intercostal space is
    entirely filled (see also Figs. 72*b* and 103). The same artery can be seen in Fig. 108, which shows the intercosto-pulmonary
    flow as well.
b: Multiple notches on the lower side of the ribs and also notches on the upper side of the proximal parts of the ribs (arrows).
    See also Fig. 107*a*.

1 See under Tetralogy of FALLOT, fig. 108.

DISCUSSION

Most of the intercosto-pulmonary anastomoses in our material were localized at a high level in the thorax. It is concievable that they form there more easily as a result of the smaller amount of movement in this region during the respiration. This might also explain the numerous intercosto-pulmonary anastomoses in almost all of our cases with tuberculous lesions in apices and upper lung fields.

In agreement with the literature we saw the most striking intercosto-pulmonary shunts after surgical treatment of the tetralogy of FALLOT; the massive filling of the pulmonary vessels on our intercostal arteriograms indicates an important amelioration of the pulmonary circulation. The relatively large difference in pressure between the systemic and the pulmonary circulations in the tetralogy of FALLOT offers, in our opinion, the explanation of the rapid dilation of these connections.

A patient with a bullous destruction of the right lung in histiocytosis X also showed very wide anastomoses and a very heavy intercosto-pulmonary flow post-operatively (Figs. 10 and 72b). For this finding there was no explanation, since the pulmonary artery received a sufficient amount of blood. The gas exchange in the destroyed lung was, however, severely disturbed so that an ample supply of oxygenated blood in the pulmonary circulation on the diseased side, protected the patient from desaturation of the peripheral blood. This patient showed a very thin bronchial artery (white arrows, Fig. 72b) and consequently no broncho-pulmonary shunts, which otherwise might have brought about a similar effect. The massive intercosto-pulmonary flow is of hemodynamic importance, just as it is, for instance, in cases of a cardiac defect with a left-right shunt.

CONCLUSIONS

1. Intercosto-pulmonary anastomoses can only form in the presence of pleural adhesions and often occur after pleurisy. They are wider, the older the adhesions, the more the difference in pressure between the systemic and the pulmonary circulations increases (e.g. in tetralogy of FALLOT), and the more the lung function decreases without a proportional decrease of the pulmonary flow.
2. Most of the intercosto-pulmonary anastomoses were localized cranially in the thorax. They were encountered most often in tuberculous lesions situated in the upper lobes.

IV.2.1.4 INTERCOSTO-BRONCHIAL ANASTOMOSES

LITERATURE

Under intercosto-bronchial anastomoses is understood arterial communications between the proximal parts of the bronchial and the intercostal arteries. These rare shunts are almost completely neglected in the literature. The only authors in whom we found an indication for the existence of these anastomoses are SNELLEN ET AL. (1950) and COLLISTER (1952) in their studies on the collateral circulation in the presence of a stenosis of the pulmonary artery and SCHOENMACKERS AND VIETEN (1958), FLORANGE (1960), and PETELENZ (1967) in their investigation of the arterial connections of the bronchial arteries with arteries outside the lungs. These anastomoses are also visible on a few figures in DONKERS's thesis (1968).

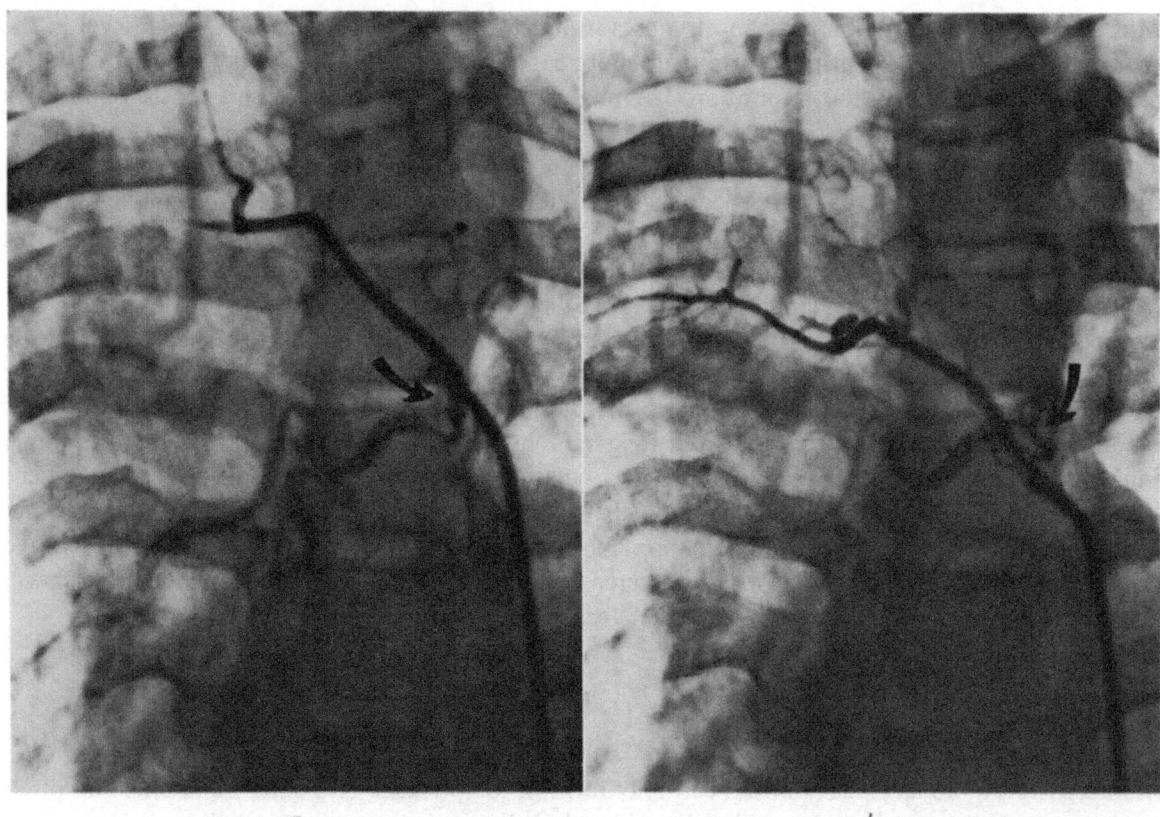

Fig. 74. Intercosto-bronchial anastomoses. Arteriograms of the 4th (*a*) and 5th (*b*) right intercostal arteries. Via thin and tortuous anastomoses (arrows) the contrast medium reaches the right inferior bronchial artery originating directly from the aorta (Fig. 104*b*).

FINDINGS IN ARTERIOGRAPHY

Intercosto-bronchial anastomoses were demonstrated in four patients: two with tetralogy of FALLOT (Figs. 74 and 75), one with a congenital bronchogenic cyst (Fig. 76), and one young patient with severe bronchiectasis that had probably developed at an early age or was perhaps of a congenital nature.

DISCUSSION

In three of these patients there were certainly and in the fourth possibly, congenital anomalies. In all of them the bronchial bloodflow was markedly increased. In the patients with acquired lesions, no such anastomoses were seen. It is tempting to conclude that intercosto-bronchial anastomoses are present in the fetal period and obliterate after birth unless there is an important augmentation of the bronchial circulation.

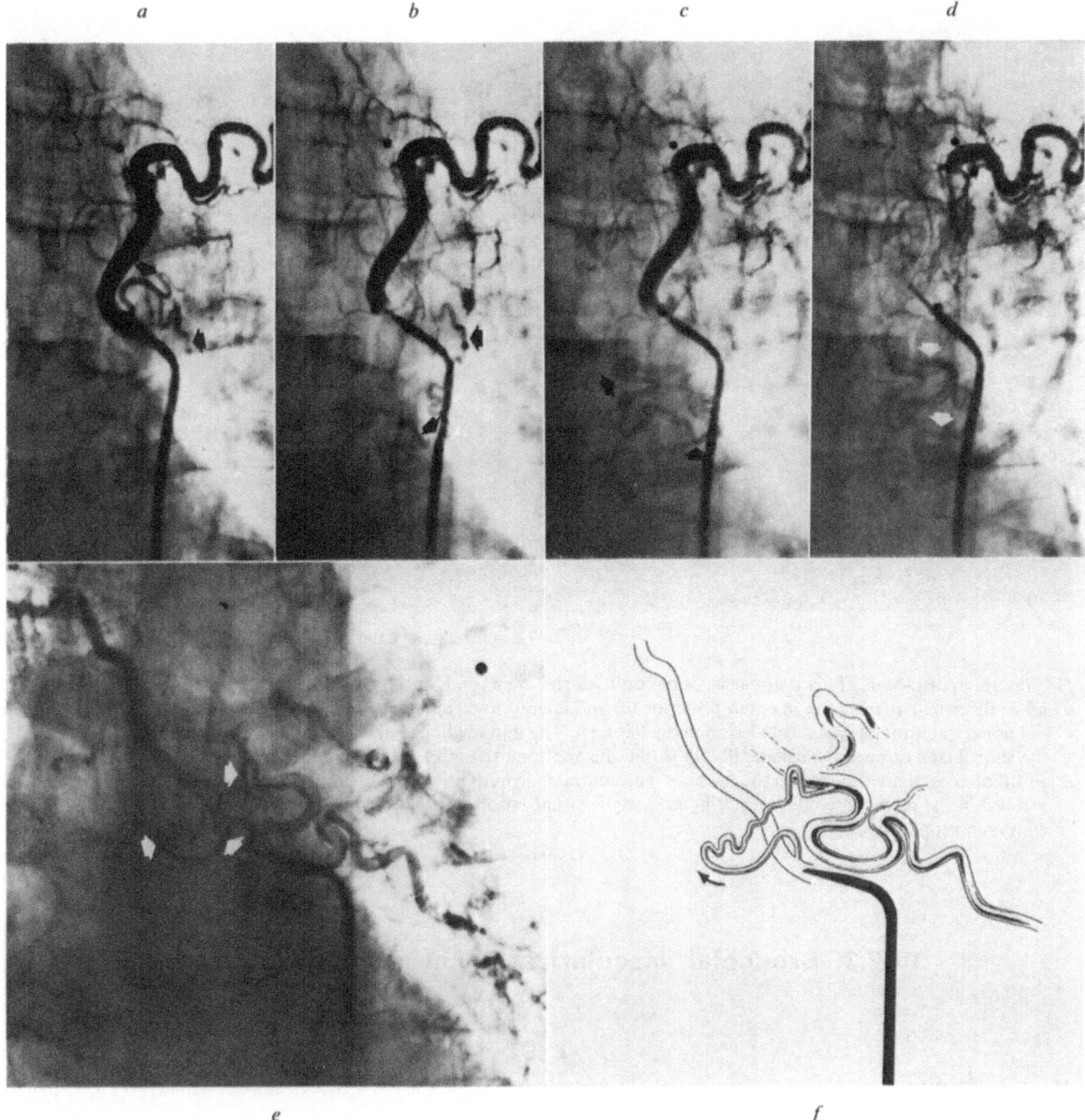

Fig. 75. Intercosto-bronchial anastomoses between two contralateral intercostal arteries and one bronchial artery.

a, b, c, and *d*: The contrast medium gradually fills a long intercosto-bronchial anastomosis (black arrows) connecting a right intercostal artery with a wide left bronchial artery.

e: Intercosto-bronchial anastomosis (white arrows) from another right intercostal to the same bronchial artery.

f: Schematic representation of *e*.

CONCLUSION

Intercosto-bronchial anastomoses are rare and probably indicate the existence of a congenital anomaly.

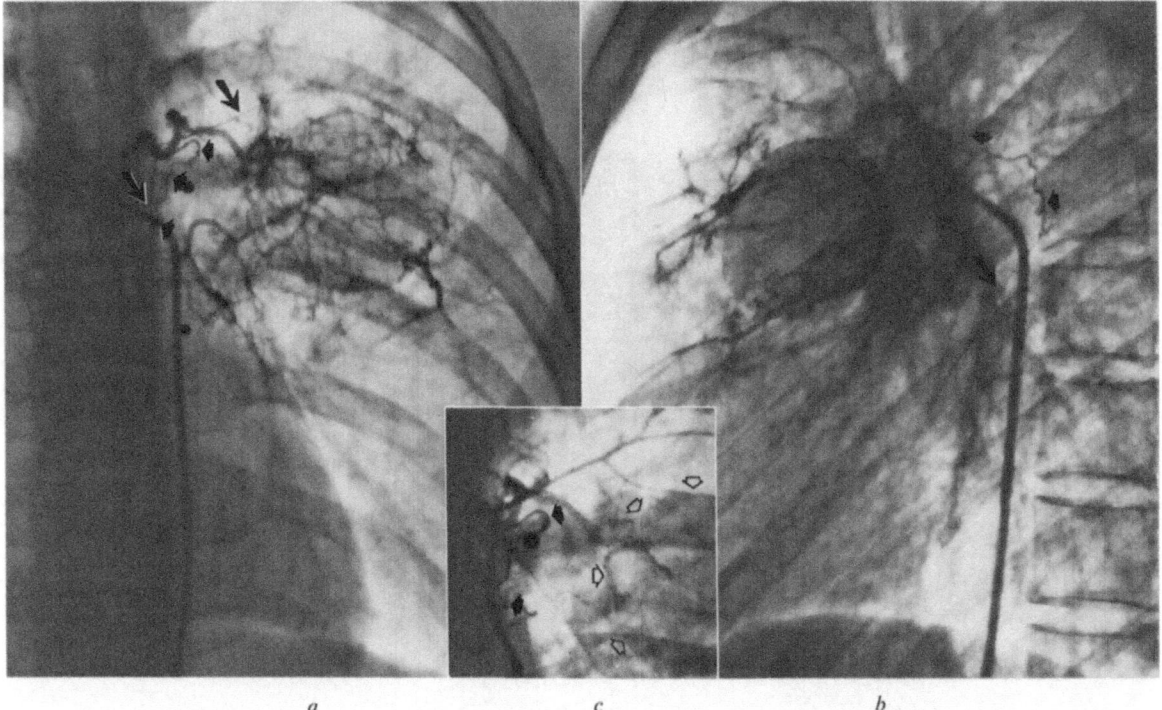

Fig. 76. Intercosto-bronchial anastomosis visible on both the intercostal and the bronchial arteriogram.
a and *b*: Bronchial arteriogram in anteroposterior (*a*) and lateral (*b*) direction. Rich vascularization with numerous broncho-
    pulmonary anastomoses of a coin lesion in the left lung. The thin tortuous intercosto-bronchial anastomosis is indicated by
    the short black arrows; the collaterally filled (via the anastomosis) 5th left intercostal artery by the long black arrows.
c: Fifth intercostal arteriogram on the left side. The contrast medium now passes the intercosto-bronchial anastomosis (solid
    arrows) in the reverse direction, resulting in a vague visualization of the bronchial artery which can be followed into the
    coin lesion (open arrows).

IV.2.2. Bronchial vascularization in pulmonary disease

IV.2.2.1. TUMORS

LITERATURE

In 1938, WOOD AND MILLER communicate that primary lung tumors are vascularized by the bronchial
arteries, whereas metastases do not show bronchial vascularization. They thought that a hemorrhage
in the presence of a malignant process in the lung indicated a primary tumor. From their publication
was deducted that metastases are avascular. WRIGHT concluded in the same year, however, that both
primary tumors and metastases are supplied by bronchial arteries, only very small metastases being
supplied by the pulmonary arteries.

WOOD AND MILLER'S theory has been generally accepted for many years and was supported by
CUDKOWICZ AND ARMSTRONG (1953b) and NAKAMURA ET AL. (1961). NAKAMURA ET AL. found an
increased bronchial flow in a patient with pulmonary metastases, but attributed this finding to a
concurrent pneumonia.

In 1965, NOONAN and co-workers demonstrated a bronchial circulation in the majority of pulmonary metastases, thus confirming WRIGHT's findings, but their illustrations show no bronchial vascularization in peripherally localized metastases. BOIJSEN AND ZIGMOND (1965), NEWTON AND PREGER (1965), and BOREK (1967) also saw vascularization of pulmonary metastases on bronchial arteriograms. VIAMONTE (1964) and HALLER ET AL. (1966), on the other hand, state that an avascular coin lesion is indicative of a metastasis or a benign lesion.

In 1967, MILNE introduced a new element with respect to the vascularization of malignant pulmonary processes. In a micro-angiographic investigation he demonstrated the considerable pulmonary contribution to the vascularization of these lesions and arrived at the following conclusions. Primary lung tumors have a bronchial vascularization, but in most of the cases there is an pulmonary contribution to the vascularization, the bronchial artery vascularizing the medial and the pulmonary artery the lateral portion of the tumor (Fig. 77a). The pulmonary contribution becomes greater and the bronchial contribution accordingly smaller, the more peripheral the location of the tumor (Fig. 77b).

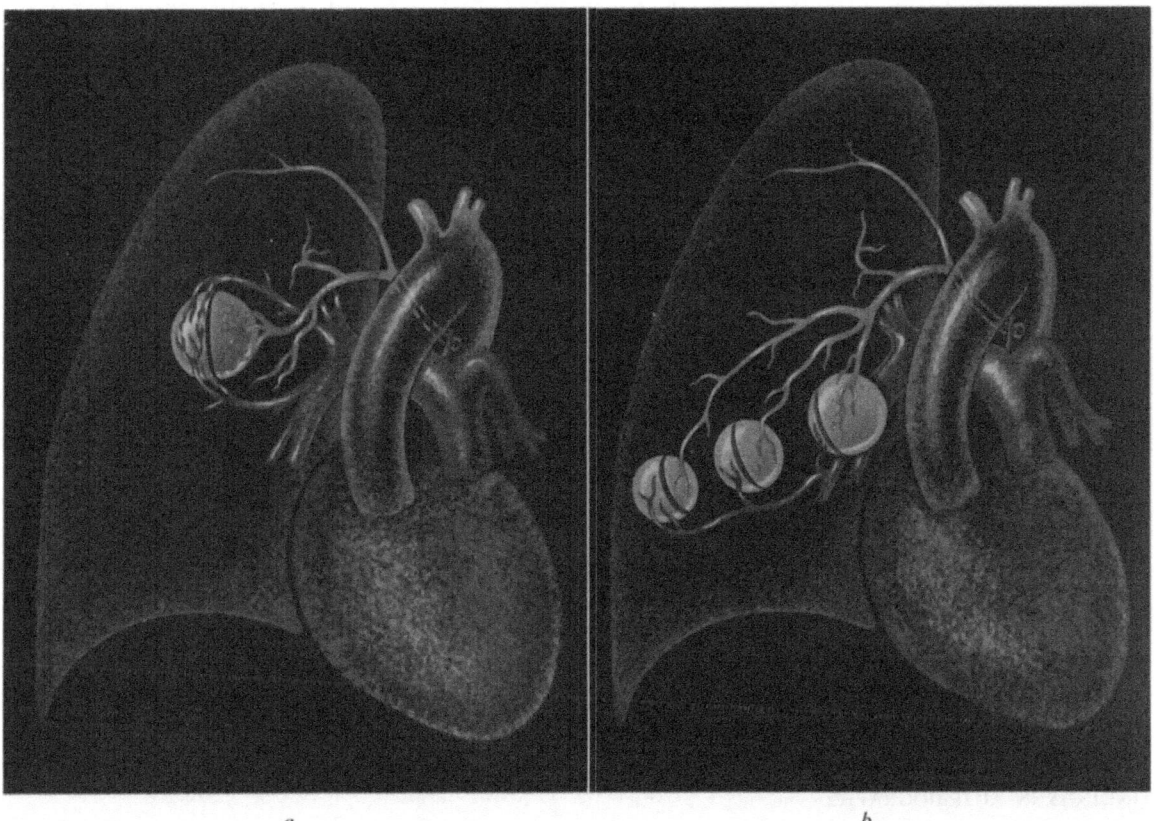

a   *b*

Fig. 77. Schematic representation of the vascularization of space-occupying processes in the lung.
a: The bronchial artery vascularizes the medial and the pulmonary artery the lateral portion of the tumor.
b: The bronchial contribution decreases from the center to the periphery and the pulmonary contribution correspondingly increases.

Metastases, however, always show an important pulmonary contribution to the vascularization, some of them also being supplied by the bronchial arteries. In metastases an analogous decrease of the bronchial contribution occurs from the center to the periphery. MILNE concludes that all the avascular lesions described in the literature were in fact supplied by the pulmonary artery. The micro-angiographic investigation of MILLER AND ROSENBAUM (1967) supports MILNE's views.

These data are of great importance for all those who attempt to treat lung tumors by injection of cytostatics into the aorta (RHEINLANDER ET AL., 1962; HOCKMAN AND MARK, 1964; FRECKMAN ET AL., 1966; sometimes with the aid of a balloon-catheter: RHEINLANDER ET AL., 1962; CLIFFTON AND DHAN RAJ MAHAJAN, 1963; SODERBERG ET AL., 1964; KLEIN ET AL., 1966; SHER ET AL., 1966) or directly into the bronchial arteries (KAHN ET AL., 1965; MARK ET AL., 1965; HALLER ET AL., 1966; RHEINLANDER ET AL., 1966; NORDENSTRÖM, 1966a; STECKEL ET AL., 1967; WIRTANEN AND ANSFIELD, 1968) and for those doing research on the value of cytostatic therapy. This therapeutical method has been applied increasingly during the last few years, while before that time selective perfusion of lung tumors via the pulmonary artery was performed by many, and more recently was still used occasionally (SUZUKI, 1967). As usually occurs with new methods, both were judged favorably at first, but especially the good results reported by FRECKMAN ET AL. (1966) for cytostatics applied through the bronchial arteries in pulmonary metastases, demand critical evaluation in the light of MILNE's findings. Recently, enthusiasm about the perfusion method via the bronchial arteries has subsided, partly because of the serious complications sometimes occurring in these cases (STECKEL ET AL., 1967).

When it became known that primary pulmonary tumors are mainly – previously thought to be entirely – supplied by bronchial arteries, the possibilities of selective catheterization of bronchial arteries were explored. This method was expected to permit the distinction between benign and malignant lesions and, it was hoped, even between the various types of lung tumors, since micro-angiographical investigations had shown that certain types of tumors have a specific vascular pattern (WRIGHT, 1938; WICKBOM, 1953; MARGULIS, 1964). However, the vessels most characteristic for the various types of tumor have a diameter varying from 20 to 200 μ, whereas only vessels with a diameter greater than the focus of the roentgen tube can be demonstrated radiographically (MILNE, 1967). For the tubes presently available for arteriography, the smallest diameter would be 600 μ. This discrepancy also explains the observation of VIAMONTE AND GILSON (1966) that a number of tumors, apparently avascular at bronchial arteriography, can be visualized with the aid of 'scannography'. According to MARGULIS (1964), a tenfold increase of the present definition would be required to typify tumors by way of arteriography. With the technical means now available, this degree of refinement of the arteriographical method cannot be reached *in vivo*.

Meanwhile, the primary lung tumors proved to be visualized at bronchial arteriography. The early reports were hopeful. VIAMONTE (1964) had the impression that primary lung tumors could be differentiated from other anomalies on the basis of the vascularization pattern. In 1965 he described seven characteristic features of tumor vascularization and three types of tumor circulation. At present, however, it is generally thought that the differentiation of lung tumors on the basis of selective bronchial arteriography is not possible, and that in most of the cases it is equally impossible to distinguish between a malignant and a benign anomaly, e.g. between a tumor and a chronic inflammatory process.

This rather discouraging introduction brings us to the discussion of the present findings.

FINDINGS IN ARTERIOGRAPHY

This study comprises 23 patients with primary pulmonary tumors, 4 patients with metastases, 2 patients with a hamartoma, and 2 patients with benign pleural tumors. Fig. 78 shows several tumors in the sequence of increasing degree of vascularization.

In the analysis of the material, attention was paid to the vascularization pattern, the degree of vascularization, the vascularized part, and the localization of the tumor; to the findings at the histological examination of the tumor, the condition of the hilar glands, and the presence or absence of transpleural vascularization; and finally to the operability of the lesion and the survival time and present condition of the patient. Since most of these patients were investigated in 1966, the average follow-up period amounts to two and a half years.

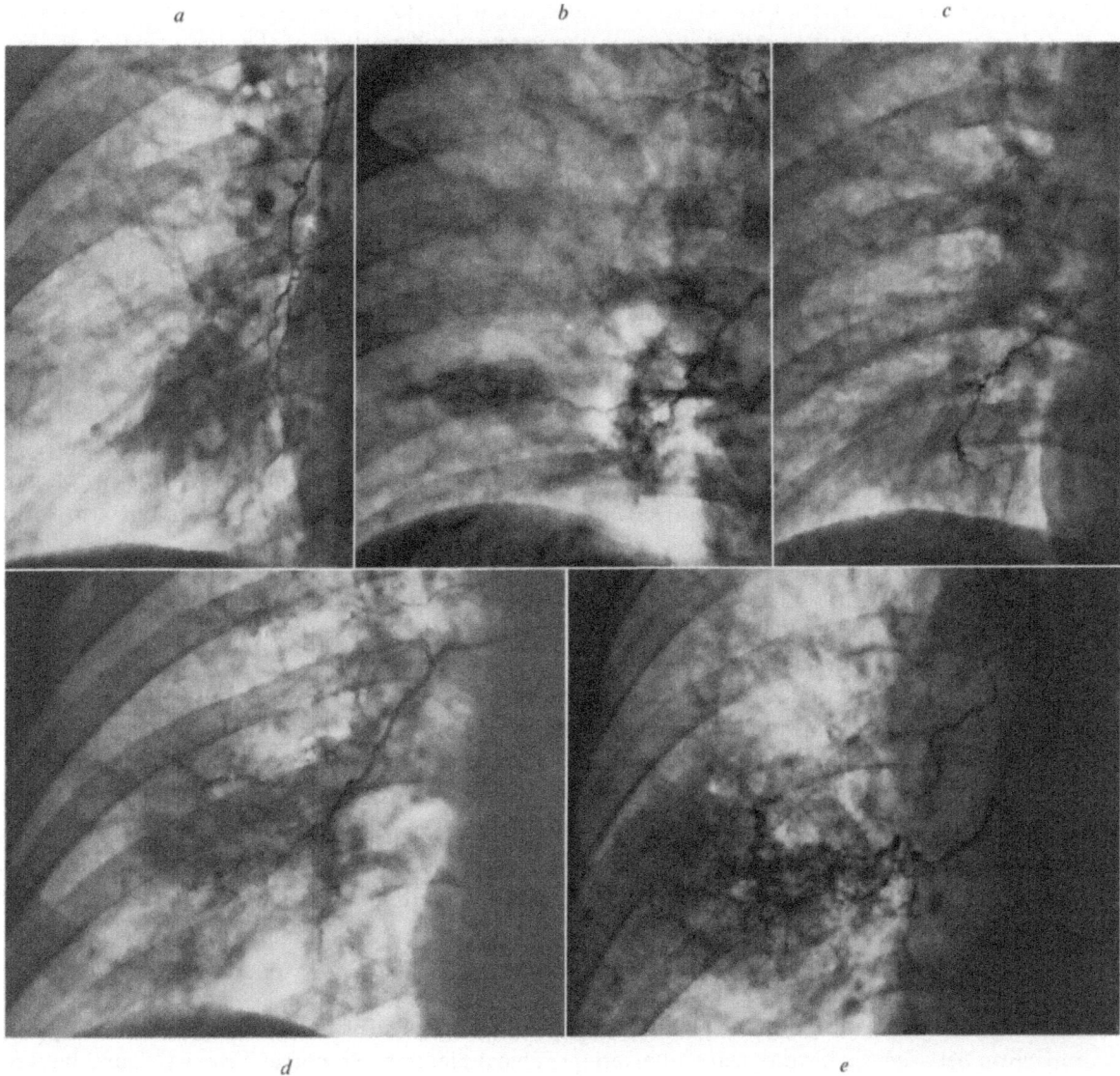

Fig. 78. Five tumors (*a-e*) showing an increasing degree of bronchial vascularization.

Localization and vascularized part of the tumor

The more peripheral the location of the tumor in the lung, the smaller the vascularized part was found to be, as table 21 illustrates.

TABLE 21.

VASC. PORTION OF THE TUMOUR	LOCALIZATION Peripheral		Parahilar		Central
NONE	3			1a	
$<\frac{1}{3}$	4	2			
$\frac{1}{3}-\frac{2}{3}$		2	3		
$>\frac{2}{3}$			4	1	1

All the tumors in our material for which the vascularized portion could be clearly distinguished are included in this table. In the vertical direction the vascularized portion of the tumor increases – via thirds – from none to almost the entire lesion. With respect to the localization, a distinction is made between peripheral, parahilar, and central. A few large tumors extended over a greater area; in the table these are shown separately and indicated by the brackets. The peripherally localized tumors are either not at all or only slightly vascularized by the bronchial arteries. When the localization is parahilar, more than one-third of the tumor shows bronchial vascularization, and when the localization is central more than two-thirds.

The bronchial share of the vascularization was always on the medial side, as fig. 79 shows. In this figure, approximately one-third of the tumors is vascularized by the bronchial arteries.

Relation to the histological findings

Since a histological investigation was performed for most of the tumors, the presence of a relationship could be established between on the one hand the vascularization pattern (a) and the richness of vascularization (b) of the tumor and on the other hand the histological findings. At the histological examination, special attention was paid not only to the classification of the tumors but also to the occurrence of connective tissue, necrosis, blood vessels, and inflammatory infiltrate.

a. No relationship was found between the vascularization pattern and the histological findings, but our material is rather small for a comparative analysis and there is no proof that such relationships would not be found in larger series.
b. In attempting to find a relationship between the richness of vascularization of the tumors and the histological findings, we were struck by the following observation. Squamous cell carcinoma and tumors with much connective tissue[1] seemed to show somewhat more vascularization, and tumors with a great deal of necrosis – understandably – less vascularization. A distinct relationship was found, however, between the inflammatory factor and the richness of vascularization of the tumors, for which comparison the tumors were classified in 5 groups according to increasing degree of vascularization. It was found that the degree of vascularization increased, the more inflammatory infiltrate was present.

Hilus

A histological examination of hilar glands was performed in most of this series of patients to permit comparison between the histological and arteriographical pictures. No correlation was found between the two. To the contrary, most arteriographically suspicious hili proved to be histologically free of metastases, and, conversely, in two cases with extensive glandular metastases an unsuspected hilus was visible on the arteriogram. The only case with agreement of both the radiological and the histological diagnoses concerned a richly vascularized tumor and well-supplied glandular metastases at the hilus.

There is another criterion that may be more reliable but with which we have had little experience. This criterion is the narrowing of bronchial arteries in the region of the hilus as an indication of the presence of glandular metastases. Fig. 30 shows a centrally constricted bronchial artery in a patient with a tumor in the right upper lobe who proved at autopsy – a few weeks after our examination – to have massive glandular metastases at the carina and the right hilus. With this picture, however, spasm cannot be excluded with certainty.

---

[1] This is in agreement with the findings in the literature. According to WRIGHT (1938), proliferation of connective tissue leads to increased bronchial vascularization, and according to CUDKOWICZ AND ARMSTRONG (1953b) and MILNE (1967), squamous cell carcinomas are richly vascularized.

Fig. 79. The bronchial contribution to the vascularization is always found on the medial side.
a: Large tumor extending from the parahilar region to the periphery.
b: Small and rather peripherally localized tumor.
c: Large tumor with necrotic cavity (marked by arrows).

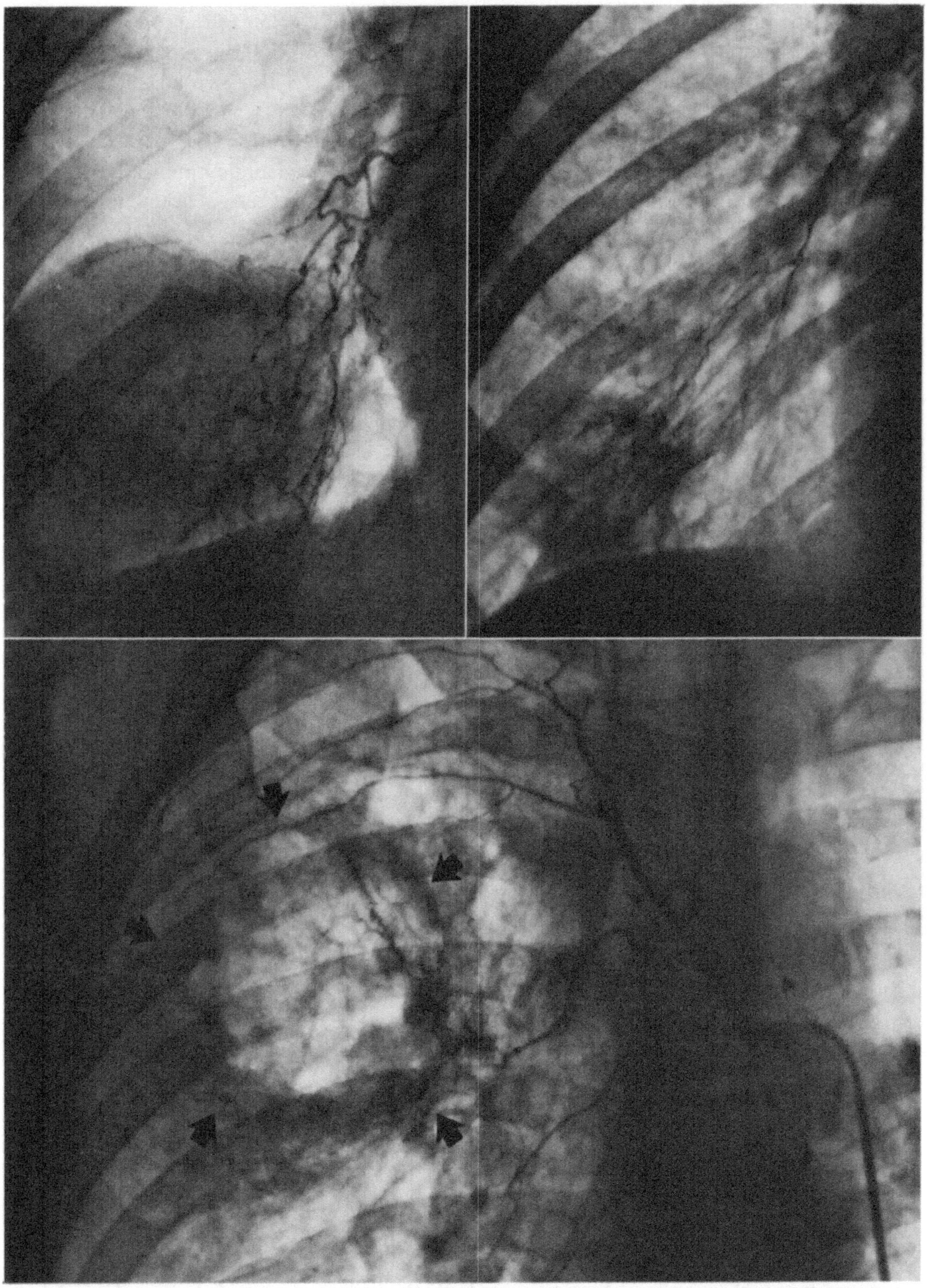

Transpleural vascularization

A number of patients showed vascularization in and around the region of the tumor, usually on an intercostal arteriogram (Figs. 80 and 81). This situation may be an indication of invasion and penetration of the pleura by the tumor. Transpleural vascularization can also be found, however, in cases of adhesions after pleuresies. Therefore, inflammation around a peripherally located tumor and leading to a local pleuritis, could also result in transpleural vascularization (Fig. 82). Nevertheless, we attempted to determine whether there was any agreement between radiographically demonstrated transpleural vascularization and penetration by the tumor. To our surprise, we found good correlation between the two.

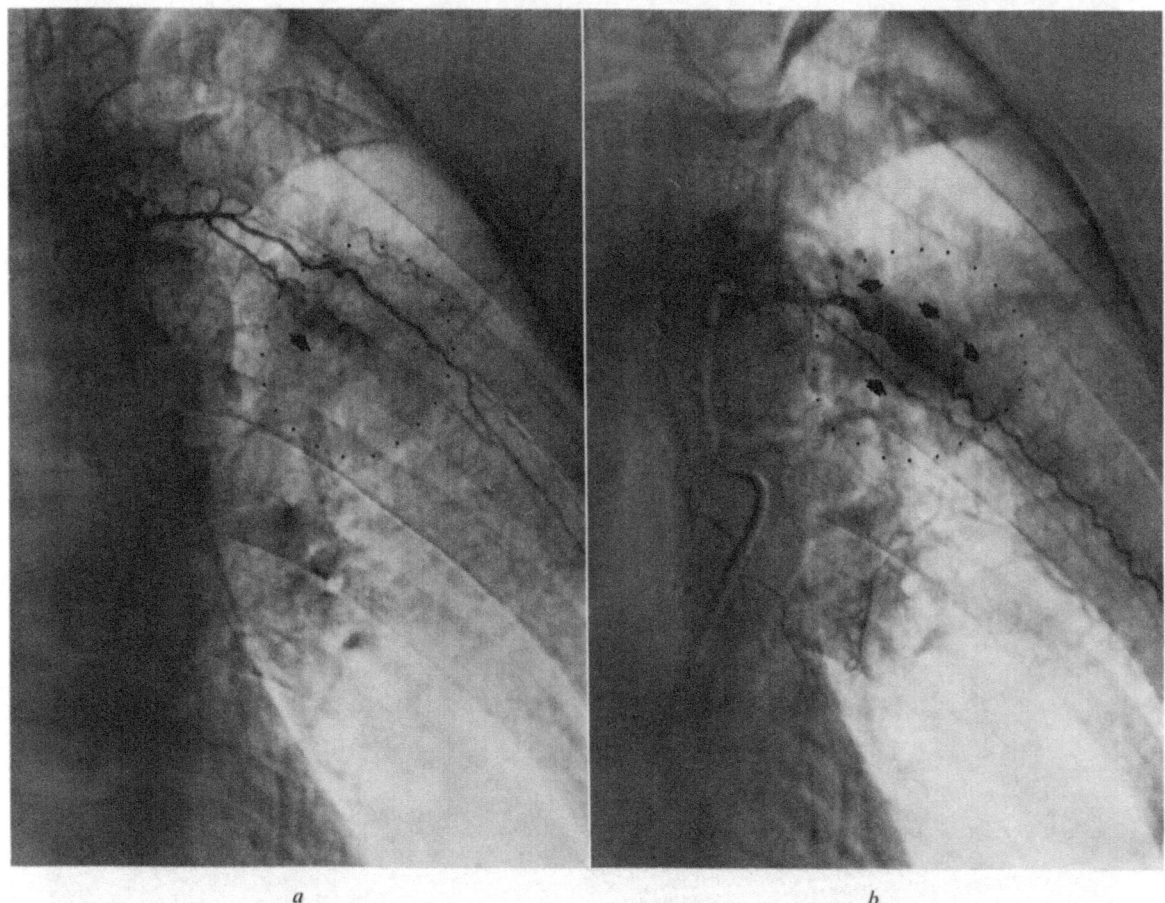

a   *b*

Fig. 80. Transpleural vascularization via intercostal arteries. Arteriography of the 4th (*a*) and 5th (*b*) left intercostal arteries. The dotted line demarcates the tumor region; the arrows indicate the region of the transpleural vascularization, in which there is a large amount of contrast medium.

In eleven patients with peripheral lung tumors, both the radiological and the histological investigations were sufficiently complete to permit evaluation of this point. In five of these patients the radiological and the histological data were negative and in five others both were positive. In the eleventh patient a distinct transpleural vascularization was seen, but the histological findings were negative (Fig. 82).

All of the five patients with pleural invasion of the tumor have died, most of them within six months of the operation. Of the six patients without histologically demonstrable pleural penetration, four are still in good condition.

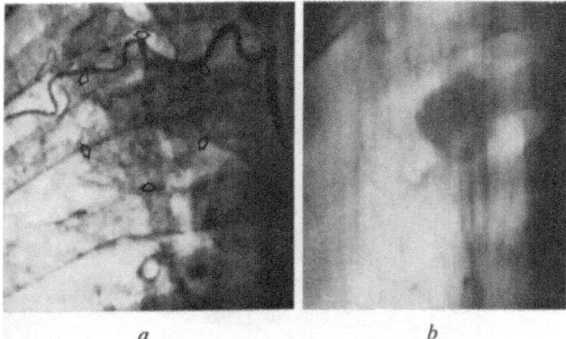

a   b

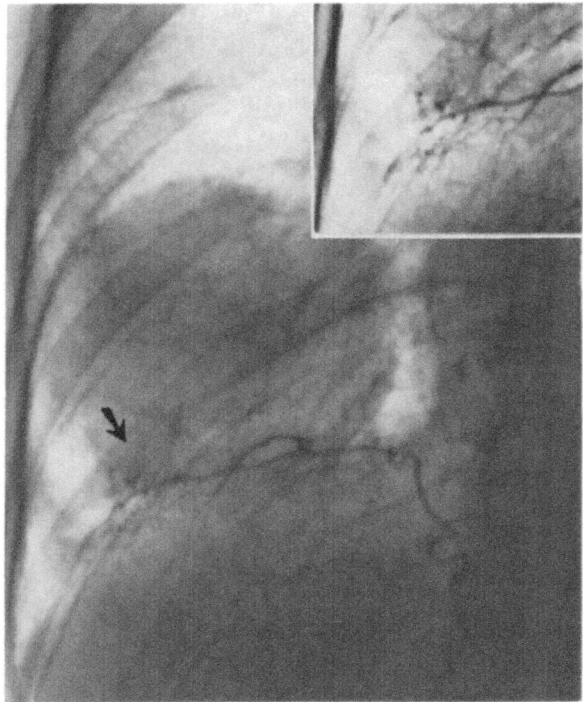

Fig. 82. Transpleural vascularization in a case with extensive adhesions found at operation, although histological examination showed no invasion of the tumor. Probably, the transpleural vascularization developed after an inflammatory infiltrate around the tumor had caused a local pleuritis.
a: Tomogram showing a tumor shadow dorsally in the right upper lobe. Histological diagnosis (biopsy): carcinoma.
b: Intercostal arteriogram showing the area of transpleural vascularization in the vicinity of the tumor. This picture is more enlarged than *a*: compare the distance between the ribs.

Fig. 81. Transpleural vascularization arising from the phrenic artery. The transpleurally vascularized part of the tumor (arrows) can be seen more clearly on the detail (inset). The bronchial vascularization of this tumor can be seen in Fig. 79*a*.

Metastases

Two patients with solitary pulmonary metastases showed a distinct bronchial vascularization, but in two others with diffuse metastases, no bronchial circulation could be demonstrated. Fig. 78*c* shows the arteriogram of a patient with a solitary and parahilary located metastasis of EWING's sarcoma.

Hamartoma

The two cases with a hamartoma did not show agreement; the first had a richly vascularized process (Fig. 83), but in the second no bronchial vascularization could be established with certainty.

a

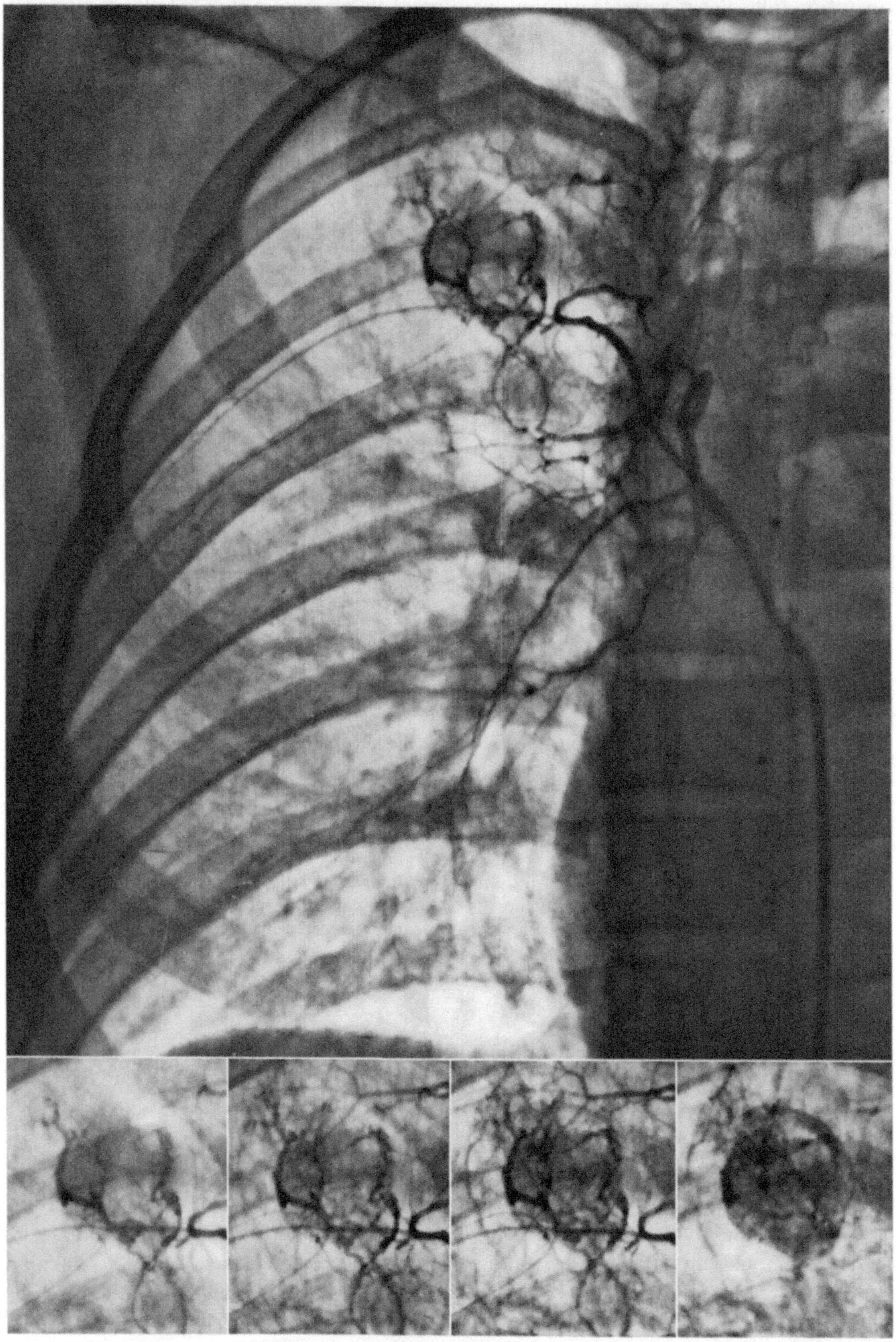

b c d e

Fig. 83. Hamartoma with abundant vascularization.
a: Arteriogram of an intercosto-bronchial trunk.
b, *c*, *d*, and *e*: Details showing the tumor during different phases of the arteriogram. Note distinct *Anfärbung* in *e*.

Pleural tumors

In the two cases with benign pleural tumors no bronchial vascularization could be demonstrated, which was not surprising in view of the peripheral location.

Irradiation

Two patients were investigated during radiotherapy (megavolt) and a third patient had already received a total tumor-dose of 6000 R. There were no obvious differences with the vascularization of non-irradiated tumors.

DISCUSSION

The standard criteria for the vascularization pattern of a neoplasm are: an irregular, sometimes chaotic, vascular network; variations in caliber (abrupt narrowing and occlusions as well as dilatations); extravasation of contrast medium, sometimes leading to pooling; and *Anfärbung*, in which the contrast medium seems to stagnate in the capillaries. We have, however, found similar features in inflammatory processes (Figs. 84 and 85). In our opinion, therefore, there is no vascularization pattern that is typical for a malignant process.

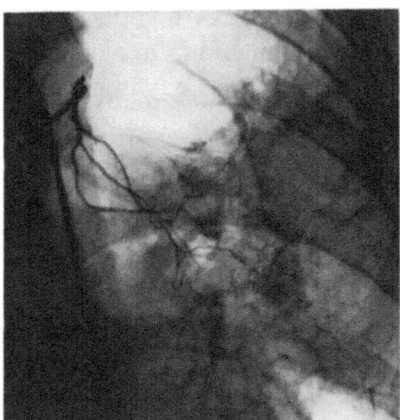 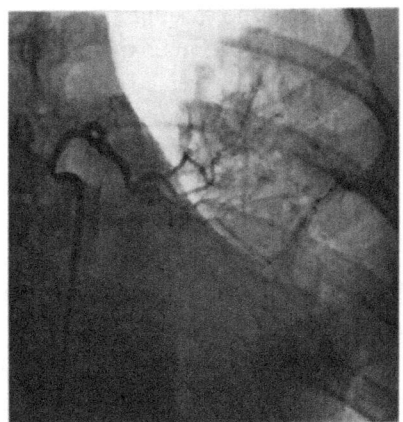

Fig. 84. Patient with infected bullae. Chaotic branching, variations in caliber, small spots of extravasation, and vague *Anfärbung*.

Fig. 85. Patient with a malignant process located in the same area as the lesions shown in Fig. 84. The vascular pictures are very similar. The vascularization pattern of the inflammatory process is even more chaotic.

But there *are* characteristic features that support the absence of a lung tumor. VIAMONTE ET AL. (1965) have put forward a number of criteria for a benign lesion, with most of which we can agree; these are distinctly dilated bronchial arteries, extensive broncho-pulmonary shunts, normal branching, gradual decrease in caliber, and a proportional distribution of the small branches However, this point requires some qualification.

We have also seen strongly dilated bronchial arteries in malignant lesions – Figs. 12*b* and 78*e* are examples – but never the combination of strong dilatation and tortuosity, as for instance in fig. 91D. Consequently, we believe that marked tortuosity of the bronchial artery is a much more important indication of benignancy than marked dilatation.

Although several broncho-pulmonary anastomoses in lung tumors have been demonstrated by TURNER-WARWICK (1963a), OUDET ET AL. (1967), and MILNE (1967) on the basis of micro-angiographical investigations and by NAKAMURA ET AL. (1961) by flow measurements, we have seen some very small shunts and then only sporadically in our cases with tumors[1], this failure apparently being due to technical deficiencies.

In addition to wide broncho-pulmonary anastomoses (Fig. 101), wide broncho-bronchial anastomoses, accessory bronchial arteries with an aberrant origin (Fig. 20), and intercosto-bronchial anastomoses (Fig. 76) also constitute evidence of a long-standing and therefore probably benign lesion.

When the presence of a coin lesion cannot be linked to a diagnosis, therefore, bronchial arteriography may provide useful information. If a thoracotomy for example, is not advisable, because of advanced age, poor heart and lung function, or for some other reason, bronchial arteriography would seem to be indicated, at least when the location of the tumor is not too peripheral.

According to VIAMONTE (1964) and HALLER ET AL. (1965), avascular (not visibly vascularized) lesions indicate a benign lesion or a metastasis. We cannot support this view. In the first place, it does not hold for peripheral carcinomas in the lung and in the second place this factor is dependent on the degree of necrosis (Table 21).

Like MILNE (1967), we found a relationship between the localization of the tumor and the bronchial contribution to the vascularization. The bronchial artery always supplies the medial part, and this part decreases from the center to the periphery.

Our material is too limited to permit conclusions concerning the possibility of differentiating and typifying tumors on the basis of bronchial arteriography. The results of our comparative analysis are very disappointing, the vascular pattern showing no specific features and the degree of vascularization appearing to be determined mainly by the amount of inflammation. On other grounds too, it is unlikely that relationships will be found in larger series, since arteriography is adequate only for arteries with a rather wide caliber (0.6 mm), whereas, as mentioned above, the vessels typifying a given tumor are much smaller (0.02–0.2 mm). In theory, tumor typification *in vivo* might be possible by applying very small and highly chargeable foci in the roentgen tubes (TAKAHASHI ET AL., 1966). Even if a multiplication of the present definition can be reached in the future, we believe that the pneumologist will still prefer not to depend solely on a diagnosis based on arteriography but will continue to want histological examination of a biopsy sample.

The degree of vascularization was found to increase with increasing amounts of inflammatory infiltrate in and around the tumor. Since an inflammatory process can show the same vascular picture as a malignant process, a large proportion of what is indicated in the literature as tumor vascularization actually depends, in our opinion, on vascularization of inflammatory infiltrate around and in the tumor.

Although the opposite opinion has been expressed (SCHOBER, 1964; BOIJSEN AND ZSIGMOND, 1965; BOREK ET AL., 1967), bronchial arteriography does not seems to be a useful investigation for the diagnostic of hilar glands. It even seems highly unlikely that favorable results are to be expected from larger series, for two reasons. In the first place, since abnormal vessels can be visualized in and around inflamed hilar glands, differentiation from a glandular metastasis is not possible. This is presumably the explanation of the false-positive results in our material, because most of the radiologically suspect hilar glands that proved to be free of tumor tissue at histological examination, did show inflammatory infiltrate. In the second place, no richly vascularized glandular metastases in the region of the hilus are to be expected in cases of very poorly vascularized tumors, which might explain the false-negative results in these cases.

Perhaps a radiologically normal hilus in the presence of a richly vascularized tumor argues against glandular metastases. This is, however, merely a hypothesis.

Narrowing of the artery due to tumor growth is possibly a more reliable criterion of pathological hilar glands (Fig. 30), but we have had little experience with this finding.

---

[1] See also under Broncho-Pulmonary Anastomoses (page 96).

BOIJSEN AND ZSIGMOND (1965), NORDENSTRÖM (1967), E COSTA (1967), and POLÁK ET AL. (1967) state that they have demonstrated narrowing and occlusion by pathological hilar glands, but their pictures are not very convincing and seem more likely to have been caused by artefacts.

Transpleural vascularization seems, more or less unexpectedly, to be a rather reliable criterion for penetration of the tumor through the pleura. In view of the very poor prognosis of these patients, all of whom died rather soon in spite of surgical treatment, arteriography would seem to be advisable when tumor ingrowth is feared. Unfortunately, the case in which a false-positive result was obtained radiologically, shows that the arteriographical findings alone are not always sufficient for the diagnosis.

Like some of the authors who have been mentioned in the discussion of the literature, we established bronchial vascularization in metastases (Fig. 78c). As in primary pulmonary tumors, the localization is of great importance. Two patients with central and parahilar metastases showed an appreciable amount of bronchial vascularization, whereas no bronchial circulation could be demonstrated in two patients with diffuse and peripherally located pulmonary metastases. The latter two patients had been treated for some time with cytostatics, which might have exerted some influence. Our findings are in agreement with the results obtained by MILNE (1967), and we therefore believe that there is no real difference between the vascular supply of metastases and of primary tumors, because the location determines the size of the bronchial share to be expected at arteriography. According to MILNE (1967), however, the average contribution of the pulmonary artery is larger in metastases than in primary pulmonary tumors.

Of two cases of hamartoma, one showed an abundant vascularization (Fig. 83) and the other no vascularization at all. In the latter case, however, the tumor was localized extremely peripherally. Three cases of hamartoma investigated by means of bronchial arteriography have been described in the literature. VIAMONTE ET AL. (1965) and HALLER ET AL. (1966) did not observe vascularization; KAHN ET AL. (1965), on the contrary found a considerable supply. Therefore, no conclusion can be reached on this matter, but we agree with KAHN ET AL. (1965) that the rich vascularization is above all a result of inflammation.

Our results do not confirm the ample vascular supply reported for carcinoids. In one case we saw a slight vascularization (Fig. 78b) and in the other case hardly any vascularization.

As for the three patients who had undergone radiotherapy with no obvious change in the bronchial vascularization, it may be noted that according to NEWTON AND PREGER (1965) radiation may influence the bronchial vascularization of tumors but that according to experimental results of WOLFE ET AL. (1967), this is not the case for the bronchial vascularization of the normal tissue.

The question might arise as to whether the degree of vascularization of the tumor could give an impression of its radiosensitivity. According to experiments done by MC ALISTER AND MARGULIS (1963), there is no correlation between the two, so that there seems to be no indication for further investigation.

CONCLUSIONS

1. There is no essential difference between the vascularization of primary pulmonary tumors and metastases. Primary lung tumors show a vascularization in which both the bronchial and the pulmonary arteries participate. The bronchial contribution decreases the more peripheral the location of the tumor. In metastases the pulmonary contribution is relatively more important.
2. The standard criteria concerning tumor vascularization are not specific.
3. Identification of tumors on the basis of bronchial arteriography does not seem to be possible.
4. Since there are a number of criteria for the bronchial vascularization pattern of long-standing pulmonary lesions, it is usually possible to distinguish between benign and malignant processes.
5. The degree of vascularization of a tumor is determined mainly by the inflammatory reaction.
6. Transpleural vascularization is a fairly reliable indication for penetration of the pleura.

7. Bronchial arteriography does not provide conclusive evidence concerning the presence of hilus-gland metastases.

INDICATIONS

In summarization of the foregoing it may be said that bronchial arteriography is not to be recommended as a routine investigation in cases of pulmonary tumors, because its diagnostic contribution is too limited. In cases of peripheral tumors it gives no information at all. In our opinion, there are two indications for arteriography.

1. In cases of a coin lesion without diagnosis, at least when the lesion is not located too peripherally, a bronchial arteriogram should be made because it may be possible to differentiate between benign and malignant processes and thus spare the patient a thoracotomy.
2. In view of the poor prognosis of patients suffering from tumors with pleural invasion, intercostal arteriograms should be made when such invasion is suspected, because the demonstration of trans-pleural vascularization may mean that the patient should not be treated surgically.

IV.2.2.2. TUBERCULOSIS

LITERATURE

The vascularization of tuberculous lesions is effected by the bronchial arteries. It is consistently reported that the pulmonary arterial branches in the vicinity of these anomalies showed thrombosis or were occluded by intimal proliferation.

Opinions concerning the bronchial vascularization of the various forms of tuberculosis differ. FLORANGE (1960) states that early exudative tubercle processes do not show vascularization but that it is present in older processes in which fibrotic demarcation has begun. A more differentiated description was provided as early as 1938 by WRIGHT, according to whom there is no vascularization of proliferative caseating lesions or in rapidly developing granulomatous tuberculosis, but that it occurs in fibrocaseous anomalies, fibrotic scars, and, to the highest degree, in the walls of tuberculous cavities. The last of these observations is supported by all the authors. WOOD AND MILLER (1938) state that the dilation and tortuosity of the bronchial arteries increases with increasing chronicity of the lesions. According to some authors, including DELARUE ET AL. (1953), there is only limited vascularization of caseous focal lesions and tuberculomas, but FLORANGE (1960) states that tuberculomas are heavily vascularized and CUDKOWICZ (1952a) gives examples of highly vascularized caseous tuberculous lesions.

Around the tubercle foci there are numerous small broncho-pulmonary anastomoses (WOOD AND MILLER, 1938; MARCHAND ET AL., 1950; DELARUE ET AL., 1953; LATARJET, 1954; CAMARRI AND MARINI, 1965; OUDET ET AL., 1967) formed, according to CUDKOWICZ (1952a), by recanalization of the occluded pulmonary arteries. Most of these shunts were found in the cavity walls. (DELARUE ET AL., 1953; OUDET ET AL., 1967). OUDET ET AL. attempted to determine the fate of the multiple anastomoses in inflamed tuberculous tissue more exactly, but their observations were conflicting: in some cases sporadic fine anastomoses were seen around old healed tuberculous foci and in others there were extensive broncho-pulmonary shunts around tuberculous fibrotic scars.

ROOSENBURG AND DEENSTRA (1954), CUDKOWICZ ET AL. (1959), FRITTS ET AL. (1961), and NAKAMURA

ET AL. (1961) measured the broncho-pulmonary flow in tuberculosis, for which CUDKOWICZ ET AL. and FRITTS ET AL. calculated an average value amounting to 5.4 and 3.2 times the normal flow, respectively. These calculations were based on comparison of the output of the right and left ventricles, the difference in output representing the blood returning to the left atrium via the left ventricle→ bronchial artery→pulmonary artery→pulmonary vein. In our opinion, these authors inadvertantly measured mainly the appreciable transpleural[1] flow that, according to DAUSSY AND ABELANET (1956), BRUWER (1966), VACCAREZZA ET AL. (1966), PINET ET AL. (1966), and PADOVANI ET AL. (1966), occurs so often in tuberculous diseases and can become greatly augmented, especially in cases with extensive fibrosis.

Several authors have attempted to establish a relationship between the bronchial vascularization and the development of the tubercle process. DELARUE ET AL. (1953) thought that some tuberculous lesions could be formed as a result of the changes in the bronchial circulation, but the other authors state that the bronchial circulation undergoes only secondary changes. According to WRIGHT (1938), the connective-tissue proliferation occurring during the formation of tubercles and other tubercle lesions is the most important cause of the expansion of the bronchial circulation, and according to CUDKOWICZ (1952a) and LATARJET (1954) infection is also an important factor in this increase.

It is evident that a study of the literature does not lead to a clear picture of the bronchial vascularization in the various tuberculous lesions. The impression is obtained that acute and florid forms of tuberculosis show less vascularization than the forms with a chronic course. With the necessary reservation, the following conclusions may be drawn:

Bronchial vascularization is limited in active and rapidly developing tuberculosis and is lowest in a proliferative caseating process. The vascularization increases with increasing fibrosis or decreasing intensity of the development of the disease. Concurrently, broncho-pulmonary anastomoses develop; these anastomoses probably persist in some residual lesions and disappear in others. The highest degree of vascularization is seen in the walls of the cavities. Tuberculomas are poorly vascularized.

FINDINGS IN ARTERIOGRAPHY

To evaluate the application of arteriography in tuberculosis we compared the clinical picture with the arteriographic results in 24 patients. The clinical picture was defined on the basis of the form and developmental course of the disease, the radiological appearance of the thorax, the results of the sputum analysis (ZIEHL-NEELSEN preparations, and cultures), the duration and effect of tuberculostatic treatment, and the surgical and histological findings when available. Arteriographic factors taken into consideration were the bronchial vascularization (classified according to five grades: very limited, limited, moderately rich, rich, abundant), the presence and number of broncho- and intercosto-pulmonary shunts, the condition of the hilus, and the pattern of the bronchial network. The most important results of this study will be reported. The material was divided into three main groups, to be discussed successively.

a. Old fibrotic and fibrocaseous lesions

This group comprises ten cases in which it was virtually certain that there was no longer any activity. Radiographically, the foci showed sharply defined margins, a very limited to limited bronchial vascularization (Fig. 86), and very few broncho-pulmonary shunts (Fig. 67). A moderately rich vascularization was seeen only once, in a patient with rather extensive focal lesions and a history of prolonged treatment for tuberculosis. Two cases show a limited transpleural vascularization (intercosto-pulmonary).

---

[1] Via anastomoses between pulmonary arteries, and intercostal and other arteries running along the thoracic wall.

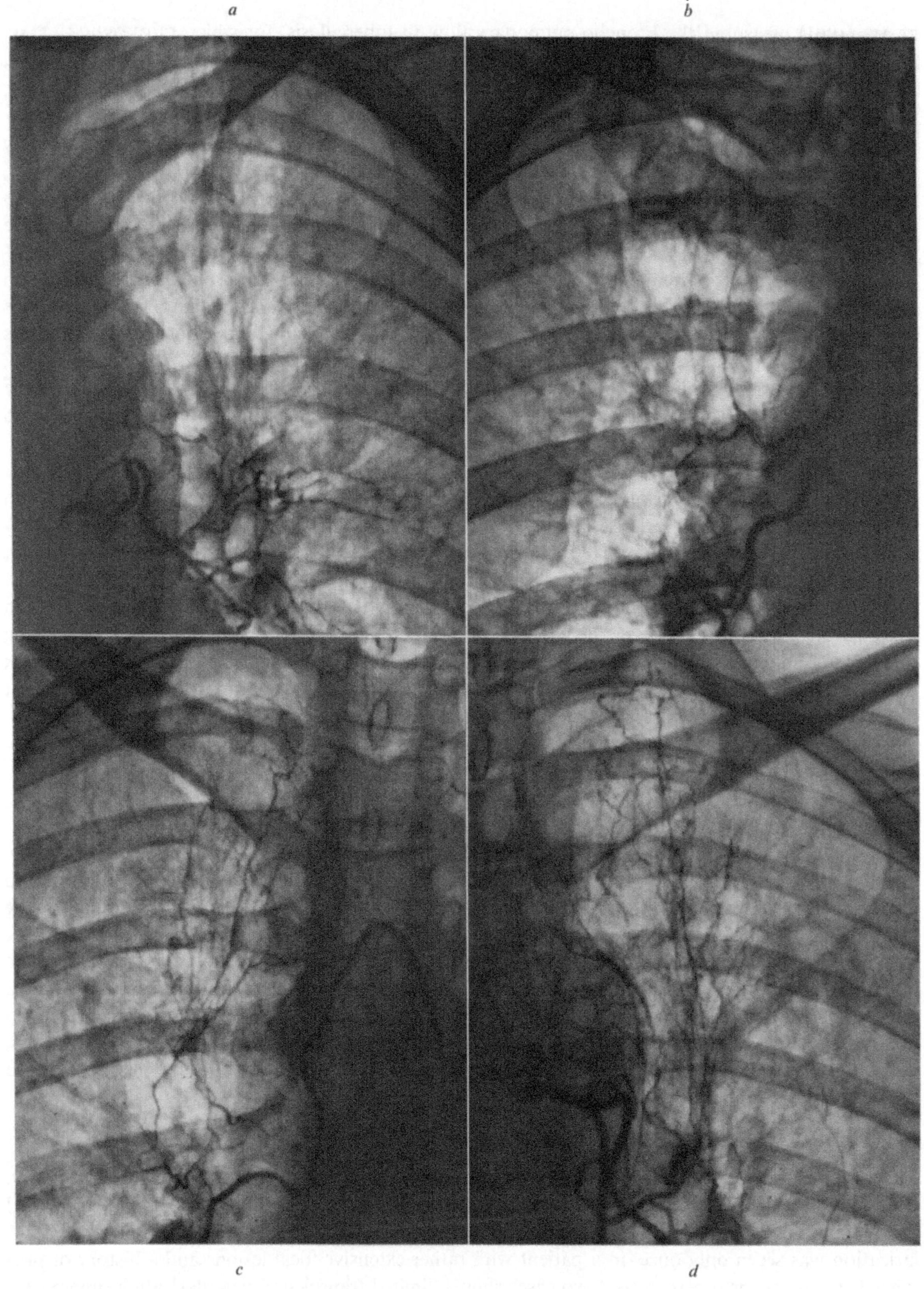

a   b

c   d

Fig. 86. Very limited to limited bronchial vascularization of old fibrotic and fibrocaseous tuberculous lesions, increasing in the sequence of the illustrations *a-d*.

b. Active fibrocaseous and caseous lesions

This group includes seven cases. Radiologically, most of the foci showed poorly defined margins. The bronchial vascularization was limited to moderately rich. There were very few to several broncho-pulmonary shunts (Figs. 87). Four patients showed a limited number of intercosto-pulmonary shunts. A few cases with old lesions and one case with a history of prolonged treatment showed the most extensive vascularization. The duration of treatment varied from two and a half weeks to four months (in one case it was two years).

One patient showed, in addition to vascularization of the radiologically demonstrated lesions in the left upper lobe, a round, pathologically vascularized solitary lesion located postero-basally in the left lower lobe (Fig. 88). Tomograms of this region failed to reveal this lesion. It therefore seems possible to use arteriography to find lesions that cannot be demonstrated by the usual radiological methods.

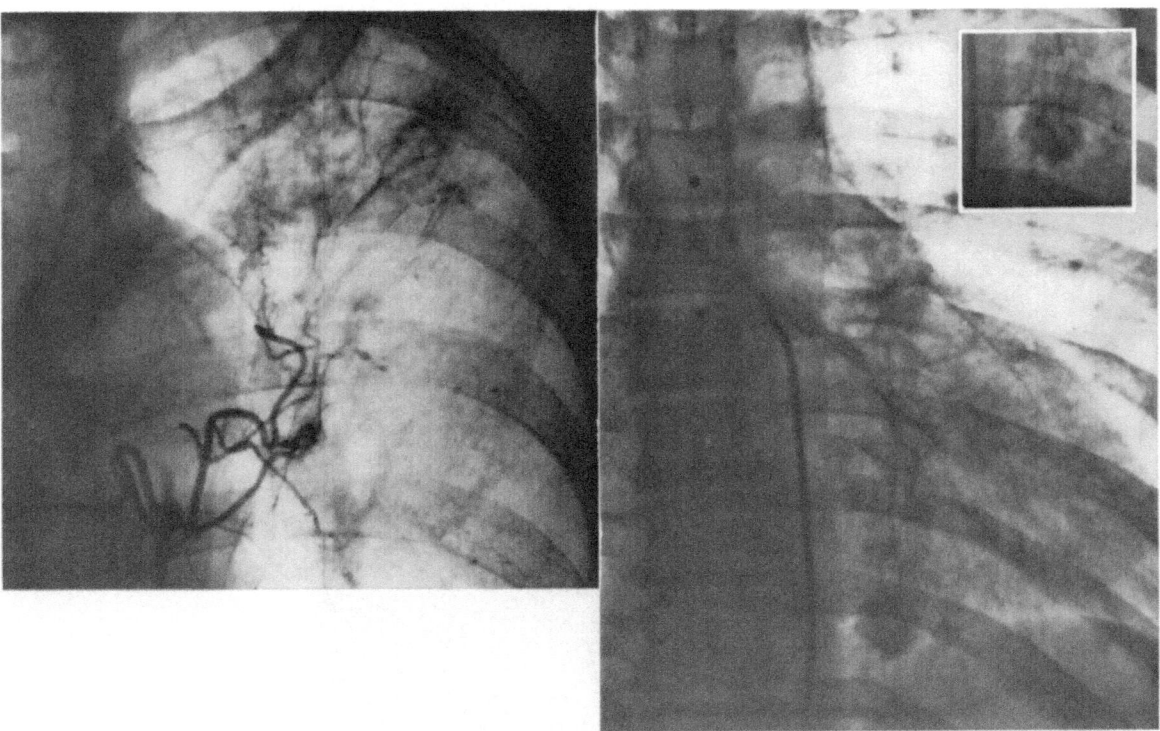

Fig. 87. Moderately rich bronchial vascularization including a few broncho-pulmonary shunts in active fibrocaseous tuberculous lesions. A case from the same group is shown in Fig. 40.

Fig. 88. Lesion in the left lower lobe that could only be demonstrated arteriographically. The round shadow projected in the left paravertebral region was shown to be localized posterobasally in the left lower lobe by the arteriogram in the lateral projection. The inset shows the lesion in an early arteriographical phase.

c. Extensive exudative caseous tuberculous lesions, with or without cavities

This group comprises five patients with a rich to abundant bronchial vascularization of the lesions, as well as dilated, slightly tortuous bronchial arteries and numerous broncho-pulmonary shunts (Fig. 89), four of the five cases also showing numerous intercosto-pulmonary shunts (Fig. 71). The lesions with the most vascularization were those which had been treated longest, some of them already showing fibrotic shrinkage.

Four of these cases showed cavitation, and in two of them clearly defined cavities had developed. Numerous vessels were seen around the cavities, but the vascularization of the walls was less extensive than the reports in the literature had led us to expect.

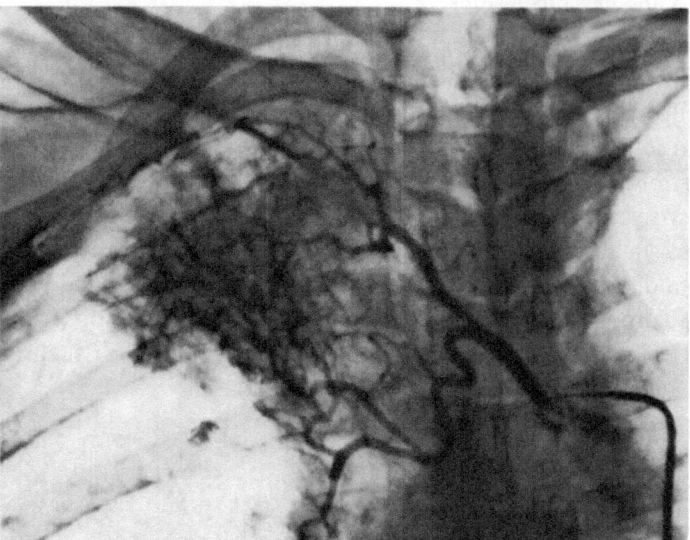

Fig. 89. Abundant bronchial vascularization in cavernous tuberculosis. Strongly dilated intercosto-bronchial trunk bifurcating in a wide, slightly tortuous bronchial artery and a dilated intercostal artery. Rich vascularization in the area of the lesion, i.e. the apical and dorsal segments of the right upper lobe. The later phases of the arteriogram showed extensive parahilar broncho-pulmonary shunts.

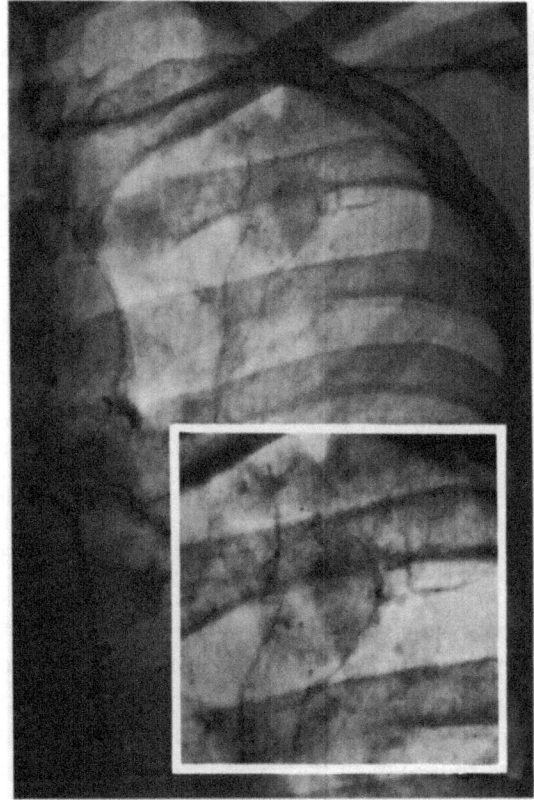

Fig. 90. Tuberculoma showing a limited bronchial vascularization. Surrounding the lesion there are small broncho-pulmonary shunts which can be seen more distinctly in the enlargement (inset).

Tuberculoma

Of two cases of tuberculoma, one showed a very limited and the other a limited bronchial vascularization (Fig. 90). The latter case also showed a minimal number of broncho-pulmonary shunts.

Remarks

In five cases unusual 'looping' arteries were seen on the intercostal arteriograms (Fig. 48a). In our material arteries of this kind were seen only in cases of tuberculosis. In two of the patients a connection with bronchial arteries seemed to be achieved via these loops. It seems possible that these structures are the anastomoses described by CUDKOWICZ (1952a) in tuberculosis, which according to him are formed during recanalization of thrombosed bronchial arteries (by intercostal arteries).

In several cases vascularization of hilus glands was demonstrated (Fig. 40); and histological investigation showed these glands to be inflamed. In these cases it was therefore possible to establish a correlation between the arteriographical and histological findings.

DISCUSSION

From the findings in our material it follows, firstly, that the degree of bronchial vascularization of tuberculous lesions corresponds with the severity and extent of the inflammatory process. This conclusion is in conflict with the opinions in the literature (e.g. WRIGHT, 1938).

Secondly, in cases belonging to the same group the vascularization was heavier the longer the duration of the anomalies and the greater the chronicity of the process. The same conclusion was reached by WOOD AND MILLER (1938). Since in these cases the fibrosis usually also showed an increase, this finding also supports WRIGHT's theory (1938).

Of these two relationships, in our material the former was seen much more consistently than the latter.

In agreement with the literature, we found that the development of broncho-pulmonary anastomoses coincided with the richness and extent of the bronchial circulation. Concurrently, the transpleural intercosto-pulmonary vascularization showed an increase. This is hardly surprising, since a local pleuritis will develop sooner and more easily the more extensive the tuberculous inflammatory process.

Most of the patients with active tuberculous lesions were treated surgically, and it was therefore possible to compare the arteriographical results with the histological findings. It was found, among other things, that fibrocaseous lesions were more richly vascularized than the caseous type, which is in agreement with the conclusions of WRIGHT (1938) and FLORANGE (1960).

All of the patients with active tuberculosis had been treated for some time with tuberculostatics, which made it more difficult to draw conclusions concerning the pattern of bronchial vascularization in the various tubercle lesions, since such treatment could conceivably exert an influence in this respect. Some of the treated patients showed extensive and others only sparse vascularization. An evaluation of the effect of treatment with tuberculostatics on the vascular pattern cannot be made for our material. Our series is too small for this purpose, and therefore this point requires further investigation.

As yet, we are unable to define the indications for bronchial arteriography in tuberculosis of the lungs. In one patient arteriography demonstrated a lesion that was not revealed by the conventional radiological methods (Fig. 88). It might therefore be advisable to perform an arteriographical investigation before the surgical resection of tuberculous anomalies to determine whether any lesions are present in the radiologically normal parts of the lung. For analogous reasons, arteriography might well be carried out in patients with only clinically suggestive signs (e.g. strongly positive or turned MANTOUX reaction).

CONCLUSIONS

1. In contrast to the general opinion in the literature, the extent of the bronchial vascularization and the development of broncho- and intercosto-pulmonary anastomoses is considered to be mainly dependent on the activity and the extent of the tuberculosis and – to a lesser degree – on the nature of the process (granulomatous, caseous, fibrotic). Furthermore, the bronchial vascularization seems to increase the longer the process has existed and the more fibrosis has developed.
2. Tuberculomas and caseous foci in otherwise healthy lung tissue are poorly vascularized.
3. The effect of tuberculostatics on bronchial vascularization has not yet been determined and requires further study.
4. Indications for bronchial arteriography in tuberculosis have not been found. The fact that this method can reveal lesions that cannot be demonstrated by conventional radiological methods means that further investigation is needed. Such studies might yield indications for the application of arteriography, for instance for the pre-operative evaluation of radiologically normal parts of the lung.

IV.2.2.3. BRONCHIECTASIS

LITERATURE

Of all the diseases of the lung, dilatation of the bronchial arteries is greatest in bronchiectasis. These arteries supply the abundant vascularization of the inflammatory process. According to LIEBOW ET AL. (1949), the increased blood supply is determined by three factors: 1. the organization of the pneumonitis in the surrounding interstitial tissue, 2. the hypertrophy of smooth muscle tissue in the ectatic bronchial wall, and 3. the proliferation of lymphoid tissue in the bronchial wall. Around bronchiectatic sacculi, angiomatous networks are formed (COCKETT AND VASS, 1951; DELARUE ET AL., 1953) in which aneurysms sometimes develop. According to cast preparations made by LIEBOW ET AL. (1949) and COCKETT AND VASS (1951) the aneurysms can rupture and thus lead to copious bleeding. LATARJET (1956) has pointed out, however, that these pictures may be the result of defective preparation.

The main cause of the dilatation of the bronchial arteries is, nevertheless, the broncho-pulmonary anastomoses, which determine the vascular picture in bronchiectasis. They have been found by all authors, several of whom have demonstrated them clearly in casts (LIEBOW ET AL., 1949; MARCHAND ET AL., 1950; COCKETT AND VASS, 1951; LATARJET AND JUTTIN, 1952; DELARUE ET AL., 1953). In these casts the bronchial arteries can be followed axially along the pulmonary arteries. Before anastomosing (end-to-side or side-to-side), the bronchial artery often shows a tortuous course over a short distance, sometimes twisting around the pulmonary artery several times (LIEBOW ET AL., 1949; COCKETT AND VASS, 1951; TOBIN, 1952; CAMARRI AND MARINI, 1965; see also fig. 62). TURNER-WARWICK (1963a) also found a second type of broncho-pulmonary anastomosis in the vascular network around the bronchiectatic sacculus.

According to LIEBOW ET AL. (1949–1950) and COCKETT AND VASS (1951), the most proximal anastomoses are localized near bronchi of the 3rd and 4th order (the segmental bronchus being of the 1st order). The bloodflow through the anastomoses was determined at 11 per cent (FRITTS ET AL., 1961) and 17.9 per cent (CUDKOWICZ ET AL., 1959) of the output of the left ventricle, and was estimated by LIEBOW ET AL. (1949) to be 1 liter per minute. For a detailed discussion of the genesis, significance, and consequences of these shunts, the reader is referred to the section on broncho-pulmonary anastomoses.

According to most of the authors (e.g. COCKETT AND VASS, 1951; CUDKOWICZ AND ARMSTRONG, 1953a;

CAMARRI AND MARINI, 1965), the branches of the pulmonary arteries in the vicinity of the lesions are obliterated by thrombosis or intimal proliferation, but according to other authors this is seldom (LATARJET, 1954b) or never (KOURILSKY ET AL., 1961) the case. CAMARRI AND MARINI (1965) state that the capillary bed also often shows marked reduction, and this is supported by the observations of TAMME-LING ET AL. (1967), who found in a case of unilateral bronchiectasis that the alveolar capillary bed was not supplied with either bronchial or pulmonary blood.

According to COCKETT AND VASS (1951) and CUDKOWICZ AND ARMSTRONG (1953a), the thrombosed pulmonary arteries are recanalized by bronchial arteries, after which broncho-pulmonary anastomoses are established. CUDKOWICZ AND ARMSTRONG attribute this recanalization to abnormal bronchial branches – termed 'aberrant bronchial arteries' – since they report that the normal branches of the bronchial arteries in the bronchiectatic region are obliterated.

The obliteration of bronchial arteries was also observed by AMEUILLE AND LEMOINE (1935) who, like DELARUE ET AL. (1952) considered the bronchiectatic changes to be a result of the abnormal bronchial vascularization. These authors therefore assume a vascular pathogenesis for bronchiectasis, in conflict with all the other authors, who see the changes in the bronchial circulation as the result of the inflammatory process. Experimental confirmation of the former hypothesis has not been obtained, although ELLIS ET AL. (1951) observed bronchiectasis in one out of thirteen dogs, four months after experimental occlusion of bronchial arteries.

In cases of extensive bronchiectasis the caliber of the large branches of the pulmonary artery becomes smaller, as is seen, for instance, in the bronchiectatic cystic lung (LANDRIGAN ET AL., 1963). KOURILSKY ET AL. (1961) attribute this anomaly to hypoplasia of the pulmonary artery. According to ABELANET (1961), a distinction can be made between congenital and acquired bronchiectasis on the basis of the histological appearance of the pulmonary artery, hypoplastic pulmonary arteries being an indication of the congenital form and hypotrophic pulmonary arteries of the acquired form.

The radiological literature reports the angiographic investigation of bronchiectasis both by aortography (ALLEY ET AL., 1958; NEYAZAKI, 1964; HUTCHIN ET AL., 1967) and by selective arteriography (VIAMONTE, 1964; VIAMONTE ET AL., 1965, 1967; BOIJSEN AND ZSIGMOND, 1965; SCHOBER, 1965; E COSTA, 1967; POLÁK ET AL., 1967; DARKE AND LEWTAS, 1968). It is remarkable that the broncho-pulmonary anastomoses were consistently recognized aortographically, but selectively only by VIAMONTE ET AL., POLÁK ET AL., and DARKE AND LEWTAS.

FINDINGS IN ARTERIOGRAPHY

Bronchial arteriography was performed in 11 patients with bronchiectasis. The arteriographical data were compared with the bronchographical findings and the clinical condition of the patient. Fig. 91 gives a composite view of the most important arteriographic findings and fig. 92, in the same sequence, the corresponding bronchographic findings. The letters under the illustrations correspond with the cases in table 22. For technical reasons, only 9 of the 11 cases are included in the composite figures (A–E, G, H, J, K). For each of these patients, only the bronchial vascularization of the lung with the most severe bronchiectatic changes is shown. When several bronchial arteries participated in the vascularization, as in Case B in which the pathological region was supplied by four bronchial arteries, the most abnormal arteriogram was chosen as illustration.

Fig. 91. Bronchial arteriography in bronchiectasis. The letters under the illustrations correspond with the cases in Table 22. For cases A, C, and E the broncho-pulmonary shunts are better visualized in Figs. 69*a*, 59, and 66, respectively. The arrow in C indicates an abrupt decrease in caliber in the peripheral course of the bronchial artery.

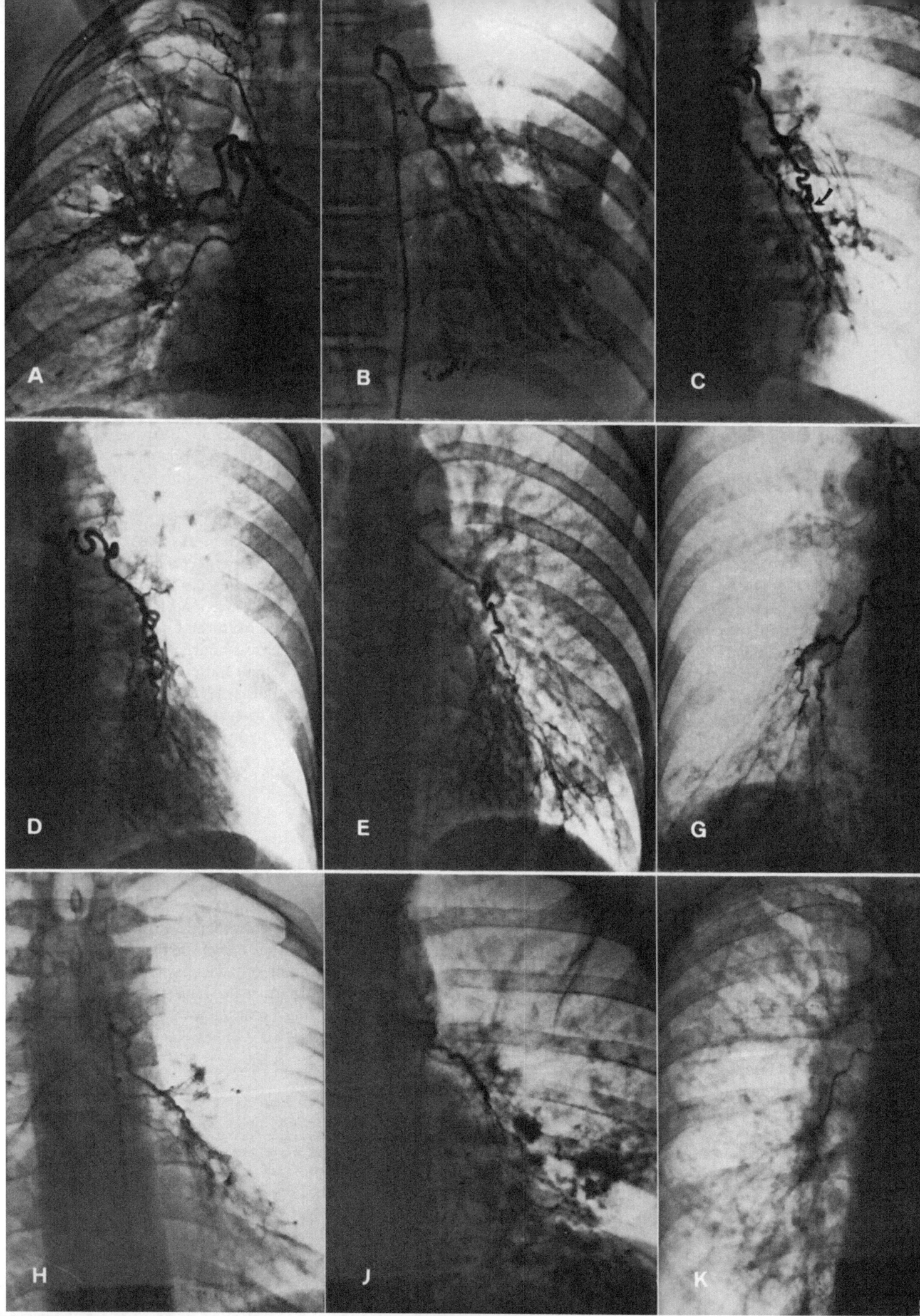

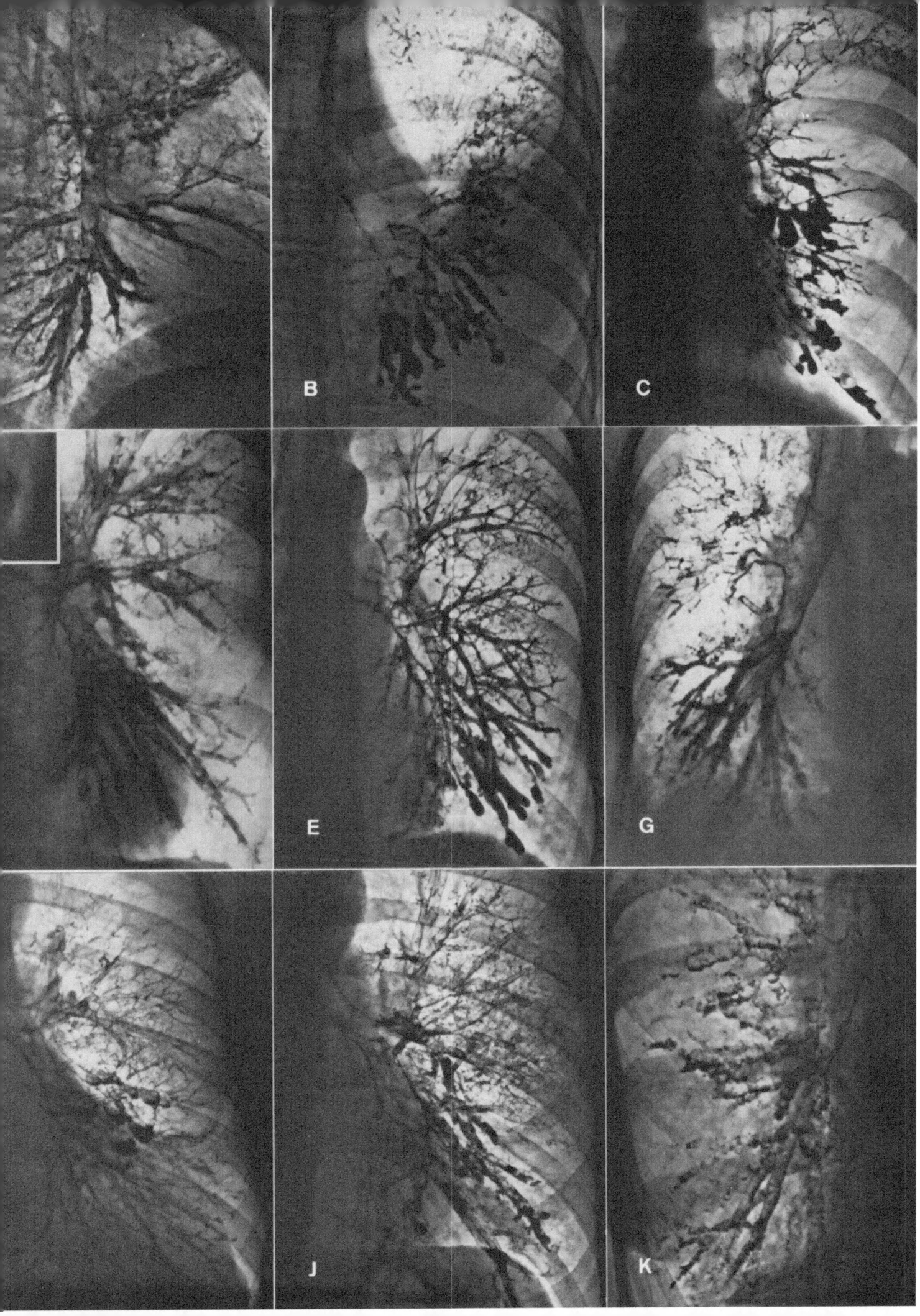

The data of these patients are shown in table 22. The sequence in which the cases are arranged is not arbitrary but in order of decreasing bronchial flow and therefore of decreasing abnormality of the arteriographic appearance. To obtain a measure for the bronchial flow, we divided, for each lung, the cross-section (in mm^2) of the supplying bronchial arteries by the number of bronchiectatic segments. Since the increase in the caliber of the bronchial arteries is determined almost exclusively by the pathological segments, the result of this calculation is a measure of the volume of the bronchial flow per bronchiectatic lung segment. When both lungs showed anomalies, we gave precedence to the lung with the most severe anomalies in determining the sequence for table 22. In summarization, for cases A–K the bronchial blood flow per ectatic bronchus decreases gradually.

The results of our investigation will be discussed, by stages, on the basis of table 22.

Type of the bronchiectasis

A distinction was made between saccular and cylindrical bronchiectasis. In some cases both forms occurred simultaneously. In the first half of the cases the saccular type predominates, in the second half the cylindrical (χ^2:7.84; p<0.01).

Between the degree of the bronchial vascularization (in the sequence A–K) and the nature of the bronchiectasis, however, no significant correlation was found (r_s:+ .33; n.s.). This is explained by the discrepancy between the nature of the changes and the bronchial vascularization in the last case (K); but this case also showed a rather severe pulmonary emphysema in which, as will be duly discussed, there is a decrease in bronchial vascularization. This situation probably clarifies much of the contradiction between the presence of generalized saccular bronchiectasis and the virtually normal bronchial circulation (Figs. 91, 92:K). If this last case is left out of consideration, there is a good correlation (r_s:+ .64; p<0.05), the bronchial arteries in saccular bronchiectasis being significantly wider than in cylindrical bronchiectasis.

Severity of the changes

The severity was rated according to five grades (0–4). Grade 0 means that a normal bronchial tree was present, and grade 4 was used for the most severely deformed bronchi. No correlation was found between the severity of the deformation and the degree of hypervascularization, as is immediately evident from a comparison of fig. 91 with 92. In case H, for instance, the bronchiectasis was very severe but there is almost no abnormal bronchial vascularization. There is also no demonstrable relationship between the deformation of the bronchi and the other factors shown in table 22, although there is of course some correlation with the type of bronchiectasis, since the saccular form gives the most deformation.

Quotient of the surface of the cross-section of the bronchial arteries in mm^2 and the number of bronchiectatic segments

This quotient – as already mentioned – is a measure for the bronchial vascularization per diseased bronchus. This value varies very widely between individuals, but since it is proportional to the square of the radius of the relevant bronchial arteries – whereas the rate of flow is, according to the law of POISEUILLE, proportional to the fourth power of the radius – the actual differences in the bronchial flow between individuals are still much greater.

Fig. 92. Bronchograms of the pathologically vascularized areas (same sequence as in Fig. 91). The bronchiectasis in case A was visualized more clearly in the lateral projection. The inset in D shows a tomogram of the posterobasal area on the left side; the saccular bronchiectasis was not filled bronchographically.

TABLE 22. Arteriographical, radiological, and clinical data in 11 patients with bronchiectasis.

	TYPE OF THE BRONCHIECTASIS	SEVERITY	DISEASED SEGMENTS	CROSS-SECTION (MM²)	QUOTIENT	BRONCHO-PULM. ANAST.	LOCALIZATION BRONCHO-PULM. ANASTOMOSES	BRONCHO-BRONCH. ANAST.	TORTUOSITY	PENETRATION	NEWLY FORMED VESSELS	ABRUPT NARROWING	HILAR GLANDS	CONDITION
A Right	saccular	3	2	32	16	+++!	1 parahilar	?	++	$\frac{1}{2}$?[4]	?[4]	-	+	poor
A Left	normal	0	0											
B Right	normal	0	0	92	15	+++	2 parahilar (-peripheral)	+++	+	$\frac{2}{3}$-1	+	±	-	poor
B LEFT	(cyl.)sacc.	4	6											
C RIGHT	saccular	(3)[1]	(3)[1]	91	13	+++	2 parahilar (-peripheral)	++	++	$\frac{2}{3}$-1	+	+	+	moderate
C LEFT	saccular	4	5	45										
D RIGHT	normal	0	0	19	8½	++	3 (parahilar-) peripheral	?	+++	$\frac{2}{3}$-1	+	-	+	moderate
D LEFT	cyl.(-sacc.)	2	2											
E RIGHT	cylindrical	1	4	22	(5½)[2]	++	3 (parahilar-) peripheral	++	-/+	$\frac{3}{3}$-1	+	-	+	moderate
E LEFT	cyl.-sacc.	3	4	33	8+									
F RIGHT	cyl.-sacc.	3	1½	13	(9-)[2]	+	4 peripheral	++/+++	+	$\frac{2}{3}$-1	+	-	±	fair
F LEFT	cylindrical	3	4	32	8									
G RIGHT	cylindrical	1	5	26	5+	+	5 very peripheral	?	+/++	1	+	-	-	fair
G LEFT	cylindrical	1	4	19	(5-)[2]									
H RIGHT	normal	0	0			±	5 very peripheral	+	-	$\frac{2}{3}$	±	-	-	fair
H LEFT	saccular	4	2	10	5									
I RIGHT	cylindrical	1	2	8	4	+	4 peripheral	?	-	$\frac{2}{3}$-1	+	-	-	good
I LEFT	normal	0	0											
J RIGHT	normal	0	0	15	3	-		-	+	$\frac{0}{3}$	±	-	-	good
J LEFT	cylindrical	2	5½											
K RIGHT	saccular	3-4	9	10	1	-		-		$\frac{1}{2}$-1	-	-	-	good
K LEFT	saccular	3	9	11	1									

1 In this case the 3 pathological segments had already been removed surgically, but the bronchial arteries were still dilated.

2 The values between brackets refer to the lung with the least severe lesions.

3 No opinion could be expressed on broncho-bronchial anastomoses, because only the bronchial arteries directly involved in the vascularization of the process were visualized.

4 The large number of parahilar broncho-pulmonary anastomoses constituted a predilection route for the flow of the contrast medium, so that peripheral bronchial arterial branches were not filled.

Broncho-pulmonary anastomoses

The number of broncho-pulmonary anastomoses per case was classified into four groups: very many (+ + +), many (+ +), few (+), and none (—). Fig. 91 A–E show these anastomoses in order of decreasing number. For cases A, C, and E, however, these anastomoses can be seen more clearly in figs. 69, 59, and 66, respectively.

There is a strikingly good agreement between the number of anastomoses and the amount of the bronchial bloodflow. This is hardly surprising, in our opinion, since the bronchial flow increases when the resistance of the capillary bed is no longer encountered, permitting the blood to enter unimpeded a region with a lower arterial pressure.

Localization of the broncho-pulmonary anastomoses

In most of these cases the anastomoses per case were found at a similar distance from the pulmonary hilus. When anastomoses were present at different distances from the hilus, only the location of the most centrally situated anastomoses was determined. For all cases this varied from a parahilar location to one close to the visceral pleura. Five locations were distinguished. The site of the anastomoses showed a distinct correlation with the bronchial bloodflow, the flow increasing the closer the anastomoses were to the hilus. There is a simple hemodynamic explanation for this finding. The difference in pressure between the two arterial systems is smaller, the more peripheral the site of an anastomosis, because at the capillary level, there is virtually no difference between the systemic and pulmonary blood pressure.

Broncho-bronchial anastomoses

Four gradations were distinguished (+ + +, + +, +, —) on the basis of the number and caliber of these shunts. A reasonably good correlation was found with the quantity of the bronchial flow and therefore also with the number and localization of the broncho-pulmonary anastomoses. However, this correlation was not as good as we had expected, since we had originally thought that the dilatation of broncho-bronchial anastomoses would keep pace with the increase in the bronchial flow. We now have the impression, however, that the broncho-pulmonary anastomoses develop more rapidly than the broncho-bronchial shunts.

In the illustrations in fig. 91 few broncho-bronchial anastomoses are visible because these shunts fill best during arteriography of the bronchial arteries vascularizing normal or almost normal parts of the lungs. They can be clearly seen, however, in fig. 57 (Case B), fig. 54 (Case C), and fig. 53 (Case F) in the section on broncho-bronchial anastomoses.

Tortuosity

The tortuous course of the bronchial arteries is rather typical of bronchiectasis. Fig. 91, A and D give the best illustration of this situation. No distinct relationship between tortuousity and the volume of the bronchial flow was found.

Penetration

The values shown in table 22 indicate how far peripherally in the lung bronchial arteries were demonstrated arteriographically. Under normal conditions no bronchial arteries are visible in the lateral half of the lung, but in bronchiectasis they can be followed far into the lung and sometimes as fas ar the pleura (Figs. 91G and 94a). Exceptions are formed by patients A and K, but these are unusual cases. In patient A the large number of wide parahilar shunts formed a more direct route for the contrast medium, so that peripheral bronchial arteries were probably not filled. The special case of patient K has already been mentioned.

Formation of new vessels

Almost all these cases showed a few unusual vessels with a course deviating from that of bronchial arteries. An example is shown in fig. 91 C (lateral of the arrow). In agreement with the view of others[1], we are of the opinion that these were newly formed vessels. For the reasons mentioned above, the first and last cases occupied an exceptional position in this respect too.

Abrupt narrowing

In arborizing, the bronchial arteries showed a gradual decrease in caliber. Two cases, however, showed an abrupt decrease in caliber for which a satisfactory explanation could not be found; an example of this is shown in fig. 91C (arrow). It is conceivable that this stenosis could have been caused by a pathological gland at the site of bifurcation of a segmental or lobular bronchus.

Hilar glands

Inflammation of hilus glands was suspected when a pathological vascularization of the hilar region (Fig. 93) or a stenosis in the central segment of the bronchial arteries (Fig. 94) was visible on the arteriogram. In four of the five cases in which inflamed hilus glands were suspected, histological findings were available and indeed showed highly active or chronic inflammatory phenomena in the hilus glands.

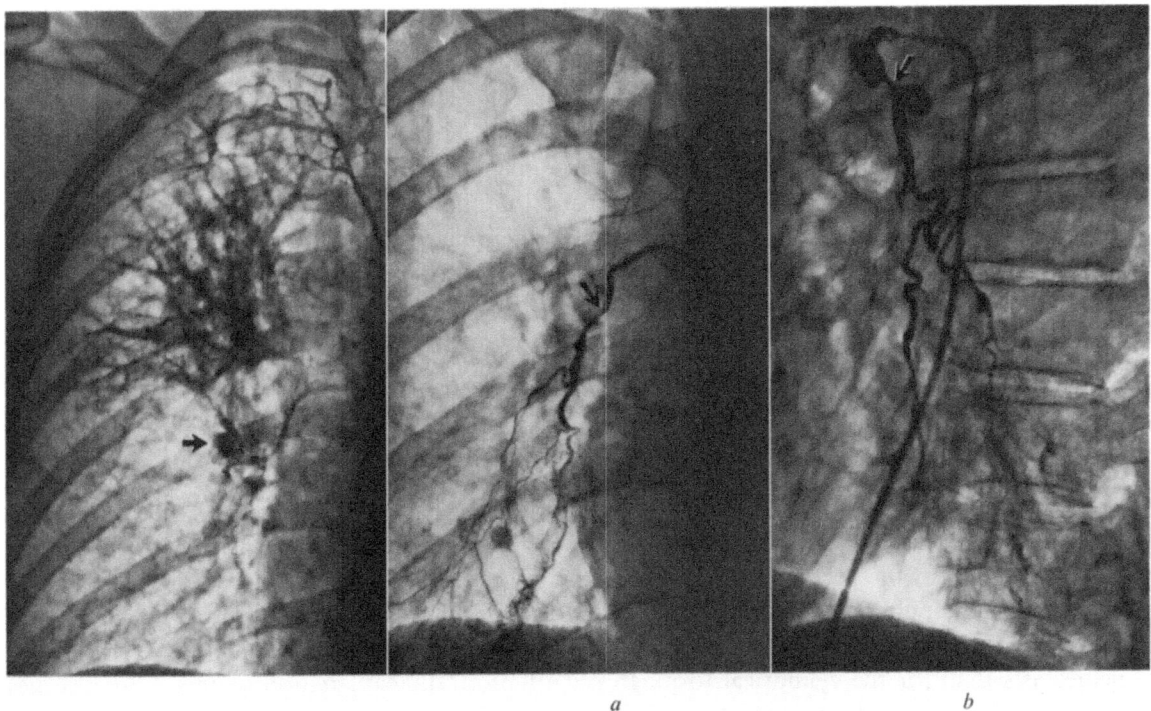

Fig. 93   a   Fig. 94   b

Fig. 93. Pathologically vascularized hilar gland (arrow) in case A. Figs. 69a and 91A show an earlier phase of the same arteriogram, but the massive broncho-pulmonary flow is better illustrated here.

Fig. 94. The constriction in the central part of the bronchial artery (arrows) constitutes a possible indication of inflamed hilar glands.

a: Bronchial arteriogram on the right side in case E.

b: Arteriogram in the lateral projection, case D. The dorsal shadow is caused by the wide saccular bronchiectasis (see also Fig. 92D: inset).

---

[1] e.g. WOOD AND MILLER (1938) and CUDKOWICZ AND ARMSTRONG (1953a).

Condition of the patient

The patient's condition was determined on the basis of a number of data obtained from the hospital record (temperature, malaise, appetite, etc.) and the degree of illness noticed during our examination. A distinction was made between a poor, moderate, fair, and good condition. The agreement with the degree of bronchial vascularization is striking and will be discussed below.

DISCUSSION

VIAMONTE ET AL. (1965) found no correlation between the bronchographic changes and bronchial hypervascularization. They thought it likely that there is a relationship between the hypervascularization and the activity of the inflammatory process in the bronchial wall. In our opinion, this assumption is correct but requires further elucidation.

According to our study, there is a strikingly good correlation between the increase of the bronchial circulation and the patient's clinical condition. How is this to be explained?

First of all, the increase of the bronchial flow and the dilatation of the bronchial arteries are a direct result of the development of broncho-pulmonary shunts. The connective element, however, is formed by the inflammatory process accompanying the bronchiectasis. On the one hand this inflammation causes complaints and on the other hand it impedes adequate oxygenation and thus leads to the formation and dilatation of broncho-pulmonary shunts.[1]

A few of our patients were treated surgically soon enough after investigation to permit useful comparison of the arteriographic results with the histological findings of the resected tissue. In these cases there was indeed more inflammatory infiltrate the higher the number of broncho-pulmonary anastomoses.

In the section on broncho-pulmonary anastomoses[2] mention was made of two patients with bronchiectasis (Cases A and E) showing a decrease in the number of broncho-pulmonary shunts. This decrease was accompanied by diminishment of the inflammatory phenomena and the complaints of both patients. This correlation was presumed earlier by GASTAING ET AL. (1961).

All in all, there are sufficient indications to justify formulation of the following statement: *The dilation of the bronchial arteries in bronchiectasis is a result of the development of broncho-pulmonary anastomoses; this development runs parallel with the intensity of the inflammatory process and with the patient's complaints.* This statement, however, does not afford an indication for arteriography.

With respect to the opinion of VIAMONTE ET AL. (1965), that there is no relationship between the bronchographic lesion and the bronchial hypervascularization, the following may be said. It is true that we found no relationship between the severity of the deformation of the bronchi and the increase of the bronchial circulation, but we did find one between the type of bronchiectasis and the extent of bronchial circulation. In saccular bronchiectasis there were wider bronchial arteries and a greater number of broncho-pulmonary shunts than in cylindrical bronchiectasis. This is in agreement with the findings of NAKAMURA ET AL. (1961), who calculated a greater broncho-pulmonary flow for saccular bronchiectasis than for the cylindrical form. In our opinion, the explanation of this difference lies in the fact that in saccular bronchiectasis the inflammatory factor is usually more severe.

In three patients we made an interesting observation: the bronchographically normal parts of the lungs showed a bronchial vascularization with the same characteristics as that of the bronchiectatic parts of the lung. VIAMONTE ET AL. (1965) made a similar observation. The meaning of this phenomenon is not clear. These vascular changes in otherwise normal areas are certainly the result of a local inflammation. The assumption of a pre-existent condition leading to a predisposition to the development of

---

[1] See Broncho-Pulmonary Anastomoses, Discussion of the Data in the Literature (page 93).
[2] See under Developmental Course (pag. 99).

bronchiectasis is perhaps too far-reaching. These changes may be only the result of an infection due to the aspiration of infected sputum from bronchiectatic segments. In any case, bronchial arteriography is the only way in which these changes can be demonstrated. If such changes are found in a patient with bronchiectasis, it might be advisable to postpone surgery and treat the inflammatory process first.

In one patient (Case B) for whom the diagnosis long-standing, possibly congenital bronchiectasis was considered, we saw unusually thin pulmonary arteries. According to ABELANET (1961), thin hypotrophic pulmonary arteries occur in congenital bronchiectasis but these arteries can also show smaller calibers in severe acquired forms of bronchiectasis. This patient also showed a very rapid venous drainage of the contrast medium from the pathological region, suggesting the presence of arteriovenous pulmonary shunts. The fact that this was the only patient with aberrantly arising accessory bronchial arteries contributing to the vascularization of the process, might argue in favor of the presence of a congenital anomaly.

In contrast to the situation for tumors, the evaluation of the hilar glands in cases of bronchiectasis is reasonably reliable. Both primary (pathological vascularization) and secondary (narrowed bronchial arteries) indications for inflamed hilar glands were obtained. Like AMEUILLE AND LEMOINE (1935) and LATARJET (1954b), we found centrally stenosed and deformed bronchial arteries in and near chronically inflamed lymph node packages (Fig. 94).

Finally, we also performed bronchial arteriography in two patients with bleeding bronchiectasis. The data of these patients were not included in table 22 because they were investigated later than the rest of the material. It proved impossible to locate the site of the bleeding, as it had already stopped before the arteriography. We could only indicate the most highly vascularized region as the most probable location. SWIERENGA (1968) has pointed the severe form these hemorrhages can take. Despite our limited experience, we think that these cases should be considered to offer an indication for bronchial arteriography until it becomes certain that the clinical value is too limited to justify its application. Only data obtained in larger series can show whether the arteriographic supplementation of the bronchoscopic findings can increase the chance that the part of the lung that is or has been bleeding can be located with certainty.

CONCLUSIONS

1. The dilatation of the bronchial arteries in bronchiectasis is a result of the development of bronchopulmonary anastomoses. This development runs parallel with the intensity of the inflammatory process and with the condition of the patient.
2. There is no correlation between the bronchial circulation and the severity of the bronchiectasis, but there is a relation with the type of bronchiectasis, the bronchial flow being greater in the saccular than in the cylindrical forms.
3. The bronchial vascularization in bronchiectasis shows a typical picture with wide tortuous bronchial arteries which seem to penetrate deeply into the lungs. There are broncho-pulmonary and often broncho-bronchial shunts, and in some instances highly irregular, possibly newly formed arteries with an abnormal course. The bronchial flow shows wide differences among individuals.
4. Bronchial arteriography is the only method of investigation by which changes in the bronchographically normal parts of the lung can be demonstrated, but the clinical significance of such finding is still unclear.
5. Clearly defined indications cannot be given, but the application of arteriography seems recommendable in two situations:
   a. pre-operatively, to determine whether anomalies are present in the bronchographically normal parts of the lungs.
   b. In bleeding bronchiectasis.

IV.2.2.4. EMPHYSEMA

LITERATURE

The bronchial vascularization in pulmonary emphysema has been studied by many investigators. Several striking points of disagreement have emerged from these studies.

According to WOOD AND MILLER (1938) and FLORANGE (1960), there is usually an increase in the bronchial circulation, but according to WYATT ET AL. (1964) it is generally normal. The other authors, however, found a decrease, which they attribute to obliteration of the bronchial arteries. Hypervascularization was seen only in the presence of secondary changes in the form of infections, bronchiectasis, or extensive fibrosis.

According to CRENSHAW AND ROWLES, (1952) CUDKOWICZ AND ARMSTRONG (1953a), and REID AND HEARD (1963), obliterative changes also occur in branches of the pulmonary artery, but according to LIEBOW (1959) and HEPPLESTON AND LEOPOLD (1961) this is seldom the case. CAMARRI AND MARINI (1965) are of the opinion that there is a correlation between the severity of the emphysematous changes and the reduction of the pulmonary vascular bed.

There is also disagreement concerning the forms taken by emphysema. In the morphological studies different classifications are given, distinguishing between, for instance, panlobular, centrilobular, vesicular, focal, diffusely hypertrophic, bullous, and irregular emphysema, the vascularization differing according to the type. According to WYATT ET AL. (1962), none of the phenomena of emphysema is specific.

A number of theories have been put forward to explain the genesis of emphysema (WRIGHT, 1960; STRAWBRIDGE, 1960a & b; HEPPLESTON AND LEOPOLD, 1961; WRIGHT AND KLEINERMAN, 1963; O'LOUGHLIN, 1965). HEPPLESTON AND LEOPOLD even mention eleven possible causes and factors that could be of influence: inflammation, organic obstructions, physiological obstructions (expiratory valve mechanism), loss of elasticity, too little smooth muscle tissue in the bronchial wall, an abnormally formed thoracic skeleton, diminished ventilation, inspiratory air flow, rupture and atrophy of the connective tissue framework of the lung, loss of the normal tension of the lungs, rupture of the wall of the acinus. Several authors (KOROL, 1938; CUDKOWICZ AND ARMSTRONG, 1953a; CRENSHAW, 1954) think that emphysema is caused solely by obliterative changes in the bronchial arteries, but LIEBOW (1959), HEPPLESTON AND LEOPOLD (1961), and STRAWBRIDGE (1960a) believe these changes to be secondary.

CUDKOWICZ AND ARMSTRONG (1953a) found obliterated bronchial arteries due to medial hypertrophy and intimal proliferation beginning peripherally and sometimes reaching as far as the extrapulmonary parts of the bronchial arteries. Abnormal bronchial arteries, called 'aberrant' by these authors and possibly newly formed, penetrate deeper into the lung and anastomose with the pulmonary arteries in regions showing secondary changes, often in the form af bronchiectasis.

CRENSHAW (1954) was so strongly convinced of the vascular pathogenesis of emphysema that he advised that these patients be treated by parietal pleurectomy to promote better vascularization of the ischemic and damaged lung tissue by inducing the development of derivatives of intercostal arteries. Although this method was widely criticized, he claimed to have obtained good results.

Animal experiments have been used to investigate whether emphysema results from occlusion of the bronchial arteries. For this purpose the bronchial arteries were injected with a sclerosing liquid or a plastic, since the studies of KARSNER AND ASH (1912/1912) and MATHES ET AL. (1931/1932) had shown that no effect can be obtained by the ligation of these arteries, due to the presence of so many collaterals. After injection with a sclerosing substance, EDWARDS (1961) found emphysematous changes in the lungs of the horse, which he, unlike MCLAUGHLIN ET AL. (1961), considers to show the same bronchial vascular pattern as the human lung. ELLIS ET AL. (1951), however, found no emphysematous changes in dogs after experimental obliteration of all bronchial branches with a diameter greater than 35 μ.

MARCHAND ET AL. (1950), CUDKOWICZ AND ARMSTRONG (1953a), and LIEBOW (1959) saw broncho-pulmonary anastomoses in regions with secondary changes (especially bronchiectasis). CUDKOWICZ ET AL. (1959), FISHMAN (1961), RYAN AND ABELMANN (1961), and NAKAMURA (1961), however, observed no increase of the bronchial flow in emphysema.

In emphysema patients the bronchial veins are dilated, and via them an extracardial shunt is formed between the right and the left atrium when the pressure in right atrium increases (LIEBOW ET AL., 1953; FISHMAN ET AL., 1961). According to these authors, this explains the cyanosis seen in emphysema patients.

The radiological literature contains a report by WILLIAMS ET AL. (1963) of a reduction of the bronchial circulation in emphysema as well as markedly wide intercostal arteries with an intercosto-pulmonary circulation via pleural adhesions.

Resumé

In 'uncomplicated' emphysema the bronchial vascularization is decreased by obliteration of the artery. In regions with secondary changes – i.e. bronchiectasis, infection, fibrosis – the bronchial vascularization is increased, mainly due to the formation of broncho-pulmonary shunts. It seems unlikely that obliteration of bronchial arteries causes pulmonary emphysema, but this point is not yet entirely clear.

FINDINGS IN ARTERIOGRAPHY

In eleven patients with a severe irreversible or almost irreversible expiratory dysfunction we performed bronchial arteriography. This material was divided into eight cases with probably diffuse emphysema and three cases with a probably bullous emphysema. This division was based on the radiological findings in the thorax. When there were no radiological changes or a *volumen pulmonum auctum* with a fine but regular pattern of the pulmonary vessels, we classified the case as diffuse pulmonary emphysema. A more detailed morphological differentiation could not be made because only two cases could be investigated histologically, and moreover the material was too small to make further differentiation profitable.

Four of the eight patients with 'diffuse pulmonary emphysema' had originally been investigated for another disease, but analysis of the lung function had shown that a severe irreversible expiratory dysfunction was also present. Of the three patients with 'bullous emphysema', two showed infected bullae (Fig. 84). Three patients also suffered from asthmatic bronchitis.

In eight cases the caliber of the bronchial arteries was remarkably small, and all the cases showed a strongly reduced bronchial vascularization in the emphysematous-bullous regions. Fig. 95 illustrates the bronchial vascularization in pulmonary emphysema. Only the bronchial arteries in the hilar region are clearly visible. Three patients showed local hypervascularization, i.e. both of the patients with infected bullae and a patient with frequently recurring infections. The latter patient was one of the two for whom histological findings were available, showing the presence of marked local fibrotic changes. Broncho-pulmonary shunts were seen only in these last three patients.

DISCUSSION

Our findings are in complete agreement with the data in the literature. In uncomplicated emphysema the bronchial vascularization is very limited, whereas in normal lungs the bronchial arteries can be followed arteriographically halfway into the lung, in emphysema patients they can be followed maximally a fourth of the distance between the hilus and the pleural region (Fig. 95*b*).

In two patients with local hypervascularization, highly abnormal branches of the bronchial arteries were seen. One of these cases is shown in fig. 96. These may represent the abnormal newly formed arteries described by CUDKOWICZ AND ARMSTRONG (1953a).

We did not find the dilation of the intercostal arteries and the intercosto-pulmonary anastomoses described by WILLIAMS ET AL. (1963).

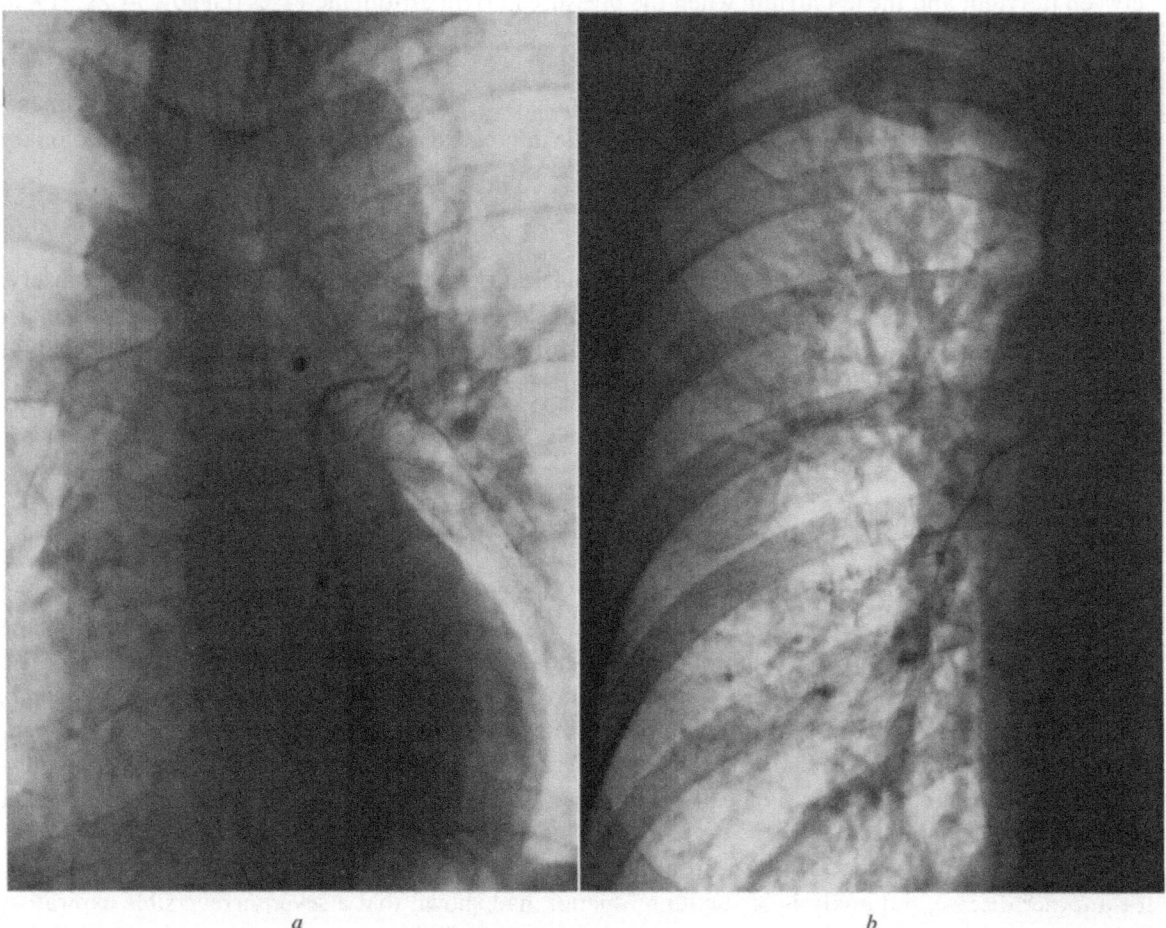

a   *b*

Fig. 95. Emphysema.
a: Abnormally small bronchial arteries. Radiologically, the vascularization remains restricted to the region the hilus.
b: Bronchial artery for the entire right lung (intercosto-bronchial trunk); its branches cannot be followed beyond the immediate parahilar region.

CONCLUSIONS

1. In pulmonary emphysema the bronchial vascularization is reduced and abnormally narrow bronchial arteries are present.
2. In the regions with secondary inflammatory changes there is local hypervascularization, often associated with broncho-pulmonary anastomoses.
3. The problem of the vascular pathogenesis due to obliteration of the bronchial arteries is not yet solved, but in all probability the vascular changes result from the emphysematous process.
4. There seems to be no indication for bronchial arteriography in patients with pulmonary emphysema.

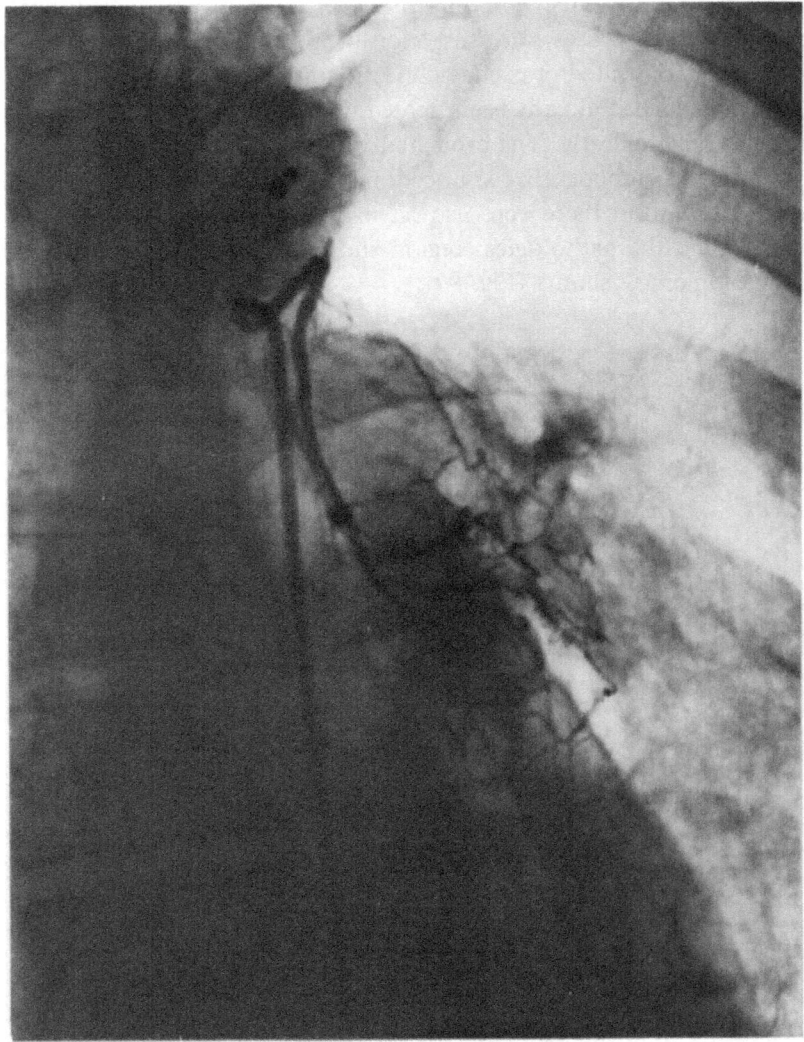

Fig. 96. Emphysema. Local hypervascularization with highly irregular branches of the bronchial artery: newly formed arteries?

IV.2.2.5. OTHER LESIONS

For the other lesions only a small number of patients was seen for each type, so that a detailed analysis of this material and a comparative study of the data in the literature are not worth-while. A brief discussion with some references to the literature will therefore suffice.

CHRONIC INFILTRATION

CUDKOWICZ (1952b) reports that after initial obstruction of the bronchial arteries in the acute pneumonic phase, patency is rather quickly restored. The bronchial arteries then become wider (FLORANGE, 1960) to a degree dependent on the severity of the inflammation (MATHES ET AL., 1931/1932) and broncho-pulmonary anastomoses develop (CAMARRI AND MARINI, 1965). If atelectasis develops, the broncho-pulmonary flow is substantial (GILROY ET AL., 1951) and measurable (RYAN AND ABELMANN, 1961).

We have investigated four patients with infiltrative changes in whom treatment did not lead to normal resorption. Since such cases raise suspicion of a lung tumor, an attempt was made to see whether this could be demonstrated or excluded arteriographically.

The first of these patients had already been treated with antibiotics for several months and showed only minimal changes radiologically. The bronchial vascularization was normal.

The second patient had a stubborn *B. coli* infection and was in a poor clinical condition at the time of our investigation. In addition, there were also extensive radiological changes. The bronchial arteries were strongly dilated and the pathological region showed marked hypervascularization and small peripheral broncho-pulmonary shunts (Fig. 97).

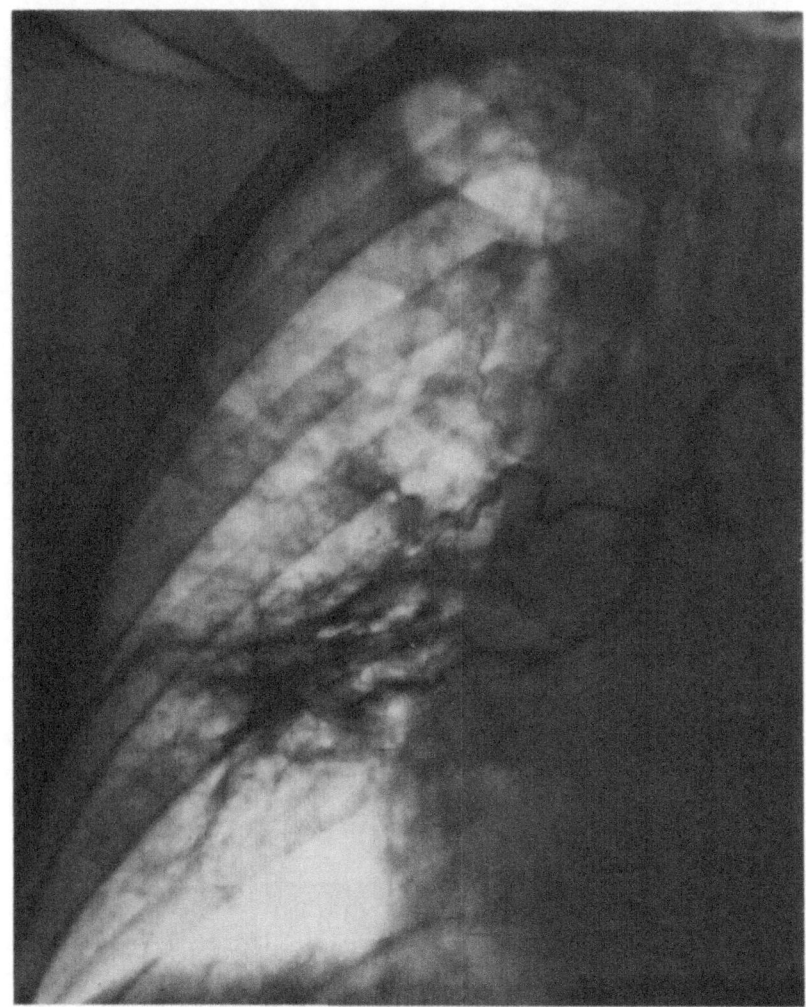

Fig. 97. Chronic infiltration, patient 2. Hypervascularization and a few broncho-pulmonary shunts.

The third patient too showed distinct residual lesions radiologically, but, like the first patient, was in good clinical condition. There was moderate local hypervascularization with a few peripheral broncho-pulmonary shunts.

The fourth patient, like the first, had undergone prolonged treatment with antibiotics, and only small residual changes were found radiologically. The bronchial arteriogram showed a limited local hypervascularization without broncho-pulmonary shunts.

NEWTON AND PREGER (1965) think that the bronchial vascularization of non-resorbing pneumonia has benign characteristics. According to VIAMONTE ET AL. (1965, 1967), arteriography is indicated in non-resorbing pneumonia to differentiate between benign and malignant processes, but no radiographic evidence is provided to support this conclusion. In our four cases we were unable to demonstrate a tumor, but neither we could exclude the possible presence of a malignant process (with the exception of richly vascularized tumors in the first and fourth patients). We are of the opinion that bronchial arteriography does not help to solve this problem, the more so since the vascular pattern of lung tumors, as already mentioned, has no specific features.

CHRONIC ASTHMATIC BRONCHITIS

Three of the four cases with chronic asthmatic bronchitis have been discussed under 'Emphysema.'
According to WYATT ET AL. (1964), the bronchial vascularization is increased in asthmatic bronchitis, but we were unable to confirm this conclusion. In two of our cases the vascularization was reduced, and in one slightly increased. No specific characteristics were found.

INFECTED CAVITIES

Two patients showed infected bullae and a third infected cysts, all three giving the same arteriographical picture. The two cases of infected bullae have already been discussed under 'Emphysema', and the arteriogram of one of them accompanies the discussion given under 'Tumors' (Fig. 84).
In all these patients the borders of the infected cavities showed local bronchial hypervascularization with broncho-pulmonary anastomoses.

DIFFUSE SMALL FOCAL LESIONS

Both cases with these changes showed small foci with bronchial hypervascularization. In one of these patients the diagnosis chronic interstitial lung fibrosis was made on the basis of a biopsy sample. In the other case the miliary lung picture was considered to be based on peribronchitis.

BRONCHOPLASTY

According to ELLIS ET AL. (1951), in the dog the bronchial circulation can be taken over by the pulmonary artery except in a small central area which comprises the main bronchus and the first few millimeters of the lobar bronchi. However, MATTHES AND FUCHS (1956) concluded that the entire canine bronchial circulation can be taken over by the pulmonary circulation. HUGGINS (1959) saw necrosis after transplantation of the lower lobe of a dog lung when the main bronchus was transected 1.5–2.0 cm proximally from the first segmental orifice of the lower lobe. In similar experiments DUVOISIN ET AL. (1964) also saw necrosis, followed by stenosis of the bronchus, the more frequently the closer the location of the anastomosis to the carina. The investigations of HUGGINS and DUVOISIN ET AL. confirmed the theory put forward by ELLIS ET AL. in 1951. According to LAUWERIJNS (1962), in man the anatomical relationships in this region are the same as in the dog.
BLANK ET AL. (1966) saw reconstitution of the bronchial arteries in dogs a year after autologous lung transplantation in which the bronchial artery had been transected. According to the results of similar experiments by STONE ET AL. (1966), the bronchial circulation recovers completely after four weeks. No similar data are available for man.

In two patients treated with bronchoplasty for small centrally situated tumors, we performed bronchial arteriography. In one, a segment of the left main bronchus had been resected around the orifice of the upper-lobe bronchus (Fig. 98a). After about 2.5 cm the bronchial artery ends abruptly, the distal portion of the artery being filled via a few tortuous collaterals (Fig. 98b). This patient also

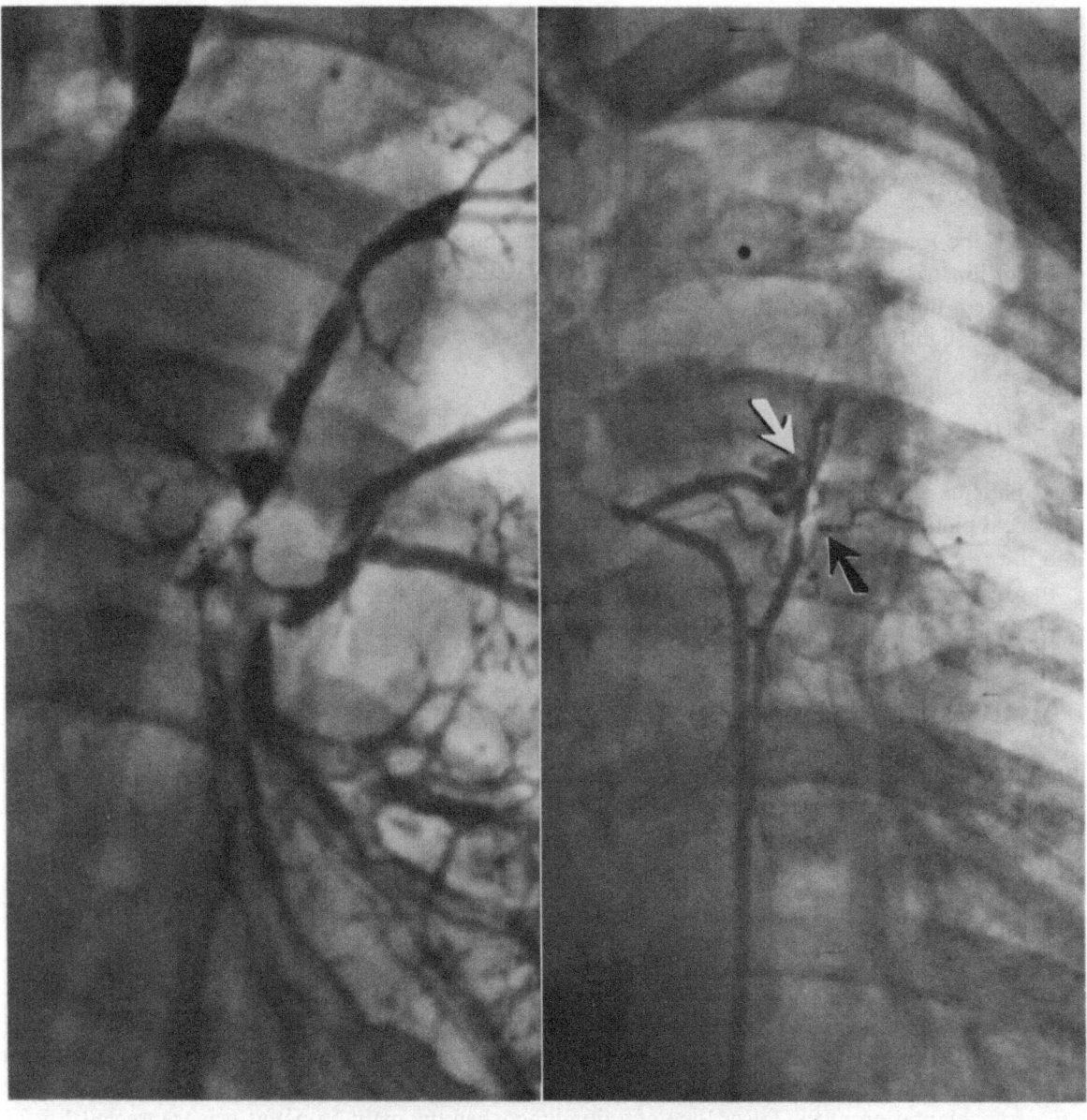

a   b

Fig. 98. Bronchoplasty.

a: End-to-end anastomosis between left main bronchus and lower-lobe bronchus. The bronchial artery in *b* appears to be occluded at the level of this anastomosis.

b: Abrupt termination of the bronchial artery after 2.5 cm (white arrow). Via thin, tortuous, probably newly formed collaterals, the contrast medium reaches the distal portion of the bronchial artery, the beginning of which is indicated by a black arrow. Fig. 39b shows a later phase of the same arteriogram and gives a better picture of this distal portion.

showed an unusual broncho-pulmonary anastomosis, probably of iatrogenic origin (Fig. 68). In the other patient the central part of the bronchial artery was intact but several of its branches terminated abruptly. These branches were connected with peripheral arterial rami of bronchial origin via broncho-bronchial anastomoses (Fig. 99). Furthermore, the arteriograms of this patient showed locally – in the region of the surgical anastomosis – a very unusual bronchial vascularization suggesting neo-formation.

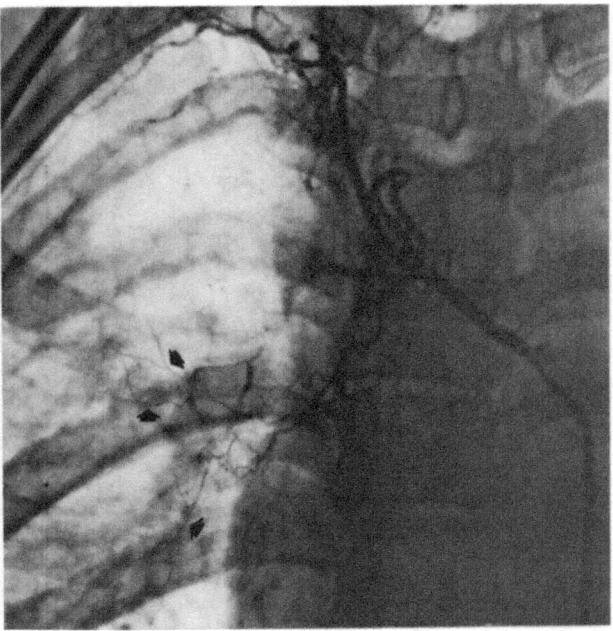

Fig. 99. Bronchoplasty. Visualization of peripheral arterial bronchial branches (arrows) filled via hilary broncho-bronchial anastomoses and newly formed vessels.

Four other cases in our material also showed pictures suggesting the reconstitution of bronchial arteries. All these patients had undergone a lobectomy or bilobectomy.

Neither of the two patients reported above showed stenosis of the bronchus after the operation, although the location of the anastomosis was sufficiently central to satisfy the criteria of ELLIS ET AL. (1951) and HUGGINS (1959). This might be explained by the fact that the bronchial circulation was restored via newly formed collaterals or broncho-bronchial anastomoses. We suspect, however, that even in the first of these patients, in whom the bronchial artery had been centrally transected or ligated, a sufficient number of rami had remained for the vascularization of the main bronchus. BLANK ET AL. (1966) considered the possibility of the development of neovascularization after severing the bronchial artery, but like these authors we are of the opinion that the reconstitution of the bron-chial circulation is effected mainly by communications to the original bronchial arteries. These communications develop, in our opinion, by neoformation (Figs. 98 and 99) or by widening of broncho-bronchial anastomoses (Fig. 99).

ASPERGILLOSIS

Two patients with an *aspergillus* infection and aspergilloma formation showed extensive long-standing tuberculous changes with retraction, destruction of lung tissue, bullous changes, and deformation of the bronchial tree. These fungus infections occur in preformed cavities.

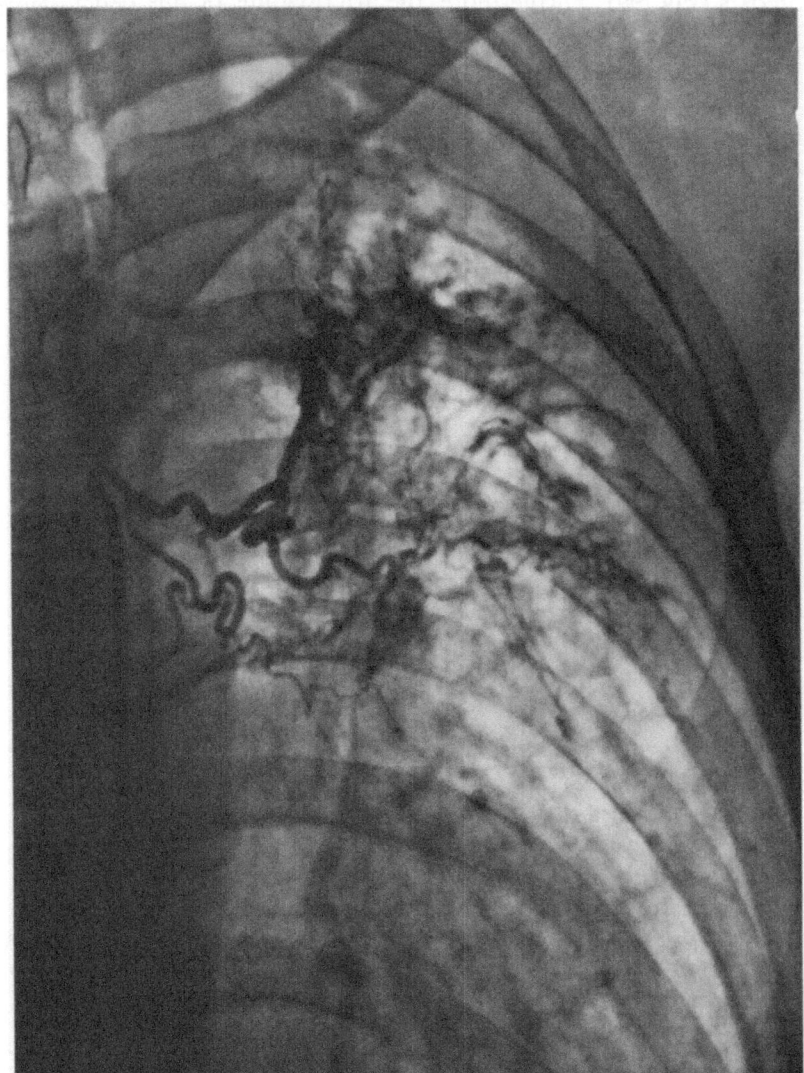

Fig. 100. *Aspergillus* infection in destroyed tuberculous lung tissue. Extremely rich bronchial vascularization.

The pathological process was extremely richly vascularized in both patients (Fig. 100), but because of the coexistent changes it would not be justifiable to assign diagnostic importance to this finding with respect to the vascularization of aspergillomas. Nevertheless, it seemed to us that the vascularization was appreciably greater than would be expected on the basis of the pre-existent anomalies alone.

VIAMONTE ET AL. (1965) give an example of vascularization in another fungus infection, actinomycosis. Here too, hypervascularization was present.

HEMOPTYSIS

The two patients with hemoptysis *e causa ignota* suffered from chronic bronchitis and BESNIER BOECK'S disease. Bronchial arteriography was done in a total of four patients with recurrent lung hemorrhages, two of whom have already been discussed in connection with bronchiectasis (page 135).

In three patients a region with local hypervascularization was demonstrated as the probable localization of the hemorrhages. Two of these patients were treated surgically, and the suspected region was resected during the operation. The fact that no more hemorrhages developed may be an indication that the bleeding part of the lung was indeed removed.

We therefore conclude that recurrent hemoptysis offers one of the best indications for selective bronchial arteriography. These cases require a *complete* bronchial arteriogram unless other investigations (e.g. bronchoscopy) have already yielded some information with respect to the site of the bleeding (e.g. right or left side).

PLEURAL TUMORS

Selective bronchial and intercostal arteriograms were made in two patients with benign pleural tumors. A histological investigation was performed in both cases, in one in a biopsy sample and in the other in resection material. In both cases the tumor proved to be benign; neurinoma, fibroma, and chondrofibroma were considered possible diagnoses. Our prior investigation had been unable to demonstrate vascularization of the lesion from either intercostal or bronchial arteries.

BRONCHOGENIC CYST

We investigated a patient with a large round shadow (diameter about 3 cm) in the anterior segment of the left upper lobe. The lesion was vascularized predominantly by a number of wide left bronchial arteries arising from two trunci communes (Fig. 101). Furthermore, four accessory, aberrantly arising bronchial arteries deriving from the left thyreocervical trunk and the left internal mammary artery also had a share in the vascularization. One of these arteries is shown in fig. 20. Around the coin lesion, parahilary and peripherally located broncho-pulmonary anastomoses were demonstrated (Fig. 101). An intercosto-bronchial anastomosis was also present (Fig. 76). Mainly on the basis of this finding, we suspected the lesion to be of a congenital nature.

The patient was treated surgically, and the pathologist found a fluid-filled infected bronchogenic cyst. The absence of pigment in the anterior segment suggests that ventilation had not occurred. According to DELARUE ET AL. (1959), this kind of anomaly is a form of intralobular sequestration.

NEWTON AND PREGER (1965) report that bronchial vascularization is normal in cases of bronchogenic cysts. According to LATARJET (1958), the bronchial arteries supplying such cysts have a normal or small caliber unless, as is often the case, there is inflammation. Apparently in our case, too, the inflammatory process was the cause of the bronchial hypervascularization and the numerous bronchopulmonary anastomoses.

SUPPURATIVE PNEUMONIA

The only case of this form of pneumonia in our material was a patient who had been treated for some time with antibiotics before our investigation. We found a slightly dilated tortuous bronchial artery, a moderate amount of local hypervascularization, and a few peripheral broncho-pulmonary anastomoses. There were, therefore, no specific features present. The vascularization pattern resembled most closely that of chronic infiltration.

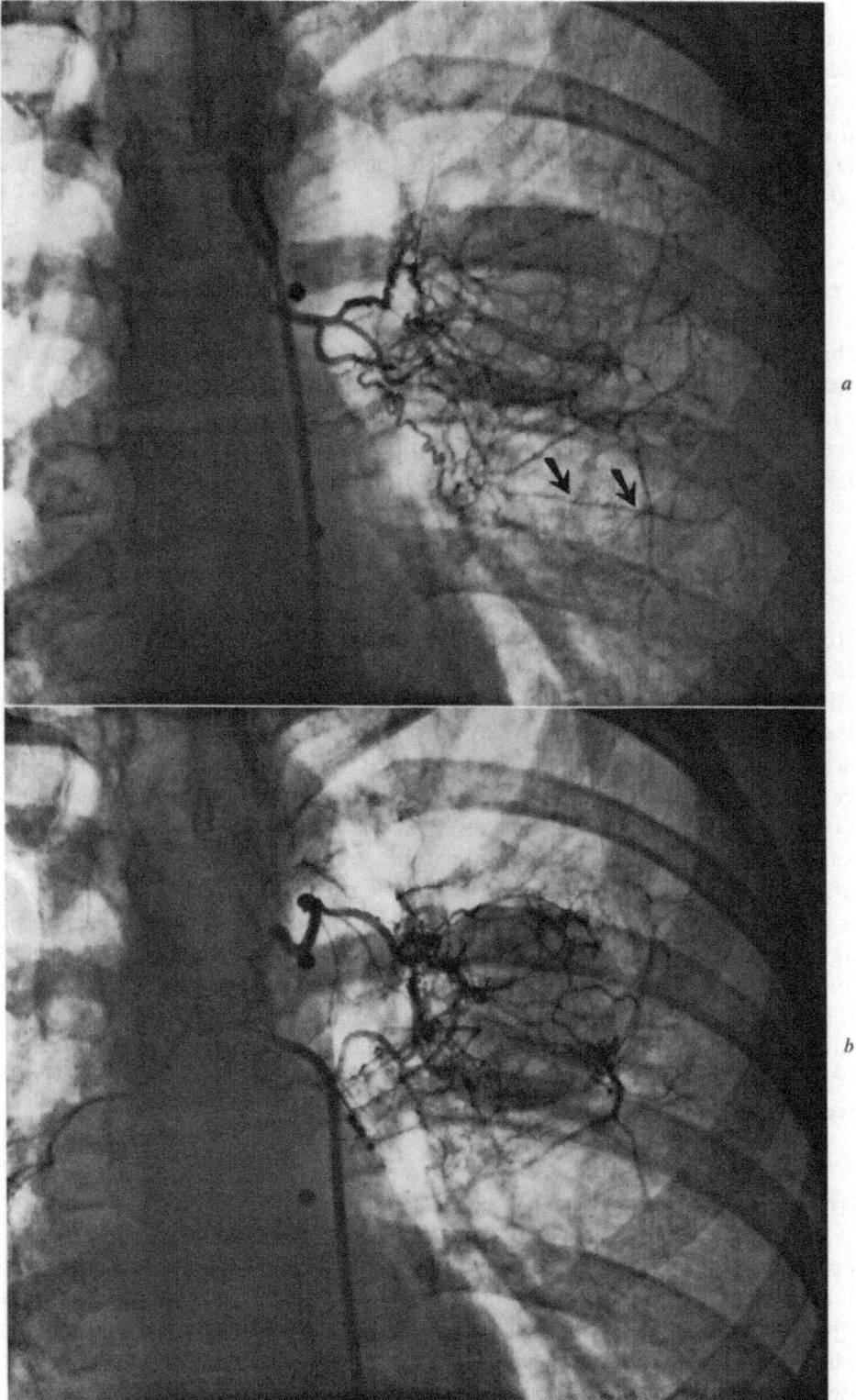

Fig. 101. Congenital bronchogenic cyst, supplied mainly by two wide left bronchial arteries (*a* and *b*). Abundant vascularization with numerous parahilar and peripheral broncho-pulmonary anastomoses around the coin lesion (see also Fig. 76). A long anastomotic canal is marked by arrows.

HISTIOCYTOSIS X

Our material included a seventeen year old girl showing severe destructive changes and cavity formation in the right lung, as well as a secondary infection of these anomalies. The bronchial artery was, however, strikingly small (Fig. 72*b*, white arrows) and even considerably thinner than in emphysema. The intercostal arteries were markedly dilated and there were numerous intercosto-pulmonary anastomoses (Figs. 10 and 72*b*). LIEBOW (1962) described identical changes in a five year old girl with histiocytosis X.

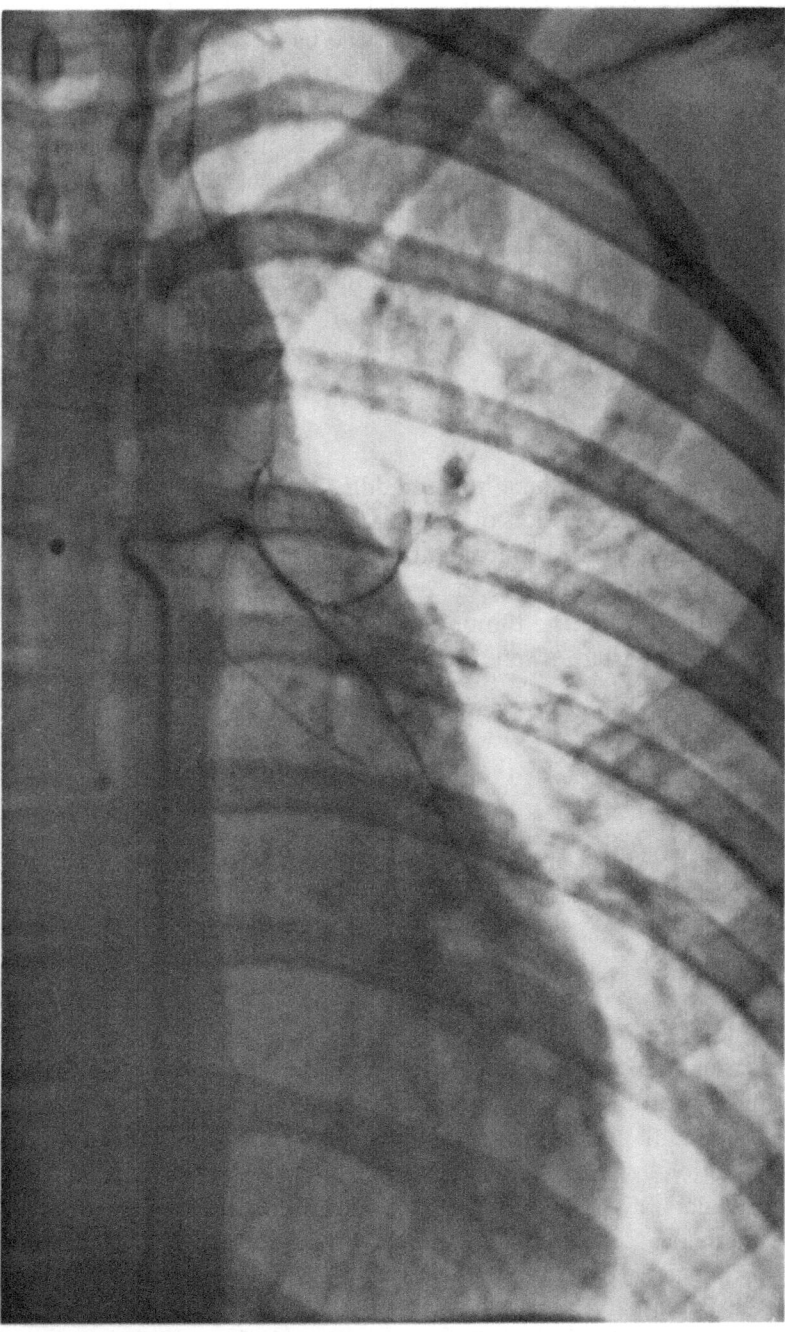

Fig. 102. Histiocytosis X. Strikingly thin left superior and inferior bronchial arteries. The left inferior bronchial artery is filled collaterally.

The left bronchial artery was also of a strikingly small caliber (Fig. 102), although the left lung showed no radiological changes and was still normal three years later.

The diagnosis histocytosis X was made on the basis of the histological evidence obtained after resection of a segment of the right upper lobe.

SUBPHRENIC ABSCESS

The material included one patient showing a right-sided subphrenic abscess with elevation of the diaphragm, pleural empyema, and compression of the basal segments of the right lower lobe. The bronchial artery was slightly dilated and tortuous, mainly in the inferior region. There were no broncho-pulmonary shunts, which in our opinion means that there were no appreciable inflammatory phenomena in the involved parts of the lung.

The arteriogram of the coeliac artery showed a dilated right inferior phrenic artery and a picture suggesting transpleural vascularization. Furthermore, an accessory bronchial artery seemed to arise from this phrenic artery. In our opinion, the dilation of the inferior phrenic artery was caused by the inflammatory process, since numerous tortuous branches arose from it, obviously serving for the supply of this process.

ESOPHAGEAL CARCINOMA

One of our patients showed a carcinoma in the middle third of the esophagus which, as mentioned in the anatomical section of the discussion of the data in the literature (page 23), is vascularized, either directly or via anastomoses, by the bronchial arteries.

Although the selective investigation of the bronchial arteries seemed to be complete in this case, our hope that vascularization of the tumor could be demonstrated in this way proved unfounded. No independent esophageal arteries were found.

IV.2.3. The bronchial circulation in heart disease

Tetralogy of Fallot

Much is known about the bronchial circulation in congenital cardiac anomalies with stenosis or atresia of the pulmonary arteries and particularly in the tetralogy of FALLOT. Most of the data on this subject are to be found in the cardiovascular and pathology literature. There are, however, almost no data on selective arteriography in these anomalies.

Most of the particulars of the bronchial circulation in the tetralogy of FALLOT have already been mentioned in the anatomical sections of the chapters 'Literature' and 'Results of the Present Study' (e.g. under Accessory Bronchial Arteries and Anastomoses) and in the section 'Anastomoses' (Broncho-Bronchial; Broncho-Pulmonary; Intercosto-Bronchial). Here, the characteristics of the bronchial circulation will be treated in the logical sequence, with as little repetition as possible. We will then discuss separately the four patients investigated, each of whom forms an individual problem.

The changes in the bronchial circulation found in the tetralogy of FALLOT are the results of a stenosis of the pulmonary artery. The bronchial arteries are strongly dilated (e.g. FATTI AND GILROY, 1949). The widest bronchial arteries have been found in the most extreme stenoses or hypoplasias of the pulmonary artery (EAST AND BARNARD, 1938) and in atresias or agenesias (MADOFF ET AL., 1952; TABAKIN ET AL., 1960; DONKERS, 1967). The number of bronchial arteries is greater than usual, because more accessory bronchial arteries are present (TAUSSIG, 1947; TYNAN AND GLEESON, 1966). The arteries often pursue an abnormal course, and they reach the lung via the pulmonary ligament (COLLISTER, 1952).

The dilation of the bronchial arteries is caused by the broncho-pulmonary bloodflow, which results from wide, usually centrally located broncho-pulmonary anastomoses (HALES AND LIEBOW, 1948; GUNTHEROTH ET AL., 1962). In cases of atresia of the pulmonary artery the prognosis is dependent on the development of the collateral pulmonary circulation (VENABLES, 1964). For hemodynamic reasons, the broncho-pulmonary flow will be greater the more severe the stenosis of the pulmonary artery. The site of this stenosis is thought to be even more important. HEIMBURG (1964) studied the broncho-pulmonary flow after experimental constriction of the main trunk of the pulmonary artery, the left or right branch, and a lobar branch. The heaviest flow developed when a lobar artery was constricted, a slightly less heavy flow after constriction of the left or right branch, and the least heavy after constriction of the main trunk. This can be explained as follows. With constriction of the main trunk, elevation of the systolic pressure in the right ventricle can re-establish the pulmonary flow. With constriction of the left or right branch, elevation of the systolic pressure in R.V. mainly increases the flow through the normal branch. Unless the peripheral resistance on the side of the normal branch is greatly increased, the pressure behind the stenosis will remain too low and a broncho-pulmonary flow will develop. For analogous reasons, this effect is even stronger when a lobar artery is constricted.

According to NAKAMURA ET AL. (1967), there is no clear correlation between the broncho-pulmonary flow on the one hand and the pulmonary flow, the pulmonary blood pressure, the oxygen saturation in the systemic circulation, the severity of the disease, and the age of the patient on the other hand.

In the tetralogy of FALLOT not only broncho-pulmonary anastomoses but also wide broncho-bronchial anastomoses are found (COLLISTER, 1952). Some cases show intercosto-bronchial anastomoses as well.

After thoracotomy, intercosto-pulmonary anastomoses develop (see under Intercosto-Pulmonary Anastomoses, Literature, page 101). The intercosto-pulmonary flow improves the pulmonary circulation. In this connection BARRETT AND DALEY proposed as early as 1949 that patients with tetralogy of FALLOT be treated with parietal pleurectomy.

FINDINGS IN ARTERIOGRAPHY

General observations

In addition to greatly dilated but otherwise normal bronchial arteries, our four patients all showed less strongly dilated accessory bronchial arteries, most of them arising from the pericardiacophrenic, internal mammary, and inferior phrenic arteries and the low thoracic aorta.

Broncho-pulmonary anastomoses had mainly a parahilar localization, although they were also found peripherally and centrally.

Broncho-bronchial anastomoses were present in all four patients. The shunts in two of these cases are illustrated in the relevant section (Fig. 52 *a* and *b*).

Three of the four patients had been treated surgically with a POTT or BLALOCK operation, after which transpleural intercosto-pulmonary anastomoses had developed.

Intercosto-bronchial anastomoses were first demonstrated *in vivo*. They occurred in two of the four patients (Figs. 74 and 75).

Case analysis

Patient 1

This patient had been operated on according to BLALOCK in 1954, at the age of six. An end-to-end anastomosis had been established between the left subclavian artery and the left branch of the pulmonary artery. This had resulted in a strong dilation of the upper left aortic intercostal artery due to its collateral supply to the axillary artery. Fig. 103 shows the arteriogram made during our catheterization in 1966. The upper combined (i.e. supplying two intercostal spaces) left intercostal artery shows marked dilation. Collaterals are visible in the intercostal region and, more laterally, contrast medium in the axillary artery, which was deprived of its blood supply by the operation. After the operation, extensive intercosto-pulmonary anastomoses had also developed. In the arteriogram shown in fig. 103, which was made six seconds after the beginning of the injection, the contrast medium can be seen vaguely in the pulmonary veins.

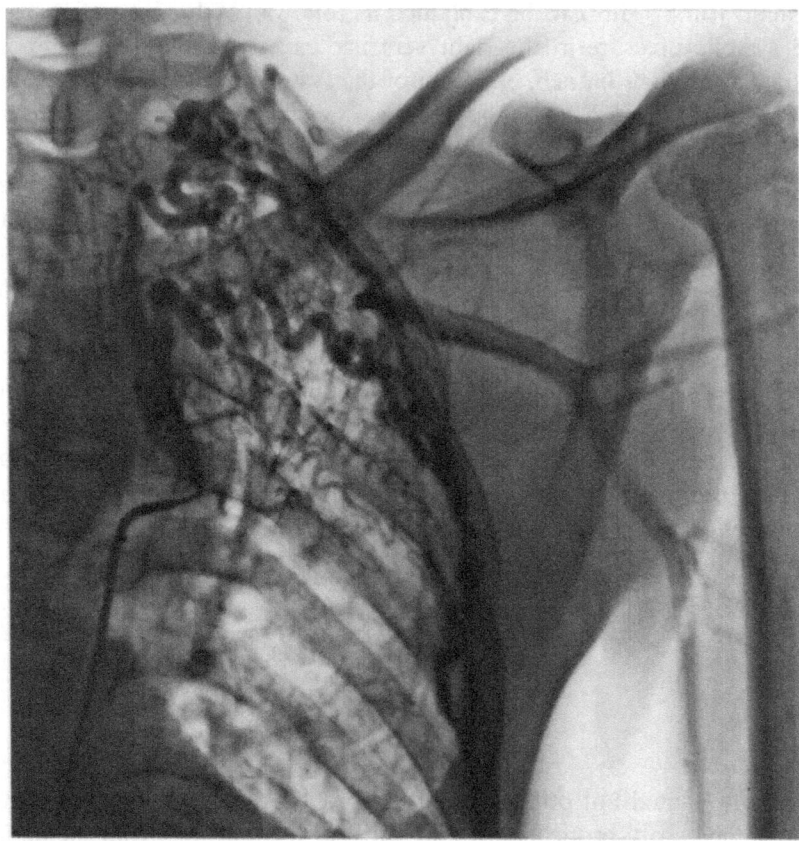

Fig. 103. Tetralogy of FALLOT, patient 1. Extreme dilation and elongation of the intercostal artery due to its collateral supply to the axillary artery. The pulmonary veins are vaguely visible, indicating the presence of intercosto-pulmonary anastomoses.

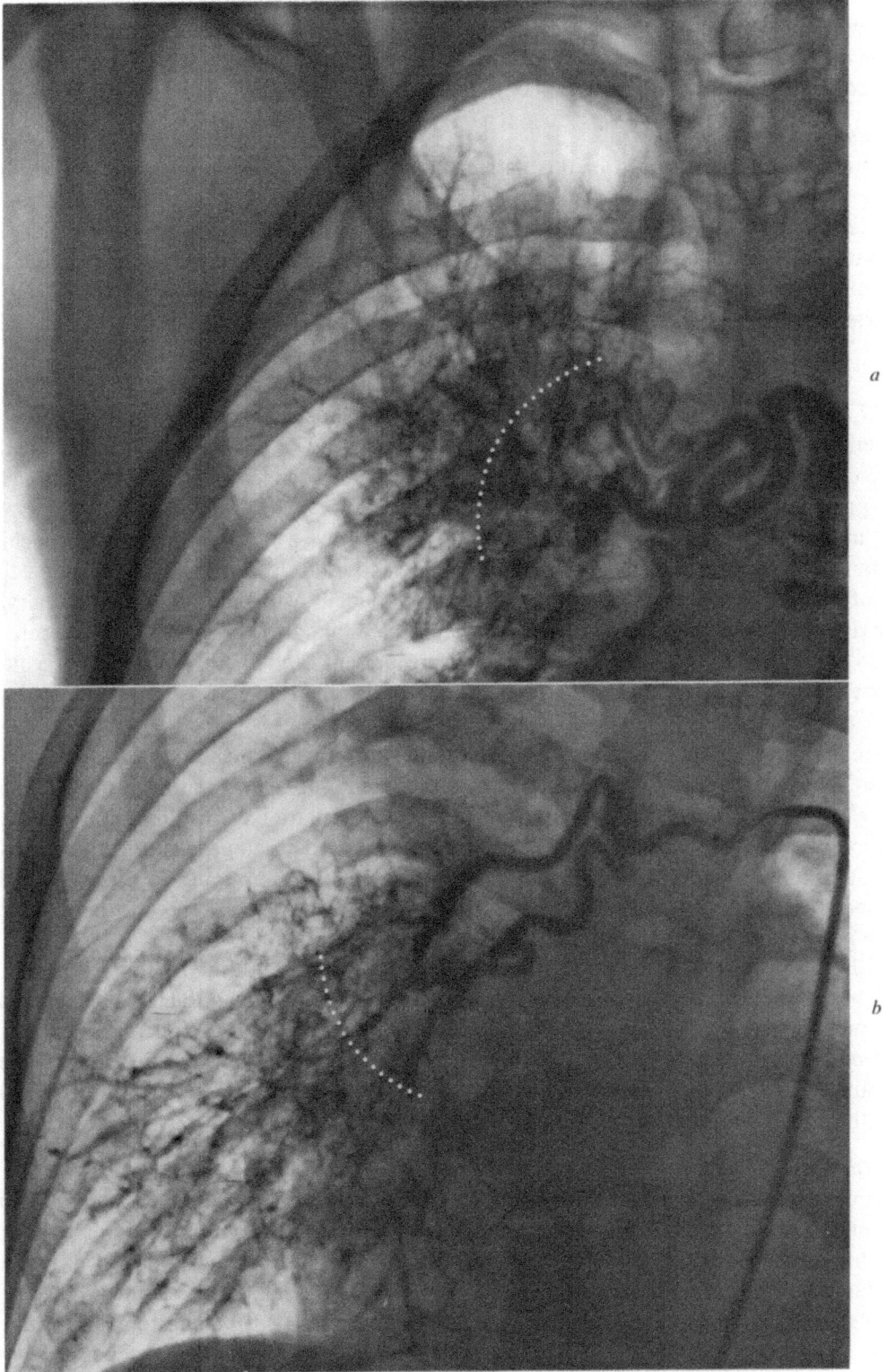

Fig. 104. Tetralogy of FALLOT, patient 1. Strongly dilated right superior (*a*) and inferior (*b*) bronchial arteries with numerous broncho-pulmonary anastomoses with a parahilar localization (dotted lines).

The bronchial arteriogram showed a widely dilated bronchial artery with large broncho-pulmonary shunts on the right side. Fig. 104 shows the right superior and inferior bronchial arteries. The shunts are located in the parahilar region, and multiple branches of the pulmonary artery are filled. On the left side the bronchial arteriogram shows almost no broncho-pulmonary shunts (Fig. 105).

The aortogram showed a patent BLALOCK anastomosis.

Discussion and conclusions

The results of the investigation of this patient permitted the following conclusion. From the small number of broncho-pulmonary shunts on the left side and the relatively small caliber of the left bronchial arteries, we were led to conclude that the BLALOCK anastomosis on the left was patent and had an unequivocal functional value, i.e. the left pulmonary artery received sufficient blood. The very wide bronchial arteries with numerous shunts on the right side, however, indicate that the right pulmonary artery did not receive sufficient blood, the deficit being reduced by the supply of bronchial blood.

Patient 2

In 1947 this patient, also at the age of six, underwent a BLALOCK operation, the anastomosis being made end-to-side. His condition remained unsatisfactory, however, and in 1963 – i.e. at the age of twenty-two – a Teflon prosthesis was inserted between the right subclavian artery and the right branch of the pulmonary artery.

Our investigation was performed in 1966. Fig. 106*a* shows a greatly dilated left bronchial artery, and many fine peripheral broncho-pulmonary anastomoses are present. Fig. 106*b* shows the venous phase of the investigation with a considerable amount of contrast medium in the pulmonary veins.

The right bronchial artery was even much more dilated than the left (Fig. 107). Numerous broncho-pulmonary shunts with a parahilar location were present, and there was retrograde flow of the contrast medium in the pulmonary artery. In the venous phase there was an abundant drainage via the pulmonary veins.

Intercostal arteriograms were also made on both sides. Fig. 108*a* shows a highly dilated tortuous fifth left intercostal artery which, in contrast to the intercostal arteries situated more cranially, does not participate in the collateral supply of the left subclavian artery. This dilation was a result of the operation performed seventeen years earlier. Rib-notching had developed. The next picture (Fig 108*b*) shows several intercosto-pulmonary shunts but an unsignificant retrograde flow in the branches of the pulmonary artery. The last picture (Fig. 108*c*), however, shows the occurrence of considerable drainage via the pulmonary veins.

Fig. 108*d* shows an arteriogram of the combined fourth and fifth intercostal arteries on the right side. These intercostal arteries are less strongly dilated than the one on the left side and show almost no tortuosity. The smaller amount of dilation is due to the fact that the operation on the right side had been performed more recently (three years earlier). Fig. 108*e* shows distinct retrograde filling of the branches of the pulmonary artery, again via multiple intercosto-pulmonary shunts. In the venous phase there is abundant filling of the pulmonary veins (Fig. 108*f*).

Discussion and conclusions

Our considerations with regard to this patient were as follows. The smaller broncho- and intercosto-pulmonary flow on the left side and the minimal retrograde flow of contrast medium in the branches of the pulmonary arteries indicated that the surgical anastomosis on the left functioned reasonably well. The abundant broncho- and intercosto-pulmonary flow on the right side indicated – together with the strong retrograde filling of the pulmonary arterial branches – that the anastomosis on the right had almost no functional value and perhaps had become occluded. On an arteriogram of the innominate artery, furthermore, no direct filling of the right pulmonary artery could be observed.

In October 1966, another operation was performed for total correction of the defect, but, unfortunately, a thorough inspection of the two anastomoses could not be performed.

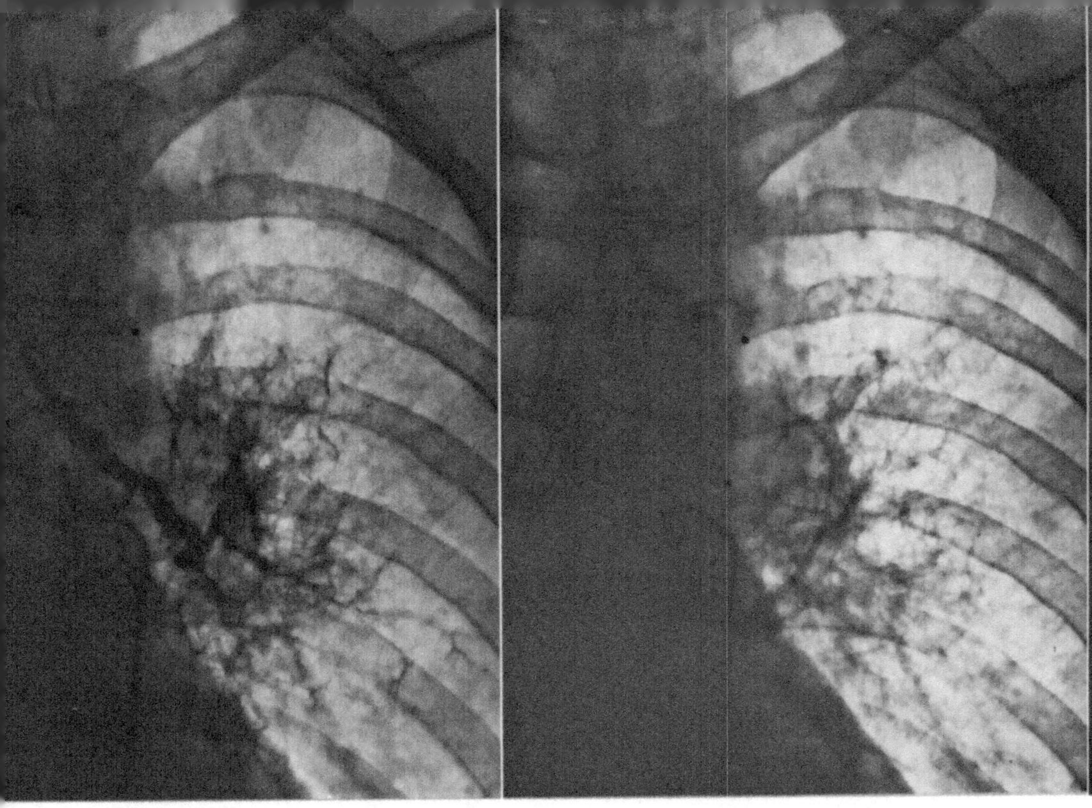

a

b

Fig. 106

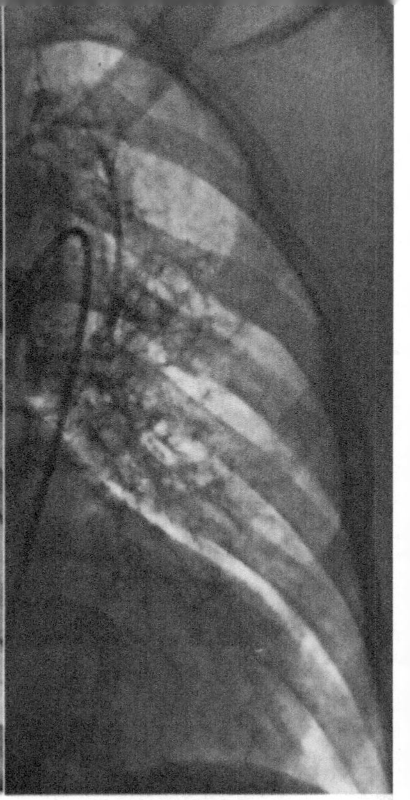

Fig. 105

Fig. 105. Tetralogy of FALLOT, patient 1. Relatively small left bronchial arteries and almost no broncho-pulmonary shunts.
Fig. 106. Tetralogy of FALLOT, patient 2.
a: Heavily dilated left bronchial artery. Multiple peripheral broncho-pulmonary shunts (see also Fig. 61).
b: Venous phase of the arteriogram.

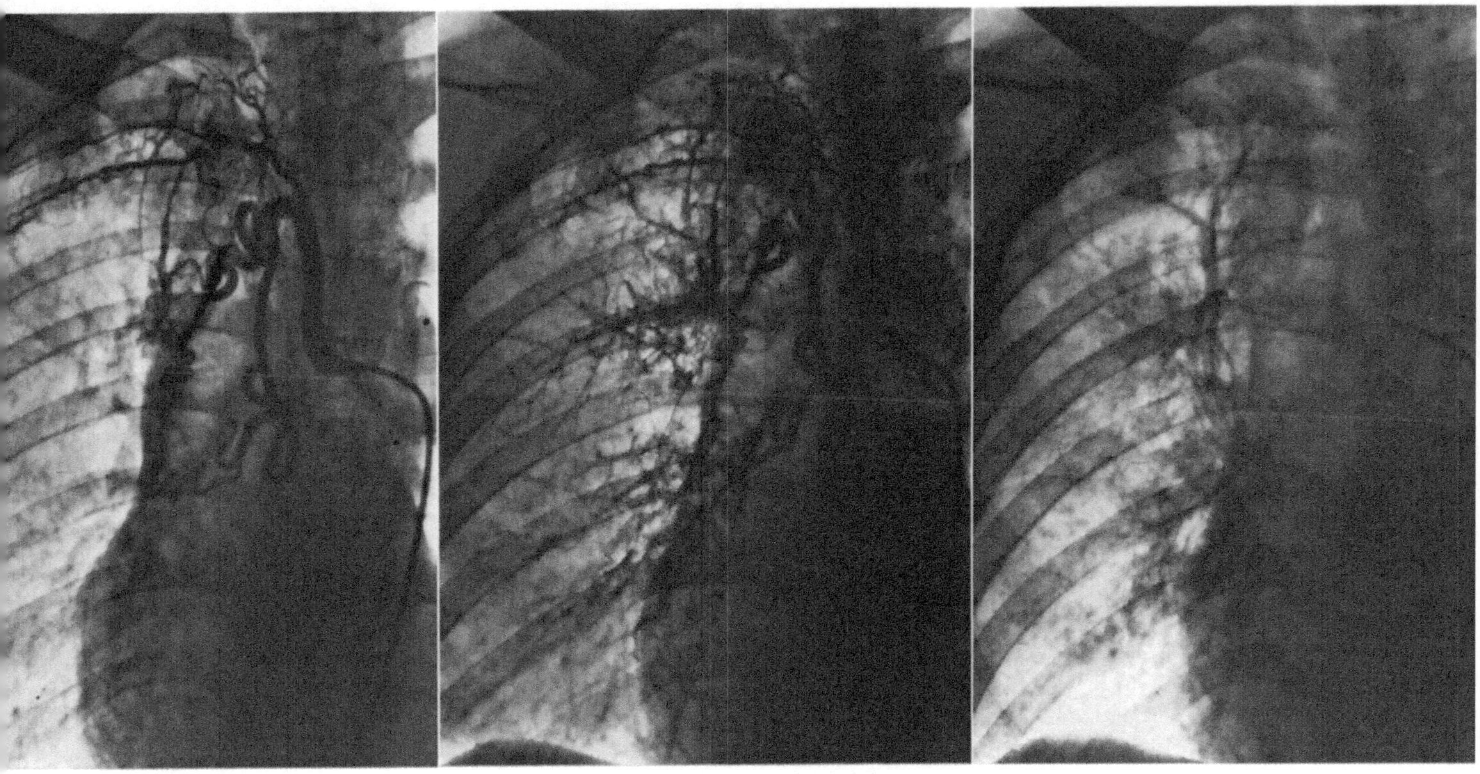

a

b

c

Fig. 107. Tetralogy of FALLOT, patient 2.
a: Very strongly dilated and tortuous right bronchial artery; beginning of the arterial phase.
b: End of the arterial phase showing multiple parahilar broncho-pulmonary anastomoses and a few intercosto-pulmonary anastomoses.
c: In the venous phase there is an abundant drainage via the pulmonary veins.

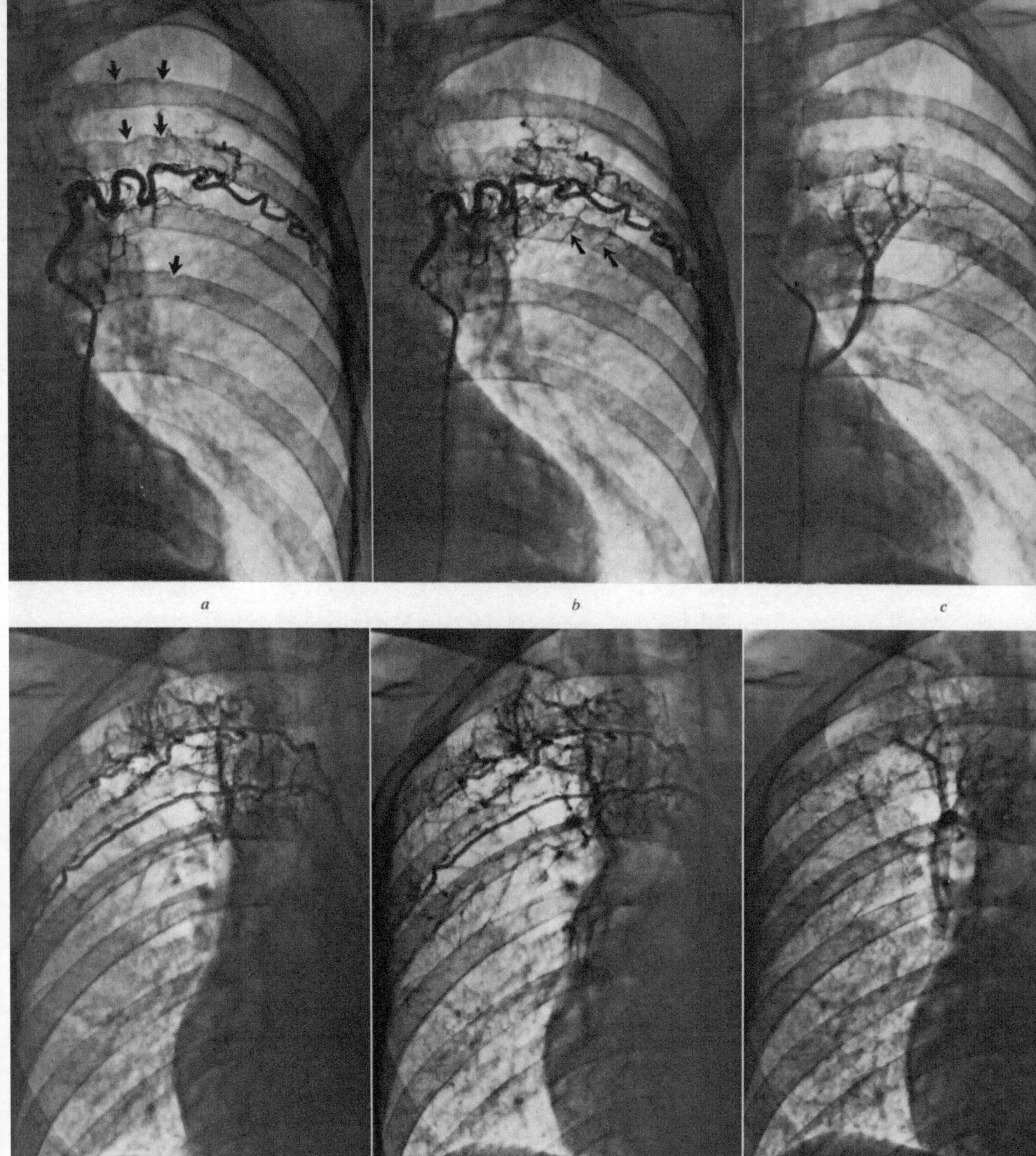

Fig. 108. Tetralogy of FALLOT, patient 2.

a, b, and c: Consecutive phases of a left intercostal arteriogram.

a: Severe dilation and elongation of the 5th left intercostal artery. Distinct rib-notching has developed (see also Figs. 73b and 103).

b: Filling via intercosto-pulmonary anastomoses of some peripheral branches of the pulmonary artery (arrows).

c: Venous phase with considerable drainage via the pulmonary veins.

d, e, and f: Consecutive phases of a right intercostal arteriogram.

d and e: Representation of the combined 4th and 5th right intercostal arteries. The intercostal arteries are less strongly dilated (as compared to the left intercostal) and show almost no tortuosity. Numerous intercosto-pulmonary shunts sometimes constituting long, parallel, anastomotic canals which traverse the projection of the ribs (especially in the lateral quadrant). Better representation of the branches of the pulmonary artery on this side than on the left, as a result of a more powerful retrograde flow, even into the right main branch.

f: Venous phase showing abundant filling of the pulmonary veins.

Patient 3

This patient was a young man of twenty-seven years who had received a POTT anastomosis in 1956 at the age of seventeen. Since then, a progressive dilation of the pulmonary artery had occurred. In 1966 the patient was largely incapacitated and for some time had had severe recurrent hemoptysis whose origin remained obscure. It was suspected that the POTT window was too wide and that pulmonary hypertension had developed.

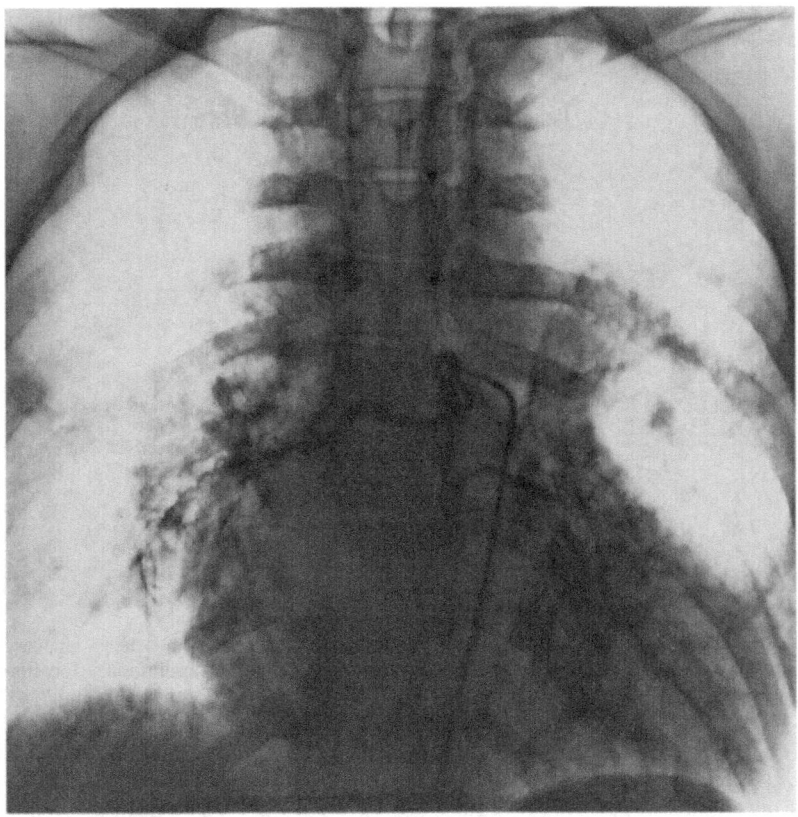

Fig. 109. Tetralogy of FALLOT, patient 3. Moderately strongly dilated bronchial artery. No broncho-pulmonary anastomoses.

We investigated this patient in 1966. The aortogram showed immediate and complete filling of the pulmonary artery (Fig. 39*d*). The fifth right intercostal artery was dilated; we shall return to this point below. During catheterization, the POTT window seemed to have a width of about 1 cm. Fig. 109 shows the selective arteriogram of the bronchial artery, which shows moderately strong dilation. No broncho-pulmonary anastomoses are present here or during the later phases of the arteriographic series.

An incidental finding was a wide collateral vascularizing a small peripheral area of the lung and arising from the fifth right intercostal artery (Fig. 110). This may have been the cause of the bleeding, since no other wide arteries or collaterals were found.

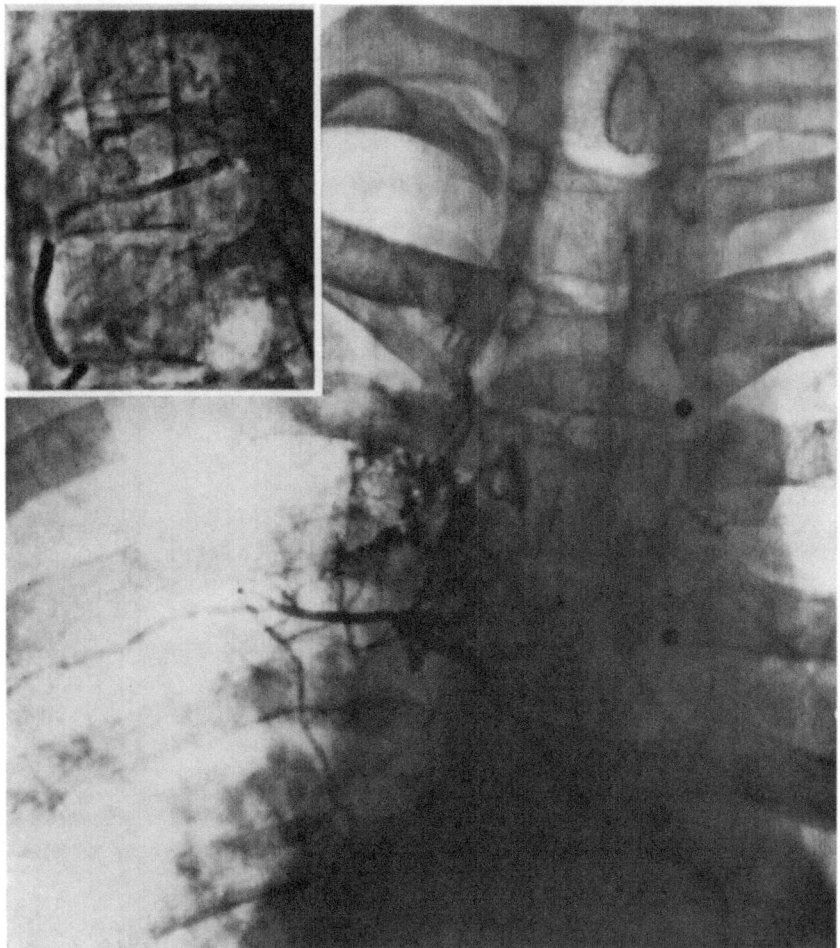

Fig. 110. Tetralogy of FALLOT, patient 3. Enlarged 5th right intercostal artery vascularizing a small area richly supplied with vessels. This area has an intrapulmonary location as appears from the lateral view (inset). Vascular bed of collateral bronchial nature?

Discussion and conclusions

We came to the following conclusions concerning this patient. The absence of broncho-pulmonary shunts indicated a very adequate blood supply of the pulmonary artery, which was in agreement with the aortographic findings. From the fact that not even one peripheral broncho-pulmonary anastomosis could be detected, it seemed likely that a high – probably exessively high – peripheral pressure was present in the branches of the pulmonary artery.

At operation, the POTT window was closed and a total correction performed. An attempt to ligate the fifth right intercostal artery proximally did not succeed.

Patient 4

This patient, a boy of seventeen years, showed a very unusual picture. There was very marked stenosis of the main trunk of the pulmonary artery. The right main branch of the pulmonary artery was atretic. Via the very narrow left branch, only the pectoral artery of the upper lobe showed filling on the angio-cardiogram. Therefore, the other branches of the pulmonary artery were probably also occluded. At bronchial arteriography, the left bronchial artery was found to be aneurysmatically enlarged showing a central anastomosis with the constricted left pulmonary artery (Fig. 65). The bronchial artery showed proximally an additional small saccular aneurysm on the lower side. Beyond the narrow central portion the segmental branches of the pulmonary artery showed post-stenotic enlargement.

The picture on the right side was even more remarkable (Fig. 111). Fig. 111*a* shows that the right bronchial artery was enormously dilated and took a tortuous course, as can be seen even more distinctly from the schematic drawing (Fig. 111*b*). The central anastomosis on the right pulmonary artery is indicated arrow. The right branch is also distinctly stenotic and here too the lobar and segmental branches show post-stenotic dilation. In this patient the main branches of the pulmonary artery therefore seemed to arise directly from the aorta, but there was interposition of the bronchial arteries.

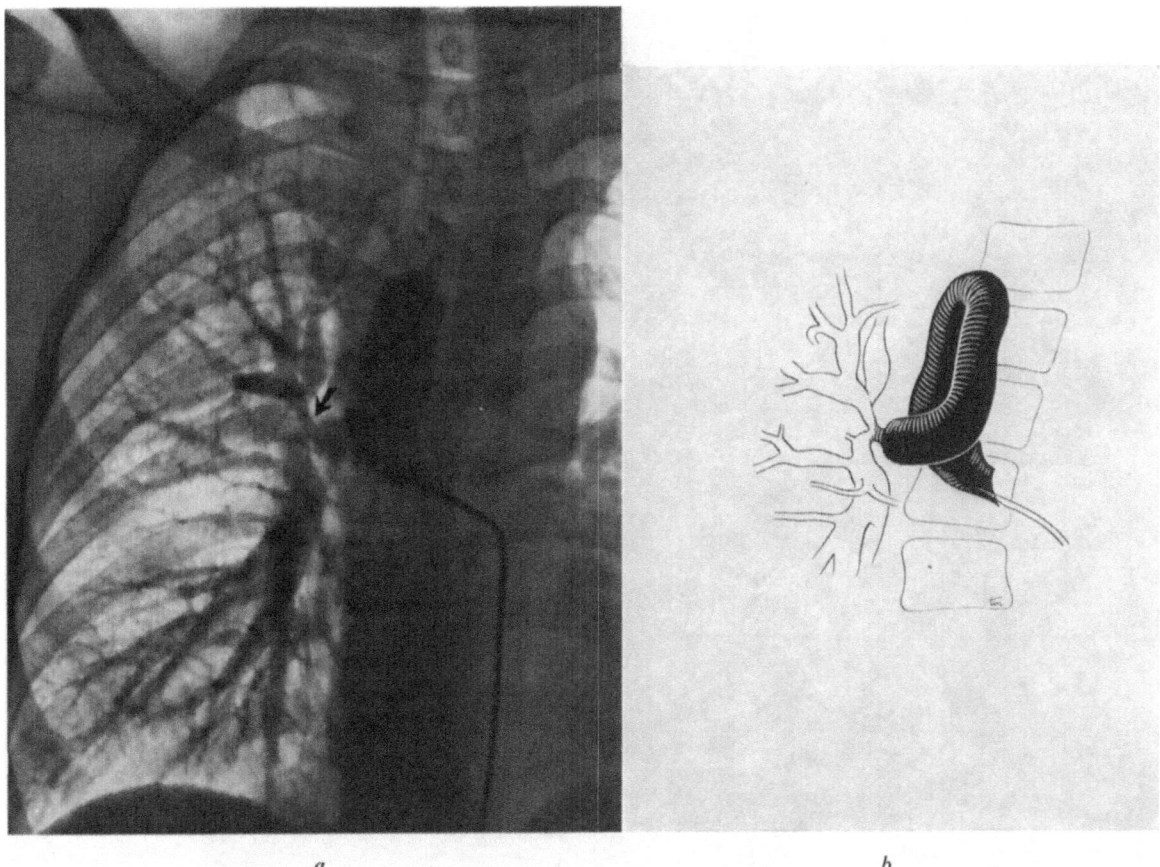

a   *b*

Fig. 111. Tetralogy of FALLOT, patient 4.
a: Enormously dilated right bronchial artery showing a central anastomosis (arrow) with the right pulmonary artery.
b: Schematic representation.

The aortogram showed that the left pulmonary artery was immediately and totally filled (Fig. 112*a*). The right side of the aorta showed a conical appendage beyond the orifice of the right bronchial artery, indicating a very severe stenosis. The right intercostal arteries were more or less strongly dilated, and one of them was also stenotic near the origin (black arrow). On the picture made 5 seconds after the beginning of the injection (Fig. 112*b*) vague contrast-medium shadows were present in the wide bronchial artery and in the branches of the pulmonary artery. The right pulmonary artery was therefore filled with a delay of 4.5 seconds as a result of the severe stenosis in the bronchial artery.

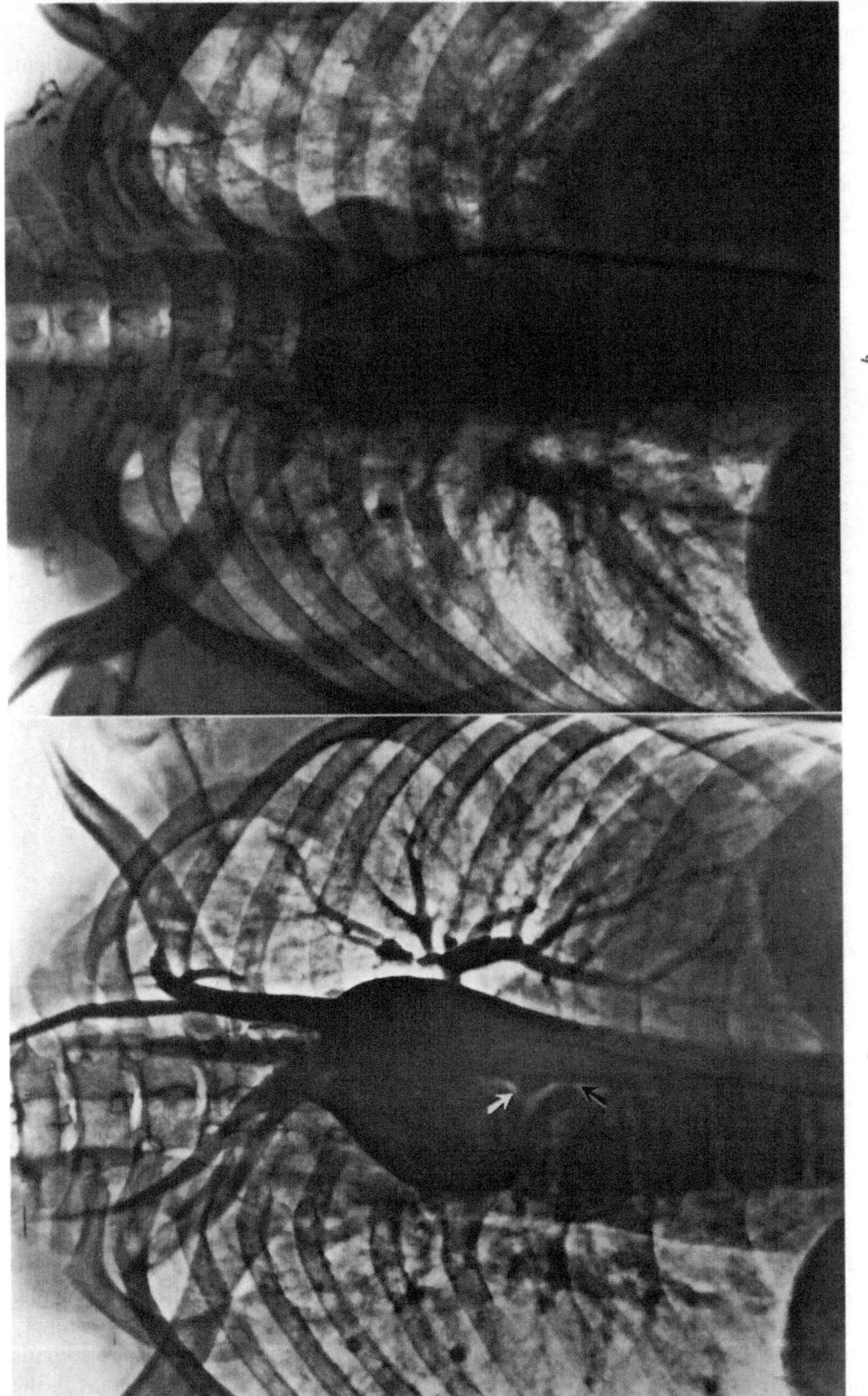

Fig. 112. Tetralogy of FALLOT, patient 4. Aortography.
a: Exposure made 0.5 seconds after the injection of contrast medium with visualization of only the left pulmonary artery. White arrow: stenosis in the right bronchial artery.
   Black arrow: stenosis in a right intercostal artery.
b: Exposure made 4.5 seconds later. Vague picture of the right bronchial and pulmonary arteries (compare with Fig. 111).

Discussion and conclusions

This investigation was important as pre-operative screening for two reasons. In the first place, it demonstrated that corrective surgery was not required on the left side. And in the second place, it showed that elimination of the stenosis in the right bronchial artery would give the patient a reasonably good pulmonary circulation on the right side.

CONCLUSION

In summarization of the foregoing, it may be said that it is advisable in cases of tetralogy of FALLOT to be informed pre-operatively about the state of the bronchial arteries if the application of a surgical anastomosis is considered. For: such important anastomoses may already have developed via the bronchial arteries, as was the case in the fourth patient, that a shunt operation would be superflous. The arteriographical findings will show what form of surgery is required.

Bronchial arteriography also has value for the evaluation of the surgical results. The amount of the broncho-pulmonary flow, and sometimes that of the intercosto-pulmonary flow as well, indicate the degree to which the corrective operation has succeeded. From the size of the retrograde flow in the branches of the pulmonary artery it can be deduced whether the antegrade flow through the surgical anastomosis is adequate. Comparison of the pictures on the right and left sides indicates which side should be chosen for a new anastomosis.

V
GENERAL CONSIDERATIONS

V.1. SUCCESS AND FAILURE OF ARTERIOGRAPHY

From the anatomical or technical point of view, an arteriographic examination of a patient may be called successful even when only a single selective bronchial arteriogram can be made, but from the pathological point of view it may be called a failure if the bronchial artery supplying the lesion is not visualized. For this discussion, the criterion of success is taken as the selective visualization of the bronchial and intercostal arteries involved in the vascularization of the lesion under study. Attention will therefore be paid to whether the arteriography was successful from the pathological point of view.

In our material, no bronchial arteries were found in seven patients (8.3 per cent). One of these patients was unable to cooperate; in two patients bronchial arteries could not be catheterized because of marked tortuosity of the pelvic arteries and the thoracic aorta; and in one case the investigation had to be cut short because of the patient's poor general condition. In three patients no demonstrable reason could be found for the failure of the catheterization, but since they were among the first fifteen, lack oif experience on our part probably played a role.

In ssx patients (7.1 per cent) arteriography failed in spite of successful catheterization of bronchial arteriet. In three of these cases the wrong bronchial artery was catheterized. In the other three the correc bronchial artery was found but insufficient information was obtained, once because spasm developed in the branch supplying the lesion and twice because uncontrollable coughing made it impossible to obtain a sharp picture.

Arteriography was partially successful in seven patients (8.3 per cent). In these patients not all the bronchial arteries involved in the circulation in and around the lesion(s) could be catheterized, which resulted in incomplete arteriographic information.

In sixty-four patients (76.2 per cent) arteriography was completely successful. In fourty-seven of these patients a complete selective arteriography of the bronchial arteries could be performed. Adequate information was obtained in all of the cases.

V.2. INDICATIONS

The indications for arteriography have already been mentioned under the various parts of the patho-logical section of the chapter 'Results of the Present Study', but a brief recapitulation will be useful here.

V.2.1. For bronchial arteriography

1. Coin lesions, undiagnosed, with the exception of the extremely peripheral locations.
2. Pre-operative exploration of the bronchographically normal parts of the lungs of patients with bronchiectasis.
3. Hemorrhaging bronchiectasis.
4. Recurrent hemoptysis of unknown cause.
5. Cases of tetralogy of FALLOT considered for a surgical anastomosis.

and possibly,

6. Pre-operative exploration of normal parts of the lungs in tuberculosis patients.

V.2.2. For intercostal arteriography

1. Suspicion of transpleural penetration of peripheral lung tumors.

V.2.3. For bronchial and intercostal arteriography

1. Post-operative check in patients with tetralogy of FALLOT when the results of corrective surgery seem doubtful.

V.3. CONTRA-INDICATIONS AND FACTORS WITH
AN UNDESIRABLE INFLUENCE

In addition to conditions making a SELDINGER catheterization inadvisable, such as complaints of dysbasia, non-pulsating leg arteries, and severe arteriosclerosis, there are other factors with an undesirable influence, particularly on bronchial arteriography. In the first place there is the maneuverability of the catheter, which severe tortuosity of the pelvic arteries and aorta may impede to such an extent, that the procedure should be terminated. In the second place there is the cooperation of the patient. This cooperation is essential: he must be able to control an urge to cough, at least during the arterial phase of the contrast injection, and to hold his breath and lie absolutely still during series exposures. When the patient will not or cannot (neurological disturbances) cooperate, it is better to discontinue the investigation. Furthermore, the results in very obese patients are often disappointing, since the small vessels register poorly or not at all. And lastly, a poor general condition must be considered a contra-indication because of the duration of the investigation, which requires a greater amount of time than other kinds of arteriography.

V.4. COMPLICATIONS

Apart from the limited risks involved in any percutaneous catheterization, intercostal arteriography involves the danger of injury to the spinal cord. The chance of this serious development will be discussed separately.

In the discussion of the other complications a distinction will be made between untoward effects for the patient and other phenomena influencing the results and the interpretation of the arteriographic examination (vascular spasm, etc.).

V.4.1. Untoward effects for the patient

Serious or lethal complications did not occur in the present series, but ten patients showed light complications.

V.4.1.1. NON-SPECIFIC COMPLICATIONS

Five patients developed light complications which in principle could occur after any percutaneous catheterization. One patient developed heavy bleeding at the site of the puncture, and required a transfusion. Another patient had a prolonged period of diminished pulsation in the posterior tibial artery and dorsal artery of the foot, on the side on which the puncture had been performed. Surgical treatment was not considered necessary, and after two days pulsation returned to normal. In one case a hematoma developed at the puncture site and the procedure had to be postponed. One patient developed a pulsating swelling at the site of the puncture; this swelling disappeared within a few days. One patient developed melena during the night after the arteriography. Since this patient had intestinal metastases and was on anticoagulant therapy (heparin), it seems possible that one or more metastases had bled during the investigation.

V 4.1.2. SPECIFIC COMPLICATIONS

Four patients showed slight complications related to the selective arteriography of bronchial and intercostal arteries, but the cause remained obscure. In all these cases 1 to 3 ml of contrast medium had been injected into very narrow arteries, whereas a dose of 0.4 ml would have been sufficient.

The first of these patients developed severe retro-sternal pain after the injection of contrast medium into a vas aortae with a small accessory bronchial branch. The pain disappeared within a few minutes.

The second patient became faint and showed differences in size between the pupils after an injection into an accessory bronchial artery arising from the aorta. These phenomena and the patient's complaints both disappeared within a few seconds.

The third patient uttered a loud shriek after injection into a very small combined artery supplying the aortic wall and hilus, and developed clonic contractions in the extremities. She recovered within a few seconds and could not remember what had happened. She reported having speech difficulties for several days afterward. The reality of this insult is doubtful. The series films made at the same time showed nothing unusual, and in particular no vessels supplying the myelum.

The fourth of these patients developed severe pain in the throat lasting for several minutes after injection of contrast medium into a small bronchial artery. These complaints were probably the result of the injection of an excessive amount of contrast medium into an esophageal branch.

V.4.2. Spasms and other artificial phenomena

Occasionally, a constriction of the contrast column near the point of the catheter was seen, apparently as a result of local irritation of the arterial wall. Two patients showed such constrictions at some distance from the tip of the catheter; in both cases, novocaine had been administered via the catheter before the injection of the contrast medium.

V.4.2.1. EFFECT OF NOVOCAINE

In an attempt to diminish the burning sensation in the back during intercostal arteriography and to prevent the coughing during bronchial arteriography, we initially administered 2–4 ml of a 2 per cent novocaine solution just before the injection of contrast medium. This practice was also applied by VIAMONTE (1964) and WIRTANEN AND ANSFIELD (1968). It sometimes resulted in arterial spasms. These spasms developed only in the arterial branches supplying a tumor, not in the normal bronchial branches. This is hardly surprising, since it is known from the pharmacological literature that tumor vessels react differently to drugs than do normal arteries. This is also mentioned in the arteriography literature, and use is made of this phenomenon in the selective arteriography of renal tumors (ABRAMS ET AL., 1962; KAHN, 1965; KAHN AND WISE, 1968). The effect of drugs on bronchial vessels has been studied by KAHN AND CALLOW (1965) and HALLER ET AL. (1966). Their results confirm the different reactions of tumor and normal vessels.

In two cases comparison made it possible to obtain an impression of the effect of novocaine injections in the bronchial arteries. These cases will be briefly described.

In one of these patients a violent bout of coughing during the antero-posterior arteriographic series resulted in a number of blurred pictures. Before the lateral series was made, therefore, 4 ml 2% novocaine was administered prior to the injection of the contrast medium. The tumor vascularization visible on the antero-posterior views could not be seen on the lateral views. The supplying arteries seemed to be occluded. The other patient began to cough violently after the test injection of contrast medium, and novocaine was administered before the injection for the first series of exposures. The cranial branch of the right bronchial artery showed an occlusion just beyond its origin (Fig. 113a). Since it was thought that the novocaine injection had resulted in spasm, a second series of exposures was made ten minutes later. These pictures showed that the occlusion had shifted in the peripheral

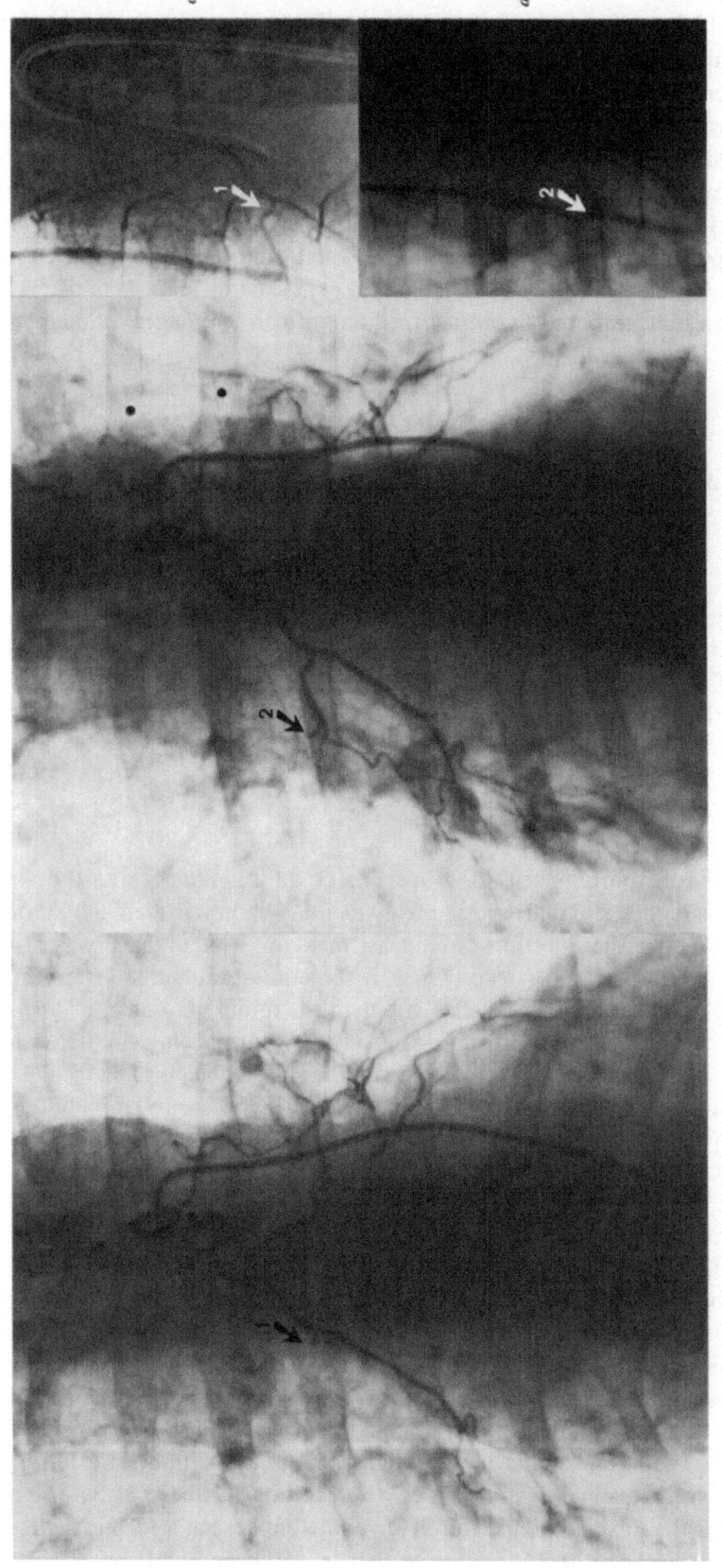

Fig. 113. Arterial spasm after injection of novocaine.

a: Arteriogram of a truncus communis (patient supine). After the first bifurcation on the right side, the cranial branch shows an apparent occlusion 4 mm from its origin (arrow).

b: Second arteriogram made 10 minutes later (patient turned 15 degrees on the right side). The proximal spasm has been abolished, but there is another occlusion in a more peripheral part of the same bronchial branch.

c: Aortogram (light print), showing the proximal portion of the right branch of the truncus communis.

d: Dark print of the same aortogram showing the further course of the occluded branch in *b*. The white arrows indicate the sites (1 and 2) of the occlusions that appeared during the selective investigation.

direction to the origin of the arterial branch supplying a mediastinal tumor (Fig. 113*b*). This branch had been visible during the fluoroscopic check of the test injection and could also be seen on an aortogram made two days before the selective arteriography was performed (Fig. 113*d*). After this second arteriographic series the investigation had to be terminated for technical reasons. On the basis of these failures we stopped the administration of novocaine through the catheter.

V.4.2.2. OTHER ARTEFACTS

In three cases the arteriogram showed small clarifications in the column of contrast medium at a short distance from the tip of the catheter. It seemed likely that small air bubbles or small clots had been responsible for these pictures. No injurious effects were observed.

V.4.3. The chance of spinal-cord lesions

To clarify the problem associated with the risk of damage to the spinal cord in intercostal arteriography, the vascularization of the spinal cord will be briefly discussed and then the possible complications in arteriography.

LITERATURE

Anatomy

The anterior part of the spinal cord is supplied by the anterior spinal artery. This artery originates from confluence of two small branches provided by the vertebral artery (SCHECHTER AND ZINGESSER, 1965). It runs in the anterior median sulcus and also receives blood from a number of segmental arteries from the aorta – intercostals and lumbars – via the anterior radicular arteries, also called the anterior medullar arteries. The most important of these latter arteries is the arteria radicularis magna, which is called after ADAMKIEWICZ, because of his thorough anatomical study, published in 1882. This artery usually arises from a segmental artery in the thoraco-lumbar region (T11, T12, L1, and L2). According to SUH AND ALEXANDER (1939), the site of origin varies from T8 to L4. In some cases the origin is situated at an unusually high level. FAURÉ ET AL. (1967) even described an arteria radicularis magna arising from the fifth left intercostal artery. The artery arises twice as often from the left segmental aortic arteries as from the right. The artery of ADAMKIEWICZ runs obliquely upward through an intervertebral foramen, after which it passes along first the lateral and then the ventral side of the myelum to reach the median sulcus. Here, the artery turns sharply in the caudal direction and continues as the descending part of the anterior spinal artery. From the top of this hairpin curve (inverted V), a smaller ascending branch arises. According to FAURÉ ET AL. (1966), the arteria radicularis magna sometimes sends a small branch for the vascularization of the posterior part of the spinal cord. CORBIN (1961) found in two out of three cases a second – accessory – anterior radicular artery in the thoraco-lumbar region, showing the same course as the first. In the thoracic region, according to FAURÉ ET AL. (1967), there is only one anterior medullar artery present at the level of T4 or T5, again with the same course as the artery of ADAMKIEWICZ. According to GILLILAN (1958), there are seven to ten anterior medullar arteries in all, and according to SUH AND ALEXANDER (1939), the anterior spinal artery represents a chain of ascending and descending branches arising from the anterior radicular arteries.

The posterior part of the cord is supplied via small posterior radicular, *sive* medullar, arteries, which according to DJINDJIAN ET AL. (1967) also form an inverted V, although the V is shorter and the angle sharper. According to GILLILAN (1958), there are ten to twenty such arteries with connecting shunts, and they arise, like the anterior radicular arteries, from intercostal and lumbar arteries.

Between the posterior and anterior vascular systems supplying the myelum there are small anastomoses which, however, cannot completely take over the supply to the anterior part of the cord after occlusion of an anterior medullar artery (GILLILAN, 1958). According to the same author, the anastomoses between the various ascending and descending parts of the anterior spinal artery are also incapable of adequately taking over the supply to the relevant parts of the anterior spinal artery after occlusion of one of the anterior radicular arteries. Intercostal and lumbar arteriography involves the risk of damage to these vulnerable arteries and can thus lead to paraplegia.

During intercostal arteriography the possibility, however rare, of a high origin of the arteria radicularis magna as well as the occurrence of another anterior radicular artery in the thoracic region, must always be kept in mind.

Arteriography

The first mention of paraplegia after abdominal aortography was made by ANTONI AND LINDGREN in 1949; later, studies were published by MC AFEE (1957), KILLEN AND FORSTER (1960), EFSEN (1966), and HUGHES AND BROWNELL (1965), the first two of these being the most detailed. The complication was seen primarily after direct puncture aortography (MC AFEE, 1957). LANG (1963), in a discussion of complications in 11,402 'SELDINGER' arteriograms, makes no mention of injuries to the spinal cord.

Paraplegia can result from a large quantity of contrast medium in the artery of ADAMKIEWICZ or in one of the other anterior radicular arteries. Since the risk is partially influenced by the composition of the contrast medium, the choice of this material is important. The acetrizoate compounds have a particular bad name (e.g. MC AFEE, 1957; KILLEN AND FORSTER, 1960; EFSEN, 1966). According to LANCE ET AL. (1958) and KILLEN AND LANCE (1962), the damage is due on the one hand to direct toxicity of the contrast medium and on the other to the anoxia occurring after retardation of the bloodflow. The symptoms of an overdose of contrast medium in the anterior spinal artery are severe pain and clonic muscular spasm of the lower extremities (FAURÉ ET AL., 1966). The paresis develops later and, according to the observations of KILLEN AND FORSTER (1960), is usually irreversible.

With respect to intercostal arteriography, two cases of the complication have been reported, and both concerned *transient* paraplegia (FEIGELSON AND RAVIN, 1965; RÉMY ET AL., 1968). The chance of a permanent lesion due to intercostal arteriography therefore seems to be lower than could be expected from the literature on abdominal aortography. The most important factor in this difference is the development of better-tolerated contrast media (DJINDJIAN AND FAURÉ, 1967).

DATA FROM OUR MATERIAL

In our material the anterior spinal artery was visualized six times with certainty and twice with probability. Filling occurred via anterior radicular arteries arising from the following intercostal arteries: 2 and 3R, 3R, 3R, 3 and 4R, 4R, 4R, 4L, 4L.

The more frequent finding of an anterior medullar artery from a right intercostal artery does not reflect the anatomical distribution, because more arteriograms were made of right than of left intercostal arteries. In two patients the descending branch of the anterior spinal artery could be traced to the lower edge of the picture, at the level of L1 (Fig. 114*a*, *b*, and *c*). Both patients felt a burning sensation travelling slowly from high in the back downward to the sacral region; the pain was not severe. It is evident that in these patients there was a arteria radicularis magna with an abnormally high origin, arising in one patient from the fourth right intercostal artery (Fig. 114*a* and *b*) and in the other from the fourth left intercostal artery (Fig. 114*c*). As far as we have been able to determine, this unusually high origin has not previously been described. The inverted V formed by this high-origin artery is smaller than that of the normally originating artery of ADAMKIEWICZ, an example of which is shown in fig. 115.[1]

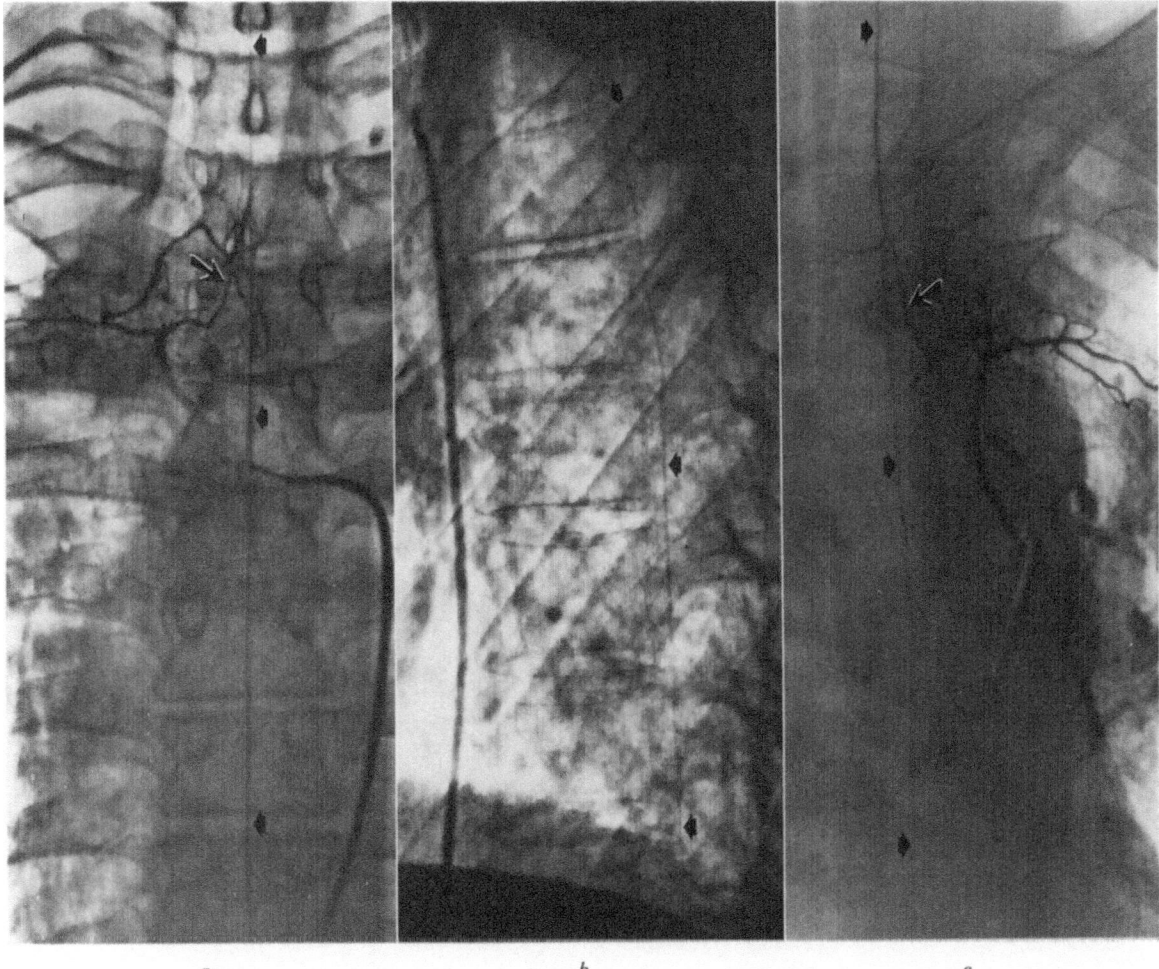

a   *b*   *c*

Fig. 114. Arteria radicularis magna originating at an unusual high level. Arteriograms of a 4th right intercostal artery in anteroposterior (*a*) and lateral (*b*) direction, and of a 4th left intercostal artery in anteroposterior direction (*c*). The radicular artery is indicated by a large arrow, and the anterior spinal artery by small arrows. Note the difference in caliber between the ascending branches in *a* and *c*.

In the other cases the supplying artery was an accessory and only a small portion of the anterior spinal artery was visualized (Fig. 116*a*). The anterior spinal artery remains filled longer and is, therefore, most easily recognized in the capillary and early venous phases of the investigation (Fig. 116*b* and *c*).

[1] According to GILLILAN (1958), this is a consequence of the relative ascent of the spinal cord during embryonic development.

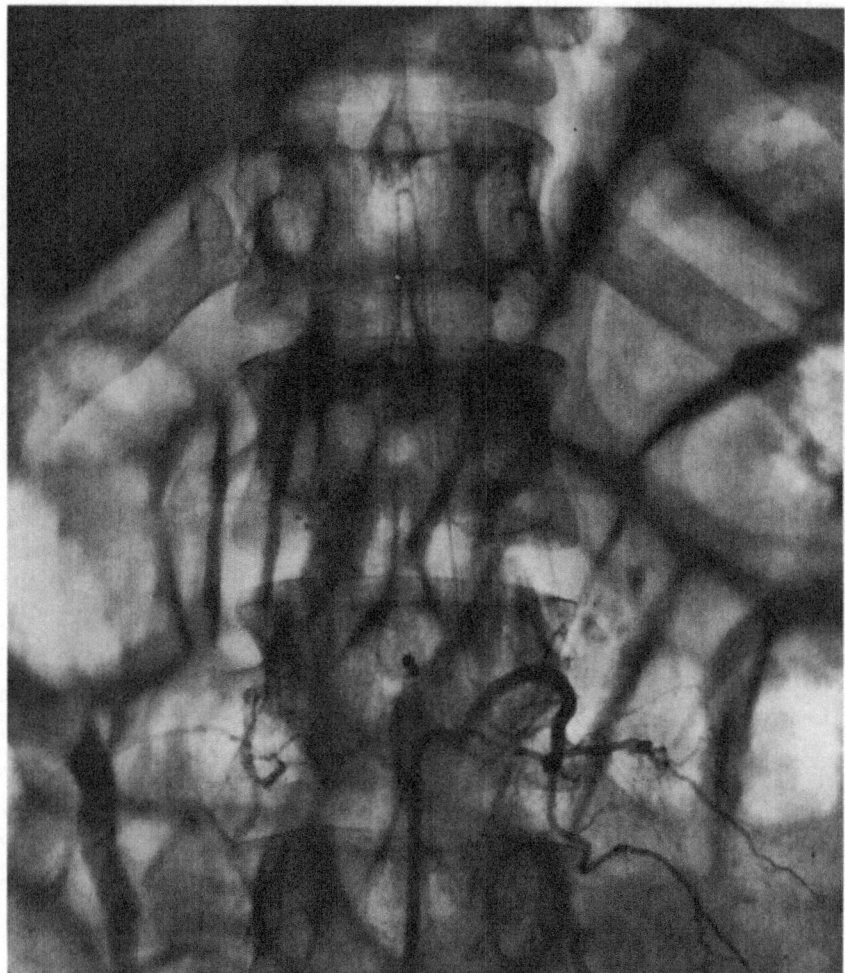

Fig. 115. The normally originating arteria radicularis magna (artery of ADAMKIEWICZ) forms a larger inverted V with a scharper hairpin curve.

Untoward effects of injection of contrast medium into the spinal-cord arteries were not observed in our material. A burning sensation was felt at a site located outside the usual extent of the region supplied by the catheterized intercostal arteries. Furthermore, the location of this burning sensation tends to shift. Loss of motor or sensibility reactions was not observed. After the completion of arteriography, the normal reflexes were present.

In four patients a possible visualization of a posterior medullar artery was obtained. These patients had no unusual sensations during the injection of contrast medium.

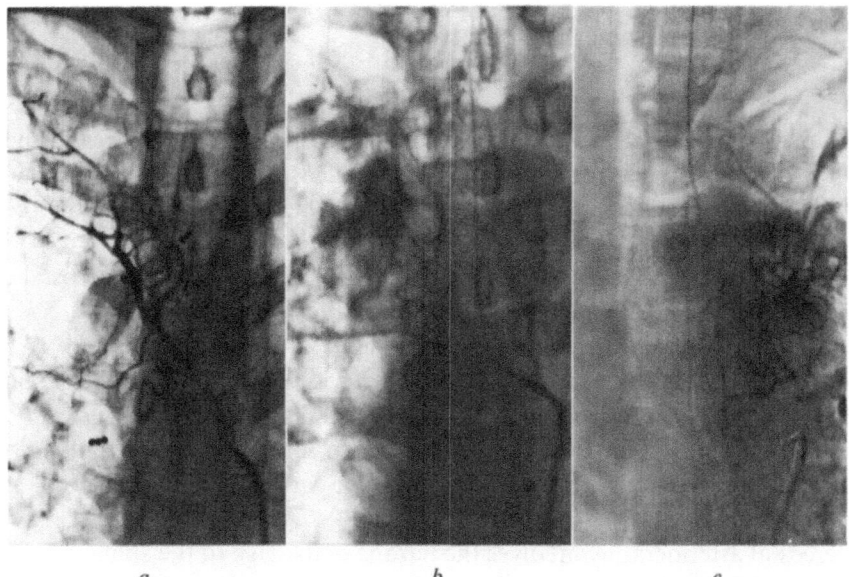

Fig. 116. Other anterior radicular arteries.

a: Anterior radicular artery in the high thoracic region supplying only a small part of the anterior spinal artery.

b and *c*: The anterior spinal artery is most easily recognized in the capillary and early venous phases of the arteriographic series.

DISCUSSION

Although a rather large number of anterior spinal arteries were visualized, we are of the opinion that they represent only a small proportion of the total number of anterior spinal arteries that had received contrast medium during our arteriography. But since we did not observe even the phenomena considered by DOPPMAN AND DI CHIRO (1968) to precede paraplegia, such as clonic contractions in the lower extremities, we think that the risk of this complication in selective intercostal arteriography is not great.

In this respect the position of the catheter is very important. If the point occludes the vessel, as in the cases described by FEIGELSON AND RAVIN (1965) and RÉMY ET AL. (1968), compensation for the deficient supply cannot be made rapidly enough to prevent hypoxia and a toxic effect of the contrast medium. The position of the catheter must therefore be carefully checked each time it is introduced. The use of catheters with a very thin tip has always enabled us to avoid occlusion.

If neurological symptoms occur in spite of all these precautions, the catheter should be withdrawn immediately. Catheterization may be continued under very strict observation if only a burning sensation occurs. Because of such signs, we share the opinion of other authors (e.g. MC AFEE, 1957; DJINDJIAN AND FAURÉ, 1967) that arteriography should not be performed under general anaesthesia; the need to observe the patient's reactions means that only local anaesthesia should be applied.

NORDENSTRÖM (1967) observed a slight positive BABINSKI reaction in one case after intercostal arteriography. On the basis of this report we carried out a brief neurological examination of the lower part of the body in our patients after catheterization. No anomalies were found.

V.4.4. Conclusions

1. From the pathological point of view (i.e. adequate information about the area of the lesion(s)), 15 per cent of the arteriographies can be said to have failed in our material, and in an additional 8 per cent of the cases insufficient information was obtained. More than 75 per cent were completely successful.
2. According to our results, there are eight indications for bronchial and intercostal arteriography.
3. There are a few specific contra-indications for bronchial arteriography.
4. There have been no serious complications in our series.
5. The injection of contrast medium into very small arteries must be done with great care, and to avoid undesirable reactions the amount must not exceed 0.4 ml.
6. The administration of novocaine through the catheter to control reactions to the contrast medium may induce vascular spasm in the branches supplying a pathological process, and is therefore not advisable.
7. Selective intercostal arteriography involves the hazard of damage to the spinal cord via an anterior radicular artery or via the arteria radicularis magna, which may be followed by paraplegia. The danger of this serious complication can be eliminated by the use of a catheter with a thin point, well-tolerated contrast media, and local anaesthesia.

SUMMARY

The present study was performed in an attempt to answer two questions.

1. Could increased anatomical information and improved catheterization techniques reduce the failure rate sufficiently for selective bronchial arteriography to be performed with a fair chance of success?
2. Is it possible to define indications for selective bronchial and intercostal arteriography?

Careful comparison of the data in the literature concerning the variable origin and different types of bronchial arteries made it possible to arrive at a simplified classification as well as to formulate a number of standard criteria, which are particularly useful for the selective investigation.

The use of catheters having very thin tips and adapted to the anatomical situation (e.g. different shapes for right and left bronchial arteries) made it possible to reduce the number of unsuccessful catheterizations. Despite a higher proportion of failures among the initial cases, the over-all percentage of completely successful investigations (visualization of all the bronchial arteries in and around the lesion or lesions) was over 75.

The analysis of 143 bronchial arteriograms and 120 intercostal arteriograms yielded some new facts about the anatomy of bronchial and intercostal arteries and several specific recommendations for the catheterization of each type of bronchial artery.

Correct interpretation of the arteriographic pictures requires becoming thoroughly familiar with the different types of arterial anastomoses. Their identification too must offer no difficulties. These shunts comprise broncho-bronchial, broncho-pulmonary, intercosto-pulmonary, and intercosto-bronchial types, each of which has diagnostic significance. The author's observations include several new findings concerning these shunts.

To estimate the value of bronchial and intercostal arteriography, the findings were analysed in cases of the following diseases: primary lung tumor (23), tuberculosis (24: comprising 18 with focal lesions, 4 with cavities, and 2 with tuberculoma), bronchiectasis (11), emphysema (11), tetralogy of FALLOT (4), chronic infiltration (4), metastases (4), chronic asthmatic bronchitis (4), infected cavities (3), diffuse small focal lesions (2), bronchoplasty (2), hamartoma (2), aspergillosis (2), hemoptysis (2), pleural tumor (2), bronchogenic cyst (1), suppurative pneumonia (1), histiocytosis X (1), subphrenic abscess (1), and esophageal carcinoma (1). Although, generally speaking, the results with respect to indications were meagre, some could be formulated:

Indications for bronchial arteriography: 1. coin lesions, undiagnosed, with exception of the extremely peripheral locations; 2. pre-operative exploration of the bronchographically normal parts of the lungs of patients with bronchiectasis; 3. hemorrhaging bronchiectasis; 4. recurrent hemoptysis of unknown cause; 5. cases of tetralogy of FALLOT considered for a surgical anastomosis; 6. and, possibly, pre-operative exploration of normal parts of the lungs in tuberculosis patients.

Indications for intercostal arteriography: suspicion of transpleural penetration of peripheral lung tumors.

Indications for bronchial and intercostal arteriography: Post-operative check in patients with tetralogy of FALLOT when the results of corrective surgery seem doubtful.

The most serious complication associated with this kind of arteriography is paraplegia resulting from damage to the myelum via anterior radicular arteries deriving from intercostals, but with adequate technical skill this risk can be eliminated.

REFERENCES

ABELANET M. (1961). Discussion lecture R. Gastaing J. *Franç. Méd. Chir. Thor.* **15**, 652.

ABRAMS H. L., BOIJSEN E., BORGSTRÖM K. (1962). Effect of epinephrine on the renal circulation. *Radiology* **79**, 911–922.

ADAMKIEWICZ A. (1882). Die Blutgefässe des menschlichen Rückenmärkes. II. Die Gefässe der Rückenmarksoberfläche. *S.-B. Akad. Wiss. Wien, math.-nat. Kl.* **85**, 101–130.

AINSWORTH J. (1958). Anomalous blood supply to lung demonstrated by aortography. *Brit. J. Radiol.* **31**, 448–449.

ALLEY R. D., STRANAHAN A., KRAUSEL H. W., FORMEL P., MIEROP L. H. S. v. (1958). Demonstration of bronchial-pulmonary artery reverse flow in suppurative pulmonary disease. *Clin. Res.* **1**, 41.

ALLEY R. D., MIEROP L. H. S. v., PECK A. S., KAUSEL H. W., STRANAHAN A. (1961). Bronchial arterial collateral circulation. *Amer. Rev. Resp. Dis.* **83**, 31–37.

AMEUILLE P., LEMOINE J. M. (1935). Bronchiectactasie et thrombose de l'artère bronchique. *Presse Méd.*, 873–877.

ANTONI N., LINDGREN E. (1949). Steno's experiment in man as complication in lumbar aortography. *Acta Chir. Scand.* **98**, 230–247.

ARAMENDIA P., LETONA J. M. L. de, AVIADO D. M. (1962a). Responses of the bronchial veins in a heart-lung-bronchial preparation (with special reference to a pulmonary to bronchial shunt). *Circulat. Res.* **10**, 3–10.

ARAMENDIA P., LETONA J. M. L. de, AVIADO D. M. (1962b). Exchange of blood between pulmonary and systemic circulations via bronchopulmonary anastomoses. *Circulat. Res.* **11**, 870–879.

ARNOULD P., PERNOT C., SIMON A. (1957). l'Occlusion unilatérale temporaire de l'artère pulmonaire chez l'homme. *Rev. Nancy Méd.* **82**, 113–128.

ARVIDSSON H., MOBERG A. (1966). Extracardiac anastomoses to the myocardium. *Acta Radiol.* **4**, 385–394.

AVERILL K. H., WAGNER W. W. jr., VOGEL J. H. K. (1962). Studies on bronchial arterial flow and bronchopulmonary anastomoses. *Med. Thorac.* **19**, 598–608.

AVIADO D. M., DALY M. DE BURGH, LEE C. Y., SCHMIDT C. F. (1961). The contribution of the bronchial circulation to the venous admixture in pulmonary venous blood. *J. Physiol. (Lond.)* **155**, 602–622.

BARRETT N. R., DALEY R. (1949). A method of increasing the lung blood supply in cyanotic congential heart disease. *Brit. Med. J.* **49**, 699–702.

BELL A. L. L., SHIMOMURA S., GUTHRIE W. J., HEMPEL H. F., FITZPATRICK H. F., BEGG C. F. (1959). Wedge pulmonary arteriography. *Radiology* **73**, 566–574.

BELTRAMI V., MARCHEGIANI C., STELLA S., FRANCESCHINI R. (1965). In tema di arteriografia bronchiale selettiva. Proposta di una nuova metodica sperimentale. *Ann. Ital. Chir.* **42**, 325–337.

BENNET J., CHALUT J., PROT D. (1966). Anomalies complexes de la vascularisation pulmonaire. *Ann. Radiol.* **9**, 495–513.

BENNET J., DEBRUN G., LABRUNE M., PLAINFOSSÉ M. C. (1967). l'Hypervascularisation systémique de poumon de l'enfant. *Ann. Radiol.* **10**, 667–674.

BERRY J. L., DALY I. DE BURGH (1931–1932). The relation between the pulmonary and bronchial vascular systems. *Proc. Roy. Soc. Med. Lond.* **109**, 319–336.

BERRY J. L. (1935). The relation between bronchial and pulmonary circulations in the human lung, investigated by radiopaque injections. *Quart. J. Exp. Physiol.* **24**, 305–313.

BING R. J., VANDAM L. D., GRAY F. D. jr. (1947). Physiological studies in congenital heart disease. II. Results of preoperative studies in patients with tetralogy of Fallot. *Bull. Johns Hopk. Hosp.* **80**, 121–141.

BJÖRK L. (1966). Anastomoses between coronary and bronchial arteries. *Acta Radiol.* **4**, 93–96.

BJÖRK L. (1966). Angiographic demonstration of extracardial anastomoses to the coronary arteries. *Radiology* **87**, 274–277.

BLALOCK A. (1951). A consideration of some of the problems in cardiovascular surgery *J. Thorac. Surg.* **21**, 543–571.

BLANK N., LOWER R., ADAMS D. F. (1966). Bronchial dynamics and the reconstitution of bronchial artery supply in the autotransplantated lung. *Invest. Radiol.* **1**, 363–370.

BLOOMER W. E., HARRISON W., LINDSKOG G. E., LIEBOW A. A. (1949). Respiratory function and blood flow in the bronchial artery after ligation of the pulmonary artery. *Amer. J. Physiol.* **157**, 317–328.

BOREK Z., MACHOLDA F., POLÁK J. (1967). Selektivní bronchiální arteriografie u bronchogenního karcinomu. *Sborn. Lék.* **69**, 99–107.

BOTENGA A. S. J. (1968). The role of bronchopulmonary anastomoses in chronic in flammatory processes of the lung. Selective arteriographic investigation. *Amer. J. Roentgenol.* **104**, 829–837.

BOTENGA A. S. J. (1969). The significance of bronchopulmonary anastomoses in pulmonary anomalies: a selective angiographic study. *Radiol. Clin. Biol.* **38**, 309–328.

BOIJSEN E., ZSIGMOND M. (1965). Selective angiography of bronchial and intercostal arteries. *Acta Radiol.* **3**, 514–528.

BOIJSEN E., REUTER S. R. (1966). Subclavian and internal mammary angiography in the evaluation of anterior mediastinal masses. *Amer. J. Roentgenol.* **98**, 447–450.

BROCK R. C. (1949). The surgery of pulmonary stenosis. *Brit. Med. J.* **2**, 399–406.

BRUNER H. D., SCHMIDT C. F. (1947). Blood flow in the bronchial artery of the anesthetized dog. *Amer. J. Physiol.* **148**, 648–666.

BRUNI A. C. (1954). La circolazione del sangue nei bronchi prima e dopo la nascita. *Bronches, les* **4**, 126–144.

BRUWER A. J. (1966). Systemic-pulmonary vascular communication arising from axillary artery. *Med. Radiogr. Photogr.* **42**, 146–151.

CALABRESI P., ABELMANN W. H. (1957). Porto-caval and portopulmonary anastomoses in Laennec's cirrhosis and in heart failure. *J. Clin. Invest.* **36**, 1257–1265.

CAMARRI E., MARINI G. (1965). *La circulation bronchique a l'état normal et patthologique.* Éditon française par M. LATARJET. Édit. Doin, Paris.

CAMPBELL M., GARDNER F. (1950). Radiological features of enlarged bronchial arteries. *Brit. Heart J.* **12**, 183–200.

CAULDWELL E. W., SIEKERT R. G., LININGER R. E., ANSON B. J. (1948). The bronchial arteries; an anatomic study of 150 human cadavers. *Surg. Gynec. Obstet.* **86**, 395–412.

CHAVEZ C. M. (1967). Selective arterial catheterization. A field of increasing dimensions. *Surgery* **61**, 634–643.

CHRISTELLER E. (1916). Funktionelles und Anatomisches bei der angeborenen Verengerung und dem angeborenen Verschlusz der Lungenarterie, insbesondere über die arteriellen Kollateralbahnen bei diesen Zuständen. *Virchows Arch. Path. Anat.* **223**, 40–57.

CICERO R., CARDOSO J. M., DEL CASTILLO H., KUTHY J. (1968). Selective angiography of the bronchial arteries in pulmonary tuberculosis. *Amer. Rev. Resp. Dis.* **98**, 623–633.

CLARKE J. A. (1965). An X-ray microscopic study of the postnatal development of the vasa vasorum in the pulmonary trunk and arteries. *Thorax* **20**, 348–356.

CLIFFTON E. E., DHAN RAJ MAHAJAN (1963). Technique for visualisation and perfusion of bronchial arteries: suggested clinical and diagnostic applications. *Cancer* **16**, 444–452.

COCKETT F. B., VASS C. C. N. (1950). The collateral circulation to the lungs. *Brit. J. Surg.* **38**, 97–103.

COCKETT F. B., VASS C. C. N. (1951). A comparision of the role of the bronchial arteries in bronchiëctasis and in experimental ligation of the pulmonary artery. *Thorax* **6**, 268–275.

COLLISTER R. M. (1952). *Collateral circulation in stenosis of the great vessels.* Thesis, Leiden.

COLUMBUS R. (1559). *De re anatomica libri XV.* Lib. XI, Cap. II, Venetiis.

CORBIN J. L. (1961). *Anatomie et pathologie artérielles de la moelle.* Masson Édit., Paris.

COSTA M. FREITAS E (1966). Visualização das artérias brônquicas. *J. Soc. Cien. Med.* **130**, 196–204.

COSTA M. FREITAS E (1967). Enige aspecten van selectieve broncho-arteriografie. *Camera Radiologica (Dagra)*, 49–63.

COURNAND A. (1947). Recent observations on the dynamics of the pulmonary circulation. *Bull. N.Y. Acad. Med.* **23**, 27–50.

CRENSHAW G. L., ROWLES D. F. (1952). Surgical management of pulmonary emphysema. *J. Thorac. Surg.* **24**, 398–410.

CRENSHAW G. L. (1954). Degenerative lung disease. *Dis. Chest* **25**, 427–442.

CSÁKÁNY G. (1964). Das Röntgenbild des hypertrophischen kollateralen Bronchialkreislaufs. *Fortschr. Röntgenstr.* **100**, 622–629.

CUDKOWICZ L., ARMSTRONG J. B. (1951). Observations on the normal anatomy of the bronchial arteries. *Thorax* 6, 343–358.

CUDKOWICZ L. (1952a). The blood supply of the lung in pulmonary tuberculosis. *Thorax* 7, 270–276.

CUDKOWICZ L. (1952b). Some observations of the bronchial arteries in lobar pneumonia and pulmonary infarction. *Brit. J. Dis. Chest* 46, 99–102.

CUDKOWICZ L., ARMSTRONG J. B. (1952). Injection of the bronchial circulation in a case of transposition. *Brit. Heart J.* 14, 374–378.

CUDKOWICZ L. (1953). Leonardo da Vinci and the bronchial circulation. *Brit. J. Tuberc.* 47, 23–25.

CUDKOWICZ L., ARMSTRONG J. B. (1953a). The bronchial arteries in pulmonary emphysema. *Thorax* 8, 46–58.

CUDKOWICZ L., ARMSTRONG J. B. (1953b). The blood supply of malignant pulmonary neoplasms. *Thorax* 8, 152–156.

CUDKOWICZ L., ARMSTRONG J. B. (1953c). Finger clubbing and changes in the bronchial circulation. *Brit. J. Dis. Chest* 47, 227–232.

CUDKOWICZ L., WRAITH D. G. (1957). An evaluation of the clinical significance of clubbing in common lung disorders. *Brit. J. Tuberc.* 51, 14–31.

CUDKOWICZ L., CALABRESI M., NIMS R. G., GRAY F. D. jr. (1959). The simultaneous estimation of right and left ventricular outputs applied to a study of the bronchial circulation in patients with chronic lung disease. *Amer. Heart J.* 58, 743–749.

CUDKOWICZ L., ABELMANN W. H., LEVINSON G. E., KATZNELSON G., JREISSATY R. M. (1960). Bronchial arterial blood flow. *Clin. Sci.* 19, 1–15.

CUDKOWICZ L. (1962). Bronchial arterial blood flow in man. A review. *Med. Thorac.* 19, 582–597.

DALY I. DE BURGH (1936). The physiology of the bronchial vascular system. *Harvey Lect.* 32, 235–255.

DARKE C. S., LEWTAS N. A. (1968). Selective bronchial arteriography in the demonstration of abnormal systemic circulation in the lung. *Clin. Radiol.* 19, 357–367.

DAUSSY M., ABELANET R. (1956). Modifications circulatoires de certains poumons pathologiques. *J. Franç. Méd. Chir. Thor.* 10, 305–313.

DAUSSY M., DAUMET PH. (1960). Bilan hémodynamique des affections pleuro-pulmonaires chirurgicales. Son intérêt pré-opératoire. *Le Poumon* 16, 349–362.

DEENSTRA (1967). De solitaire haard in de longen. *Ned. T. Geneesk.* 111, 1003–1004.

DELARUE J., PAILLAS J., SORS CH. (1952). Présence de segments d'arrêt et de glomi dans la paroi des bronches ectasiées. *J. Franç. Méd. Chir. Thor.* 6, 249–259.

DELARUE J., SORS CH., MIGNOT J. (1953). Les modifications vasculaires au cours des bronchiectasies. *J. Franç. Méd. Chir. Thor.* 7, 225–238.

DELARUE J., SORS CH., MIGNOT J. (1953). Étude comparée de la vascularisation des cavernes tuberculeuses et des foyers caséeux circonscrits. *Rev. Tuberc., Paris* 17, 609–640.

DELARUE J., PAILLAS J., ABELANET R., CHOMETTE G. (1959). Les broncho-pneumopathies congénitales. *Bronches, les* 9, 114–211.

DESILETS D. T., RUTTENBERG H. D., HOFFMAN R. B. (1966). Percutaneous catheterization in children. *Radiology* 87, 119–122.

DJINDJIAN R., HURTH M., JULIAN H. (1967). Arteriographie normale et pathologique de la moelle dorso-lombaire. *J. Belge Radiol.* 50, 214–221.

DJINDJIAN R., FAURÉ C. (1967). Accidents médullaires de l'aortographie. *J. Belge Radiol.* 50, 207–213.

DONKERS B. (1968). *Een anatomisch onderzoek van pulmonalis-atresie, mede in verband met de collaterale bloedvoorziening van de longen.* Proefschrift, Leiden.

DOPPMAN J., DI CHIRO G. D. (1968). The arteria radicularis magna: radiographic anatomy in the adult. *Brit. J. Radiol.* 41, 40–45.

DUSSAUT M.-A. (1966). *l'Angiographie des artères bronchiques. Applications en pathologie thoracique.* Thèse, Lyon.

DUVOISIN G. E., FOWLER W. S., PAYNE W. S., ELLIS F. H. (1964). Reimplantation of the dog lung with survival after contralateral pneumonectomy. *Surg. Forum* 15, 173–175.

EAST T., BARNARD W. G. (1938). Pulmonary atresia and hypertrophy of the bronchial arteries. *Lancet, the* I, 834–837.

EDWARDS D. W. (1961). A summary of the third conference on research in emphysema: Air pollution and chronic pulmonary insufficiency. Answer to question no. 5. *Amer. Rev. Resp. Dis.* 83, 581–582.

EFSEN F. (1966). Spinal cord lesion as a complication of abdominal aortography. *Acta Radiol.* 4, 47–61.

ELBERT P. A., ALLGOOD R. J., JONES H. W. III, SABISTON D. C. (1967). Hemodynamics during pulmonary artery occlusion. *Surgery* **62,** 18–24.

ELLIOTT F. M., REID L. (1965). Some new facts about pulmonary artery and its branching pattern. *Clin. Radiol.* **16,** 193–198.

ELLIS F. H., GRINDLAY J. H., EDWARDS J. E. (1951). The bronchial arteries. I. Experimental occlusion. *Surgery* **30,** 810–826.

ENNABLI M. E. (1966). Situation et rapport des artères intercostales aortiques. *Presse Méd.,* 2113.

FALKENBACH K. H., ZHEUTLIN N., DOWDY A. H., O'LOUGHLIN B. J. (1959). Pulmonary hypertension due to pulmonary artery coarctation. *Radiology* **73,** 575–590.

FATTI L., GILROY J. C. (1949). Thoracoscopy as an aid to diagnosis in congenital heart disease. *Brit. Heart J.* **11,** 398–406.

FAURÉ C., DJINDJIAN R., LEFEBVRE J. (1966). A propos du risque médullaire de l'aortographie abdominale. *Ann. Radiol.* **9,** 523–530.

FAURÉ C., LEFEBVRE J., DEBRUN G., DJINDJIAN R. (1967). La vascularisation artérielle normale et pathologique du renflement lombaire de la moelle épinière chez l'enfant: l'artère d'Adamkiewicz. *Ann. Radiol.* **10,** 129–140.

FEDOROVA V. V. (1965). Ramifications of bronchial arteries in human pleura (In russian). *Tr. Kuibyshevsk. Med. Inst.* **35,** 32–37.

FEIGELSON H. H., RAVIN H. A. (1965). Transverse myelitis following selective bronchial arteriography. *Radiology* **85,** 663–665.

FERGUSON F. C., KOBILAK K. E., DEITRICK J. E. (1944). Varices of the bronchial veins as a source of hemoptysis in mitral stenosis. *Amer. Heart J.* **28,** 445–456.

FESANI F., PELLEGRINO F., ROSSI L. (1966). Study of the bronchial circulation in pulmonary affections by means of thoracic aortography. *Ateneo Parmense* **37,** 277–288.

FISHMAN A. P., TURINO G. M., BRANDFONBRENER M., HIMMELSTEIN A. (1958). The effective pulmonary collateral blood flow in man. *J. Clin. Invest.* **37,** 1071–1086.

FISHMAN A. P. (1961). The clinical significance of the pulmonary collateral circulation. *Circulation* **24,** 677–690.

FLORANGE W. (1960). Anatomie und Pathologie der Arteria bronchialis. *Ergeb. Allg. Path. u. Path. Anat.,* 152–224.

FOX I. J., CROWLEY W. P., GRACE J. B., WOOD E. H. (1966). Effects of de Valsalva maneuver on blood flow in the thoracic aorta in man. *J. Appl. Physiol.* **21,** 1553–1560.

FRECKMAN H. A., MENDEZ F. L., MAURER E. R., FRY H. L. (1966). Chemotherapy for lungcancer by intra-aortic infusion. *J. Amer. Med. Ass.* **196,** 5–10.

FRITTS H. W. jr., HARRIS P., CHIDSEY C. A., CLAUSS R. H., COURNAND A. (1961). Estimation of flow through bronchial-pulmonary vascular anastomoses with use of T-1824 dye. *Circulation* **23,** 390–398.

FROMENT R., GALY P., TOLOT F., COHEN P., GARDÈRE J., UGNAT F. A. (1954). Hypertension ou dilatation artérielle pulmonaire primitive et communications entre artères bronchiques et pulmonaires. *Rev. Lyon Méd.* **3,** 255–269.

GAHAGAN T., MANZOR A. (1966). Reestablishment of pulmonary-artery flow after prolonged complete occlusion. *J. Amer. Med. Ass.* **198,** 639–640.

GARDÈRE J. (1953). *Hypertension artérielle pulmonaire primitive et communications entre artères bronchiques et pulmonaires.* Thèse, Lyon.

GARUSI G. F. (1961). Opacification of the bronchial arteries in the living. *Radiol. Clin.* **30,** 65–75.

GASTAING R., FREOUR P., CHEVAIS R., GERMOUTY J. (1961). Étude hémodynamique des bronchiectasies. *J. Franç. Méd. Chir. Thor.* **15,** 645–653.

GEBAUER P. W., MASON C. B. (1959). Intralobar pulmonary sequestration associated with anomalous pulmonary vessels: a nonentity. *Dis. Chest* **35,** 282–288.

GERARD F. P., LYONS H. A. (1958). Anomalous artery in intralobar bronchopulmonary sequestration. Report of two cases demonstrated by angiography. *New Engl. J. Med.* **259,** 662–666.

GERNEZ-RIEUX CH., RÉMY J., VOISIN C., ROUSELLE J.-M., WALLAERT C. (1967). l'Artériographie bronchique sélective. *J. Franç. Méd. Chir. Thor.* **21,** 463–475.

GHOREYEB A. A., KARSNER H. T. (1913). A study of the relation of pulmonary and bronchial circulation. *J. Exp. Med.* **18,** 500–506.

GILLILAN L. A. (1958). The arterial blood supply of the human spinal cord. *J. Comp. Neurol.* **110,** 75–103.

GILROY J. C., WILSON V. H., MARCHAND P. (1951). Observations on the haemodynamics of pulmonary and lobar atelectasis. *Thorax* **6,** 137–144.

GIORDANI M., PINNA C. D. (1956). l'Origine delle arterie bronchiali (Ricerca di anatomia chirurgica). *Gazz. Int. Med. Chir.* **61**, 2733–2751.

GOETZ R. H., ROHMAN M., STATE D. (1965). The hemodynamics of bronchopulmonary anastomoses. *Surg. Gynec. Obstet.* **120**, 517–529.

GOFFRINI P. (1967). Bronchial arterial system and bronchial arteriography in lung diseases. *J. Cardiovasc. Res.* **8**, 501–509.

GROEN A. S., ZIEDSES DES PLANTES B. G., WESTRA D. (1965). Angiography of the bronchial circulation in bronchial carcinoma by means of subtraction technique: its value in regional infusion. *Dis. Chest* **48**, 634–640.

GROEN A. S., ZIEDSES DES PLANTES B. G., JONG J. DE, WESTRA D. (1966). Angiografie van de bronchiale arteriën met toepassing van de subtractiemethode. *Ned. T. Geneesk.* **110**, 2201–2210.

GUNTHEROTH W. A., ARCASOY M. M., PHILLIPS L. A., FIGLEY M. M. (1962). Demonstration of collateral circulation to the lung with angiocardiographic studies in congenital heart disease. *Amer. J. Cardiol.* **62**, 293–300.

HALES M. R., LIEBOW A. A. (1948). Collateral circulation to the lungs in congenital pulmonic stenosis. *J. Tech. Meth.* **28**, 1–22.

HALLER J. D., BRON K. M., WHOLEY M. H., POLLER S., ENERSON D. M. (1966). Selective bronchial artery catheterization for diagnostic and physiologic studies and chemotherapy for bronchogenic carcinoma. *J. Thorac. Cardiovasc. Surg.* **51**, 143–152.

HARRIS P., HEATH D. (1962). *The human pulmonary circulation. Its form and function in health and disease.* Livingstone, London.

HAYEK H. V. (1940). I. Über verschluszfähige Arteriën in der menschlichen Lunge. II. Über periarterielle Lymphräume in der menschlichen Lunge. *Anat. Anz.* **89**, 216–224.

HAYEK H. V. (1953a). IV. Die menschliche Lunge und ihre Gefässe, ihr Bau unter besonderer Berücksichtigung der Funktion. *Ergebn. Anat.* **34**, 144–249.

HAYEK H. V. (1953b). Die anatomischen Grundlagen des Lungenoedems. *Wien. Klin. Wschr.* **65**, 740–743.

HAYEK H. V. (1953c). *Die menschliche Lunge.* Springer, Berlin.

HAYEK H. V. (1954). La vascularisation sanguine des bronches. *Bronches, les* **4**, 110–125.

HEIMBURG P. (1964). Bronchial collateral circulation in experimental stenosis of the pulmonary artery. *Thorax* **19**, 306–310.

HEPPLESTON A. G., LEOPOLD J. G. (1961). Chronic pulmonary emphysema. Anatomy and pathogenesis. *Amer. J. Med.* **31**, 279–291.

HERTZOG P., ISRAEL R., TOTY L., PERSONNE C. (1952). Interprétation des images angiopneumographiques. Distinction entre l'amputation organique des artères et la simple raréfaction fonctionnelle de la circulation pulmonaire. *J. Franç. Méd. Chir. Thor.* **5**, 450–454.

HOCKMAN R. P., MARK J. B. D. (1964). Effect of bronchial arterial infusion of mechlorethamine on pulmonary structure in the experimental animal. *Surg. Forum* **15**, 194–196.

HORISBERGER B., RODBARD S. (1960). Direct measurement of bronchial arterial flow. *Circulat. Res.* **8**, 1149–1156.

HOVELACQUE A., MONOD O., EVRARD H. (1936). Note au sujet des artères bronchiques. *Ann. Anat. Path.* **13**, 129–141.

HUDSON C. L., MORITZ A. R., WEARN J. T. (1932). The extracardiac anastomoses of the coronary arteries. *J. Exp. Med.* **56**, 919–926.

HUGGINS C. E. (1959). Reimplantation of lobes of the lung. *Lancet, the* **I**, 1059–1062.

HUGHES J. T., BROWNELL B. (1965). Paraplegia following retrograde abdominal aortography. An example of toxis myelitis. *Arch. Neurol.* **12**, 650–657.

HURWITZ A., CALABRESI M., COOKE R. W., LIEBOW A. A. (1954). An experimental study of the venous collateral circulation of the lung: I. Anatomical observations. *Amer. J. Path.* **30**, 1085–1116. II. Functional observations. *J. Thorac. Surg.* **28**, 241–246.

HUTCHIN P., TERZI R. G. G., PETERS R. M. (1967). Bronchial-pulmonary artery reverse flow: Angiographic demonstration in bronchiectasis. *Ann. Thorac. Surg.* **4**, 391–398.

IKEDA M., NEYAZAKI T., CHIBA S., YONETI M., SUZUKI C. (1968). Bronchial vascular pattern of various pulmonary diseases, with particular emphasis on its diagnostic value in pulmonary cancer. *J. Thorac. Cardiovasc. Surg.* **55**, 642–652.

ISLEY J. K., BACOS J., HICKAN J. B., BAYUN G. J. (1962). Bronchiolar behavior in pulmonary emphysema and in bronchiectasis. *Amer. J. Roentgenol.* **87**, 853–858.

KAFKA V., BECO V. (1960). Simultaneous intra- and extrapulmonary sequestration. *Arch. Dis. Childh.* **35**, 51–56.

KAHN P. C. (1965). The epinephrine effect in selective renal angiography. *Radiology* **85**, 301–305.

KAHN P. C., PAUL R. E., RHEINLANDER H. F. (1965). Selective bronchial arteriography and intra-arterial chemotherapy in carcinoma of the lung. *J. Thorac. Cardiovasc. Surg.* **50**, 640–647.

KAHN P. C., CALLOW A. D. (1965). Selective vasodilatation as an aid to angiography. *Amer. J. Roentgenol.* **94**, 213–220.

KAHN P. C. (1967). Selective angiography of the inferior phrenic arteries. *Radiology* **88**, 1–8.

KAHN P. C., WISE H. M. jr. (1968). The use of epinephrine in selective angiography of renal masses. *J. Urol.* **99**, 133–138.

KARSNER H. T., ASH J. E. (1912–1913). II. Experimental bland infarction of the lung. *J. Med. Res.* **27**, 205–224.

KIEFFER S. A., AMPLATZ K., ANDERSON R. C., WALTON LILLEHEI C. (1965). Proximal interruption of a pulmonary artery. *Amer. J. Roentgenol.* **95**, 592–597.

KILLEN D. A., FORSTER J. H. (1960). Spinal cord injury as a complication of aortography. *Ann. Surg.* **152**, 211–230.

KILLEN D. A., LANCE E. M. (1962). Investigation of means to prevent spinal cord and renal damage incident to urokon aortography. *Surgery* **51**, 338–346.

KILMAN J. W., BATTERSBY J. S., HOOSHANG TAYBI, VELLIOS F. (1965). Pulmonary sequestration. *Arch. Surg.* **90**, 648–657.

KLEIN A., CZERWIŃSKI W., MEYZA J., WERNER H. (1966). Ocena wartości paliatywnego leczenia raka pluca metodac Clifftona-Mahajana. *Nowotwory* **16**, 151–153.

KOROL E. (1938). Pulmonary emphysema in tuberculosis. Definition and classification. *Amer. Rev. Tuberc.* **38**, 594–605.

KOURILSKY R., DECROIX G. (1960). *Les suppurations bronchiques pulmonaires et pleurales.* Baillière Édit., Paris.

KOURILSKY R., DECROIX G., PIÉRON R., KOURILSKY P., CHARLIER P., JACQUILLAT CL., VERLEY J.-M. (1961). Nouvelles observations de troubles ventilatoires et circulatoire unilatéraux. *J. Franç. Méd. Chir. Thor.* **15**, 633–644.

KOZUKA T., NOSAKI T., SATO K., IHARA K., TACHIIRI H. (1964). Single lumen balloon catheter (In japonese). *Nippon Acta Radiol.* **24**, 960–965.

LANCE E. M., DUNCAN A., KILLEN D. A., OWENS G. (1958). An exploration of factors involved in the production and prevention of paraplegia following intraaortic Urokon injection. *Surg. Forum* **9**, 728–731.

LANDRIGAN P. L., PURKIS I., ROY D., CUDKOWICZ L. (1963). Cardio-respiratory studies in a patient with an absent left pulmonary artery. *Thorax* **18**. 77–82.

LANG E. K. (1963). A survey of complications of percutaneous retrograde arteriography. Seldinger technic. *Radiology* **81**, 257–263.

LATARJET M., JUTTIN P. (1951). Données nouvelles sur la circulation dans les artères bronchiques. *Le Poumon* **7**, 35–50.

LATARJET M., JUTTIN P. (1952). Emploi des injections de matière plastique dans l'étude anatomo-pathologique pulmonaire. *Le Poumon* **8**, 459–463.

LATARJET M. (1954a). Anastomoses vasculaires dans les „séquestres pulmonaires" avec artère anormale. *Le Poumon* **11**, 33–40.

LATARJET M. (1954b). La vascularisation sanguine des bronches. *Bronches, les* **4**, 145–175.

LATARJET M. (1956). La circulation collatérale intra-pulmonaire dans les suppurations broncho-pulmonaires chroniques et dans la tuberculose pulmonaire. *Lyon Chir.* **52**, 187–197.

LATARJET M. (1958). Dispositifs vasculaires dans les kystes congénitaux du poumon humain. *C. R. Ass. Anat.* **101**, 473–482.

LAUWERIJNS J. (1962). *De longvaten. Arthitectoniek en rol bij de longontplooiing.* Proefschrift, Brussel.

LEES M. H., DOTTER C. T. (1965). Bronchial circulation in severe multiple peripheral artery stenosis. *Circulation* **31**, 759–761.

LE FORT L. (1859). *Recherches sur l'anatomie du poumon chez l'homme (Veines broncho-pulmonaires, 97).* Delahaye, Paris.

LEVINSON G. E., CUDKOWICZ L., ABELMANN W. H. (1959). Measurement of regional blood flow by indicator dilution. *Science* **129**, 840–841.

LIEBOW A. A., HALES M. R., LINDSKOG G. E. (1949). Enlargement of the bronchial arteries and their anastomoses with the pulmonary arteries in bronchiëctasis. *Amer. J. Path.* **25**, 211–233.

LIEBOW A. A., HALES M. R., HARRISON W., BLOOMER W., LINDSKOG G. E. (1949–1950). The genesis and functional implications of collateral circulation of the lungs. *Yale J. Biol. Med.* **22**, 637–650.

LIEBOW A. A., HALES M. R., BLOOMER W. E., HARRISON W., LINDSKOG G. E. (1950). Studies on the lung after ligation of the pulmonary artery. II. Anatomical changes. *Amer. J. Path.* **26**, 177–195.

LIEBOW A. A. (1953). The bronchopulmonary venous collateral circulation with special reference to emphysema. *Amer. J. Path.* **29**, 251–289.

LIEBOW A. A., HALES M. R., BLOOMER W. E. (1958). Relation of bronchial to pulmonary vascular tree. *Pulmonary circulation. An international symposion*, 79–98. Edited by W. R. Adams and I. Veith. Grune & Stratton, Ihe, New York–London.

LIEBOW A. A. (1959). Pulmonary emphysema with special reference to vascular changes. *Amer. Rev. Resp. Dis.* **80**, 67–93.

LIEBOW A. A. (1962). Recent observations on pulmonary collateral circulation. *Med. Thorac.* **19**, 609–612.

LIEBOW A. A. (1965). Patterns of origin and distribution of the major bronchial arteries in man. *Amer. J. Anat.* **117**, 19–32.

LOPO DE CARVALHO. Cited by PAPILLON ET AL. (1960).

LUDIN H. (1963). Hämodynamische Wirkungen des Vasalva-Versuches. *Med. Thorac.* **20**, 193–210.

LURUS A. G., COWEN R. L., ECKERT J. F. (1969). Systemic-pulmonary arteriovenous fistula following close-tube thoracotomy. *Radiology* **92**, 1296–1298.

LUSCHKA H. (1863). *Die Anatomie der Brust des Menschen.* I, 2, 316. Tübingen, Laupp.

MACK J. F., MOSS A. J., HARPER W. W., O'LOUGHLIN B. J. (1965). The bronchial arteries in cystic fibrosis. *Brit. J. Radiol.* **38**, 422–429.

MADOFF I. M., GAENSLER E. A., STRIEDER J. W. (1952). Congenital absence of the right pulmonary artery. Diagnosis by angiocardiography, with cardio-respiratory studies. *New. Engl. J. Med.* **247**, 149–157.

MAKSIMUK (1962). Adaptability of the bronchial arteries and the dynamics of external respiration (In russian). *Med. Inst. Stanislav.*, 68–69.

MANDELBAUM I., GIAMMONA S. T. (1966). Bronchial circulation during cardiopulmonary bypass. *Ann. Surg.* **164**, 985–989.

MARCHAND P., GILROY J. C., WILSON V. H. (1950). An anatomical study of the bronchial vascular system and its variations in disease. *Thorax* **5**, 207–221.

MARGULIS R. (1964). Arteriography of tumours: difficulties in interpretation and the need for magnification. *Radiol. Clin. N. Amer.* **2**, 543–562.

MARK J. B. D., HOCKMAN R. P., CARRINGTON C. B. (1965). Experimental bronchial arterial infusion of mechlorethamine. *J. Thorac. Cardiovasc. Surg.* **50**, 9–15.

MARTINEZ J., LETONA I. DE, MATA R. C. DE LA, AVIADO D. M. (1961). Local and reflex effects of bronchial arterial injection of drugs. *J. Pharmacol. Exp. Ther.* **133**, 295–312.

MASSUMI R. A., DONOHOE R. F. (1965a). Congenital absence versus acquired attenuation of one pulmonary artery. *Circulation* **31**, 436–447.

MASSUMI R. A., RIOS J. C., DONOHOE R. F. (1965b). The pathogenesis of angiographic nonvizualization or attenuation of a patent pulmonary artery and the role of bronchial artery-pulmonary artery anastomoses. *J. Thorac. Cardiovasc. Surg.* **49**, 772–789.

MATHES M. E., HOLMAN E., REICHERT F. L. (1932). A study of the bronchial, pulmonary and lymphatic circulations of the lung under various pathologic conditions experimentally produced. *J. Thorac. Surg.* **1**, 339–362.

MATTHES T., FUCHS U. (1956). Experimenteller Beitrag zur Frage der kollateral einspringenden pulmonalen Gefäszversorgung nach Ligatur der Bronchialarterien und Resektionen und Anastomosen am Hauptbronchus. *Ärztl. Forsch.* **10**, 577–581.

MCAFEE J. G. (1957). A survey of complications of abdominal aortography. *Radiology* **68**, 825–838.

MCALISTER W. H., MARGULIS A. R. (1963). Angiography in malignant tumours in mice following irradiation. *Radiology* **81**, 664–675.

MCLAUGHLIN R. F., TYLER W. S., CANADA R. O. (1961). A study of the subgross pulmonary anatomy in various mammals. *Amer. J. Anat.* **108**, 149–165.

MILLER W. S. (1906). The arrangement of the bronchial blood vessels. *Anat. Anz.* **28**, 432–436.

MILLER W. S. (1947). *The lung.* Second edition. Thomas Publisher, Springfield-Ill.

MILLER B. J., ROSENBAUM A. J. (1967). The vascular supply to metastatic tumors of the lung. *Surg. Gynec. Obst* et. **125**, 1009–1012.

MILNE E. N. C. (1967). Circulation of primary and metastatic pulmonary neoplasms. A postmortem microarteriographic study. *Amer. J. Roentgenol.* **100**, 603–619.

MOBERG A. (1967a). Anastomoses between extracardiac vessels and coronary arteries – I – via bronchial arteries. *Acta Radiol.* **6**, 177–192.

MOBERG A. (1967b). Anastomoses between extracardiac vessels and coronary arteries – II – via internal mammary arteries. *Acta Radiol.* **6**, 263–272.

MORAND P., LAFFONT H., VAILLAUD J.-C., HOUEL J. (1963). Étude de la circulation bronchique dans les lésions pulmonaires étendues unilatérales. Apport de l'aortographie rétrograde. *J. Franç. Méd. Chir. Thor.* **17**, 369–392.

NAKAMURA N. (1924). Zur Anatomie der Bronchial-Arterien. *Anat. Anz.* **58**, 508–517.

NAKAMURA T., KATORI R., MIYAZAWA K., OHTOMO S., WATANABE TA., WATANABE TE., MIURA Y., TAKIZAWA T. (1961). Bronchial blood flow in patients with chronic pulmonary disease and its influences upon respiration and circulation. *Dis. Chest* **39**, 193–206.

NAKAMURA T., KATORI R., MIYAZAWA K., ODA J., ISHIKAWA K. (1967). Measurement of bronchial blood flow in tetralogy of Fallot. *Circulation* **35**, 904–912.

NEYAZAKI T. (1962). A method for arteriography of the bronchial artery. *Jap. Heart. J.* **3**, 523–536.

NEYAZAKI T. (1964). An angiographic study between pulmonary and bronchial circulation in various pulmonary diseases. *Tuberc. Leprosy Cancer* **11**, 324–350.

NEWTON T. H., PREGER L. (1965). Selective bronchial arteriography. *Radiology* **84**, 1043–1051.

NOONAN C. D., MARGULIS A. R., WRIGHT R. (1965). Bronchial arterial patterns in pulmonary metastasis. *Radiology* **84**, 1033–1042.

NORDENSTRÖM B. (1960). Contrast examination of the cardiovascular system during increased intrabronchial pressure. *Acta Radiol. suppl.* **200**, 1–110.

NORDENSTRÖM B. (1962). Balloon catheters for percutaneous insertion into the vascular system. *Acta Radiol.* **57**, 411–416.

NORDENSTRÖM B. (1963). Methods of altering circulatory dynamics to improve roentgen examination of the cardiovascular system. *Amer. J. Roentgenol.* **89**, 233–253.

NORDENSTRÖM B. (1965). A preliminary report on the selective application of cytostatics and the transthoracic needle coagulation of bronchial carcinomas. *Acta Radiol.* **3**, 115–128.

NORDENSTRÖM B. (1966a). Selective catheterization with tifocyl injection of broncho-mediastinal arteries in bronchial carcinoma. *Acta Radiol.* **4**, 298–304.

NORDENSTRÖM B. (1966b). Percutaneous balloon-occlusion of the aorta. *Acta Radiol.* **4**, 365–374.

NORDENSTRÖM B. (1966c). Angiocardiography. Effect of increased intrabronchial pressure. *Stockholm. Postgrad. Med.* **40**, A-67.

NORDENSTRÖM B., TÖRNELL G. (1966). Possibilities of angiography during temporary occlusion of the aorta in man. *Acta Radiol.* **4**, 321–330.

NORDENSTRÖM B. (1967). Selective catheterization and angiography of bronchial and mediastinal arteries in man. *Acta Radiol.* **6**, 13–25.

NORTH L. B., BOUSHY S. F., HOUK V. N. (1969). Bronchial and intercostal arteriography in non-neoplastic pulmonary disease. *Amer. J. Roentgenol.* **107**, 328–342.

ÖDMAN P. (1959). The radiopaque polythene catheter. *Acta Radiol. suppl.* **52**, 52–63.

O'LOUGHLIN B. J. (1965). Experimental approaches to pulmonary emphysema. *Amer. J. Roentgenol.* **93**, 850–867.

O'RAHILLY R., DEBSON H., SUMMERFIELD K.-T. (1950). Subclavian origin of bronchial arteries. *Anat. Rec.* **108**, 227–238.

ORELL S. R., HULTGREN S. (1966). Anastomoses between bronchial and pulmonary arteries in pulmonary thromboembolic disease. *Acta Path. Microbiol. Scand.* **67**, 322–338.

OSIPOV B. K., MANEVICH V. L., EVGRAFOV V. L. (1965). Ischemia, intravascular thrombogenesis and atelectasis of the lungs in temporary bronchiovascular occlusion (In russian). *Khirurgiia* **41**, 14–18.

OUDET P., PETITJEAN R., WEITZENBLUM E. (1967). Les anastomoses artérielles broncho-pulmonaires. Étude par radiocinématographie de l'injection de pièces d'exérèse; valeur de la méthode. *J. Franç. Méd. Chir. Thor.* **21**, 147–156.

OUTURQUIN G. (1967). *Intérêt de l'artériographie bronchique sélective dans les hémoptysies en apparence inexpliquées.* Thèse, Lille.

PADOVANI J., MORAND PH., CLEMENT J., HOUEL J. (1966). Les fausses amputations de l'artère pulmonaire dans les poumons détruits. *Ann. Radiol.* **9**, 512–522.

PAPILLON J., PINET F., CHASSARD J. L. (1960). l'Angiopneumographie dans l'exploration des malformations pulmonaires. *Gaz. Med. Port.* **13**, 274–282.

PARKE W. W., MICHELS N. A. (1965). The nonbronchial systemic arteries of the lung. *J. Thorac. Cardiovasc. Surg.* **49**, 694–707.

PETELENZ T. (1965). Extracoronary shunts with coronary arteries in man. *Cardiologia* **47**, 323–336.

PETELENZ T. (1967). Non-coronary anastomoses of bronchial arteries. *Cardiologia* **50**, 43–55.

PINET F., GRAVIER J., PINET A. (1959). l'Aortographie rétrograde sous hypotension contrôlée. *J. Radiol. Électrol.* **40**, 115–126.

PINET F., NAUDIN E.-P., PINET A., WOEHRLE R., DUSSAUT M.-A. (1965). l'Angiographie des artères bronchiques. Application à la pathologie pleuro-pulmonaire. *Supplément à la Presse Méd.* **20**, 73, no. 49, 23/1–23/4.

PINET F., NAUDIN E.-P., PINET A. (1966). l'Angiographie des artères bronchiques. *Ann. Radiol.* **9**, 489–494.

POLÁK J., MACHOLDA F., BOREK Z. (1967). Metodické zkušenosti se selektivní bronchiální arteriografii. *Sborn. Lék.* **69**, 93–98.

PRYCE D. M. (1946). Lower accessory pulmonary artery with intralobar sequestration of lung: a report of seven cases. *J. Path. Bact.* **58**, 457–467.

PUMP K. K. (1963). The bronchial arteries and their anastomoses in the human lung. *Dis. Chest* **43**, 245–255.

REID J. A., HEARD B. E. (1963). The capillary network of normal and emphysematous human lungs studied by injections of Indian ink. *Thorax* **18**, 201–212.

RÉMY J., WALLAERT C., VOISIN C., GERNEZ-RIEUX Ch. (1968). Angiographie sélective des artères bronchiques. *Presse Méd.* **76**, 729–732.

REUTER S. R., OLIN T., ABRAMS H. L. (1965). Selective bronchial arteriography. *Radiology* **84**, 87–95.

RHEINLANDER H. F., MILLER H. H., MOQUIN R. B., DETERLING R. A. jr. (1962). Upper hemibody infusion with alkylating agents for advanced lung cancer. *J. Thorac. Cardiovasc. Surg.* **44**, 801–812.

RHEINLANDER H. F., TATSUZO TANABE, PAUL R. E. jr. (1966). Selective infusion of bronchial arteries with mechlorethamine in dogs. *Surgery* **60**, 1044–1050.

RICHTER K. (1965). Anomalous systemic arteries to the lung visualized by tomography. *Amer. J. Roentgenol.* **95**, 629–635.

RIBAUDO C. A., ROSSI P., COMER J. V. (1966). Intralobar bronchopulmonary sequestration demonstrated by aortography and selective arteriography of the anomalous vessel. *Ann. Intern. Med.* **64**, 381–386.

ROOSENBURG J. G., DEENSTRA H. (1954). Bronchial-pulmonary vascular shunts in chronic pulmonary affections. *Dis. Chest* **26**, 664–671.

RUBIN E. H., RUBIN M., ATTAI L., HEIMANN W. G. (1966). Intralobar pulmonary sequestration: aortographic demonstration. *Dis. Chest* **50**, 561–571.

RUYSCH F. (1732). *Observationes anatomicae.* Observatio XV, Amsterdam.

RYAN T. J., ABELMANN W. H. (1961). Response of bronchial blood flow to tissue proliferation in the human lung. *J. Clin. Invest.* **40**, 1077.

SANTY P., BÉRARD M., GALY P., NGUYEN HUU (1952). La séquestration pulmonaire kystique avec artère anormale d'origine aortique a propos de six cas. *J. Franç. Méd. Chir. Thor.* **6**, 101–139.

SCHECHTER M. M., ZINGESSER L. H. (1965). The anterior spinal artery. *Acta Radiol.* **3**, 489–496.

SCHOBER R. (1964). Selective Bronchialisarteriographie. *Fortschr. Röntgenstr.* **101**, 337–348.

SCHOBER R. (1965). *Deutscher Röntgenkongress 1965.* Teil A, 65–68. Georg Thieme Verlag, Stuttgart.

SCHOEDEL W., BALTZER G. (1962). Einstrom und Ausstrom von Blut über broncho-pulmonale Gefässverbindungen. *Pflügers Arch. Ges. Physiol.* **275**, 539–550.

SCHOENMACKERS J. (1958). Zur Anatomie und Pathologie der Coronargefäsze. *Bad Oeynhausener Gespräche II*, Berlin-Göttingen-Heidelberg (133–158).

SCHOENMACKERS J. (1960). Über Bronchialvenen und ihre Stellung zwischem groszen und kleinem Kreislauf. *Arch. Kreisl.-Forsch.* **32**, 1–86.

SCHOENMACKERS J. (1963), Über das „arterio-venöse" Schaltsystem im kleinen Kreislauf. *Z. Kreisl.-Forsch.* **52**, 313-323.

SEGERS M., BROMBART M. (1953). *l'Oesophage en cardiologie*, 163–165. Masson Édit., Paris.

SHER M. H., TRUMMER M. J., MOQUIN R. B. (1966). Palliative treatment of nonresectable lung cancer by upper hemibody perfusion of chlorimine (short-acting alkylating agent). *Amer. Surg.* **32**, 385–390.

SHERRICK D. W., KINCAID O. W., DU SHANE J. W. (1962). Agenesis of main branch of pulmonary artery. *Amer. J. Roentgenol.* **87**, 917–928.

SMITH G. T., HYLAND J. W., PIEMME T., WELLS R. E. (1964). Human systemic-pulmonary arterial collateral circulation after pulmonary thrombo-embolism. *J. Amer. Med. Ass.* **188**, 452–458.

SNELLEN H. A., DANKMEIJER J., COLLISTER R. M. (1950). Comparative clinical and anatomical investigation in tetralogy of Fallot. *Congrès de Cardiologie, Paris.*

SODERBERG C. H. jr., COLBERT M. P., LEONE L. A. (1964). Bronchial artery infusion therapy of lung neoplasms with nitrogen mustard. *Surgery* **56**, 897–904.

SOSSAÏ M. (1966). Anastomose artérielle transthoracique entre la grande et la petite circulation. *Ann. Radiol.* **9**, 711–719.

STATE D., SALISBURY P. F., WEIL P. (1957). Physiologic and pharmacologic studies of collateral pulmonary flow. *J. Thorac. Surg.* **34**, 599–608.

STECKEL R. J., DOPPMAN J. L., ROLLEY R. T., MARTOS E. J. (1967). Rupture of the aorta after mechlorethamineHCI infusion of a bronchial artery. *J. Amer. Med. Ass.* **199**, 936–939.

STEINBERG I., FINBY N. (1959). Great vessel involvement in lung cancer: angiografic report on 250 consecutive proved cases. *Amer. J. Roentgenol.* **81**, 807–818.

STONE R. M., GINSBERG R. J., COLAPINTO R. F., PEARSON F. G. (1966). Bronchial artery regeneration after radical hilar stripping. *Surg. Forum* **17**, 109–110.

STRAWBRIDGE H. G. T. (1960). Pulmonary emphysema. *Amer. J. Path.* **37**, 170–171. *Amer. J. Path.* **37**, 404.

SUH T. H., ALEXANDER L. (1939). Vascular system of the human spinal cord. *Arch. Neurol. Psychiat. (Chic.)* **41**, 659–677.

SUZUKI Y. (1965). Chemotherapy of lung cancer by means of pulmonary arterial occlusion with a balloon tipped catheter. *J. Jap. Ass. Thorac. Surg.* **13**, 995–1003.

SWEET R. H. (1950). *Thoracic Surgery.* Saunders Company, Philadelphia–London.

SWIERENGA J. (1952). *Intrapulmonale bronchuscysten.* Scheltema & Holkema Uitgevers, Amsterdam.

SWIERENGA J. (1968). Het gesprongen adertje in de keel. *Ned. T. Geneesk.* **112**, 1541–1543.

SWIGART L. V. L., SIEKERT R. G., HAMBLEY W. C., ANSON B. J. (1950). The esophageal arteries. An anatomic study of 150 specimens. *Surg. Gynec. Obstet.* **90**, 234–243.

TABAKIN B. S., HANSON J. S., ADHIKARI P. K., MILLER D. B. (1960). Physiologic studies in congenital absence of the left main pulmonary artery. *Circulation* **22**, 1107–1111.

TAKAHASHI K. (1963). Studies on the patho-physiology of the pleura: The effects of pleurisy upon intercostal and intrathoracic arterial systems with particular reference to observations on the resin-cast specimens of the systems (In japanese). *J. Jap. Soc. Intern. Med.* **51**, 1433–1446.

TAKAHASHI S., SAKUMA S., KANEKO M., KOGA S. (1966). Angiography at fourfold magnification with special reference to the examination of tumours. *Acta Radiol.* **4**, 206–216.

TALALAK P. (1960). Pulmonary sequestration. *Arch. Dis. Childh.* **35**, 57–60.

TAMMELING G. J., NIEVEEN J., SLUITER H. J. (1967). Studies on anomalous collateral systemic-pulmonary circulation: report of four cases. *Circulation* **35**, 457–470.

TAUSSIG H. B. (1947). *Congenital malformations of the heart.* The Commonwealth Fund, New York.

TOBIN C. E. (1952). The bronchial arteries and their connections with other vessels in the human lung. *Surg. Gynec. Obstet.* **95**, 741–750.

TROCMÉ P., CHEDAL J. (1958). *Le cathétérisme du coeur droit et des artères pulmonaires en pneumologie.* Masson Édit., Paris.

TURNER-WARWICK M. (1963a). Precapillary systemic-pulmonary anastomoses. *Thorax* **18**, 225–237.

TURNER-WARWICK M. (1963b). Systemic arterial patterns in the lung and clubbing of the fingers. *Thorax* **18**, 238–250.

TYNAN M. J., GLEESON J. A. (1966). Pulmonary atresia with bronchial arteries arising from the subclavian arteries. *Brit. Heart J.* **28**, 573–576.

VACCAREZZA R. F., VIOLA A. R., VACCAREZZA O. A., UGO A. V., VICARIO D. J., ZUFFARDI E. A. (1966). Verification of the collateral systemic circulation in pulmonary pathology. *Dis. Chest* **48**, 130–138.

VAILLAUD J.-C. (1962). *Contribution à l'étude de la circulation bronchique dans les poumons détruits. Apport de l'aortographie.* Thèse, Alger.

VALLE A. R., WHITE M. L. (1947). Subdiaphragmatic aberrant pulmonary tissue. *Dis. Chest* **13**, 63–68.

VENABLES A. W. (1964). The patterns of pulmonary circulation in pulmonary atresia. *Brit. Heart J.* **26**, 760–769.

VERLOOP M. C. (1948). The arteriae bronchiales and their anastomoses with the arteria pulmonalis in the human lung; a micro-anatomical study. *Acta Anat.* **5**, 171–205.

VIAMONTE M. (1964). Selective bronchial arteriography in man. *Radiology* **83**, 830–839.

VIAMONTE M. (1965a). Diagnostic and therapeutic bronchial arterial catheterization in the human. *International Congress Radiologiae, Roma,* 316.

VIAMONTE M. (1965b). Angiographic evaluation of lung neoplasms. *Radiol. Clin. N. Amer.* **3**, 529–542.

VIAMONTE M., PARKS R., SMOAK W. (1965). Guided catheterisation of the bronchial arteries. *Radiology* **85**, 205–230.

VIAMONTE M., GILSON A. (1966). Angioscanography. *Radiology* **87**, 351–352.

VIAMONTE M. (1967). Intrathoracic extracardiac shunts. *Semin. Röntgen.* **2**, 342–367.

VIAMONTE M., MARTINEZ L. O. (1967). Newer techniques in the study of the pulmonary circulation. *Angiology* **18**, 323–333.

VIDONE R. A., LIEBOW A. A. (1957). Anatomical and functional studies of the lung deprived of pulmonary arteries and veins, with an application in the therapy of transposition of the great vessels. *Amer. J. Path.* **33**, 539–571.

VOORTHUISEN A. E. V. (1967). *Ervaringen met selectieve arteriografie van de arteria coeliaca en de arteria mesenterica superior.* Proefschrift, Leiden.

WAGENVOORT C. A., HEATH D., EDWARDS J. E. (1964). *The pathology of the pulmonary vasculature.* Thomas Publisher, Springfield, Ill.

WAGENVOORT C. A. (1966). Bronchopulmonale en pulmobronchiale arteriën. *Ned. T. Geneesk.* **110**, 505–506.

WEIBEL E. R. (1960). Early stages in the development of collateral circulation to the lung in the rat. *Circulat. Res.* **8**, 353–376.

WHOLEY M. H., EISEN H. B., POLLER S. (1965). Fundamentals of angiographic techniques. *Surg. Gynec. Obstet.* **121**, 517–527.

WICKBOM I. (1953). Angiographic demonstration of tumour pathology. *Acta Radiol.* **40**, 529–546.

WILLIAMS J. R., BONTE F. J. (1962). Bronchial arteriography. *Amer. J. Roentgenol.* **78**, 234–236.

WILLIAMS J. R., WILCOX W. C., BURNS R. R. (1963). Angiography of the systemic pulmonary circulation. *Amer. J. Roentgenol.* **90**, 614–627.

WIRTANEN G. W., ANSFIELD F. J. (1968). Bronchial artery infusion in bronchogenic carcinoma. *Cancer Chemother. Rep.* **52**, 263–269.

WOLFE S. F., BENFIELD J. R., CRUMMY A. B., BRIGGS R. C. (1967). Early radiation pneumonitis. *Ann. Thorac. Surg.* **4**, 399–411.

WOOD D. A., MILLER M. (1938). The rôle of the dual pulmonary circulation in various pathologic conditions of the lungs. *J. Thorac. Surg.* **7**, 649–670.

WRIGHT R. D. (1938). The blood supply of abnormal tissues in the lungs. *J. Path. Bact.* **47**, 489–499.

WRIGHT R. R. (1960). Bronchial atrophy and collapse in chronic obstructive pulmonary emphysema. *Amer. J. Path.* **37**, 63–77.

WRIGHT G. W., KLEINERMAN J. (1963). A consideration of the etiology of emphysema in terms of contemporary knowledge. *Amer. Rev. Resp. Dis.* **88**, 605–620.

WYATT J. P., FISCHER V. W., SWEET H. C. (1962). Panlobular emphysema: anatomy and pathodynamics. *Dis. Chest* **41**, 239–259.

WYATT J. P., FISCHER V. W., SWEET H. C. (1964). The pathomorphology of the emphysema complex. Part I and II. *Amer. Rev. Resp. Dis.* **89**, 533–560, 721–735.

ZUCKERKANDL E. (1881). Über die Anastomosen der Venae pulmonales mit den Bronchialvenen und mit dem mediastinalen Venennetze. *S.-B. Akad. Wiss. Wien, math.-nat. Kl.* **84**, 110–152.

ZUCKERKANDL E. (1883). Über die Verbindungen zwischen den arteriellen Gefässen der menschlichen Lunge. *S.-B. Akad. Wiss. Wien, math.-nat. Kl.* **87**, 171–186.

GPSR Compliance

The European Union's (EU) General Product Safety Regulation (GPSR) is a set of rules that requires consumer products to be safe and our obligations to ensure this.

If you have any concerns about our products, you can contact us on ProductSafety@springernature.com

In case Publisher is established outside the EU, the EU authorized representative is:

Springer Nature Customer Service Center GmbH
Europaplatz 3
69115 Heidelberg, Germany

Batch number: 09635766

Printed by Printforce, the Netherlands